# The Foundations of Bioethics

# The Foundations of Bioethics

SECOND EDITION

H. Tristram Engelhardt, Jr.

New York     Oxford
OXFORD UNIVERSITY PRESS
1996

Oxford University Press

Oxford  New York
Athens  Auckland  Bangkok  Bombay
Calcutta  Cape Town  Dar es Salaam  Delhi
Florence  Hong Kong  Istanbul  Karachi
Kuala Lampur  Madras  Madrid  Melbourne
Mexico City  Nairobi  Paris  Singapore
Taipei  Tokyo  Toronto

and associated companies in
Berlin  Ibadan

Copyright © 1986, 1996 by Oxford University Press, Inc.

Published by Oxford University Press, Inc.,
198 Madison Avenue, New York, New York 10016

Oxford is a registered trademark of Oxford University Press

Library of Congress Cataloging-in-Publication Data
Engelhardt, H. Tristram (Hugo Tristram), 1941–
The Foundations of bioethics / H. Tristram Engelhardt, Jr.—2nd ed.
p.  cm.
Includes index.
ISBN 0–19–505736–8
1. Medical ethics. 2. Bioethics. I. Title.
R724.E54  1996
174'.2—dc20      94–25267

9 8 7 6 5 4 3 2 1

Printed in the United States of America
on acid-free paper

To the memory of
Josef Karl Tristram
and
Elsie Tristram Engelhardt,
who introduced me to philosophy—
the first in the spirit and the second in the flesh—
and in gratitude to my wife,
Susan Gay Malloy Engelhardt,
and
Herman of Alaska,
who have each, albeit in different ways, supported me
in the framing of this second edition

# Preface

This is not a book in applied ethics. More accurately, this is not a book that applies a particular, canonical, concrete, content-full moral understanding to health care. Instead, there is a swarm of alternative ethics ready to give rise to a babble of conflicting bioethics. This circumstance constitutes the foundational moral challenge of all health care policy. It brings the very field of bioethics into question.

Rather than sharing one morality, we confront strikingly different concrete moral visions and accounts of moral obligations, rights, and values. Each account asserts its own priority. Some hold that euthanasia and physician-assisted suicide are morally appropriate to health care; others hold these practices to be immoral. Some consider commercial surrogate motherhood immoral; others consider that it is a way of acknowledging the dignity of women as free moral agents. Some argue that the rich should not be allowed to buy life-saving treatment unavailable to the poor; others argue that all should be free to purchase whatever treatment they are able. When asked how to justify these diverse moral understandings, some appeal to considerations of consequences; others appeal to principles of right or wrong that are independent of outcomes. It is against this cacophonous plurality of bioethics that contemporary health care policy is framed. The diversity of moral visions and justifications challenges the coherence of maintaining that there is a secular bioethics.

This book recognizes the impossibility of discovering *the* secular, canonical, concrete ethics. *The Foundations of Bioethics* attempts instead to secure a content-less secular ethics. Given the limits of secular moral reasoning, all that is available is a means (within certain constraints) of giving moral authority to common undertakings without establishing the moral worth or moral desirability of any particular choices. The project of securing as much universality as possible for the claims of bioethics has roots in the Enlightenment project of establishing a universal content-full ethics and a moral community of all persons outside of any particular religious and cultural assumptions. This Enlightenment project, for its part, has roots in natural-law theory and Western philosophical assumptions regarding the capacities of reason. This book focuses on the failure of this project to discover a canonical, content-full ethics for bioethics to apply. The implications that follow from this failure are the focus of this volume.

Many reviewers considered *Foundations* lacking in sympathy for the moralities that sustain and frame concrete moral communities. This judgment may in great measure be a criticism born of their failure to acknowledge the arguments offered regarding the distinction between the morality that can bind moral strangers and that which binds moral friends. This book begins with the recognition that there are concrete communities within which men and women can live coherent moral lives and pursue virtue. There are devout Jews, Protestants, Orthodox Catholics, Roman Catholics, Moslems, Hindus, and others. There are fervent egalitarians and libertarians. There are capitalists and socialists of various persuasions. There still remain even Marxists. Each possesses a concrete bioethics, however informally articulated. Some constitute moral communities able to give a full and substantial content to the moral life.

The force of this book's arguments is to privatize all such moral commitments and forms of bioethics from the perspective of large-scale secular social undertakings such as those of secular states. This is the case precisely because the secular morality offered is meant to reach to individuals across diverse moral communities. However, this privatization is not a qualification or a diminution of the significance and substance of the moral commitments of particular moral communities. It is rather a recognition that the truth known by and within a particular community will not be appreciated by moral strangers as having a claim on them unless they convert and thus cease to be moral strangers.

Since the first edition was written, it has become painfully obvious that much I said was misperceived. In part, this stemmed from my own reticence. I had held back from stating many positions as forcefully as I could have. As I remarked in the first edition, I had been led to a recognition of the incapacities of philosophical moral reasoning, a recognition that I found far from appealing. Many of the conclusions to which I found myself drawn were (and still are) abhorrent. I had set upon an intellectual adventure without knowing its ultimate destination. I was forced to draw a cardinal distinction between the morality of particular communities and the secular morality that can bind the larger society. Despite my having acknowledged these circumstances, it seems that many reviewers and perhaps many readers did not take my confessions (and laments) seriously. In particular, they saw me as critical of the rich matrices of obligations and values that shape particular moral communities.

From the perspective of those who do not acknowledge the difficulties that beset the modern philosophical project of providing a justification for a canonical secular ethics, it will be hard to interpret the significance of this volume. Others will regard the book as adding yet one more ethic to the cacophony of secular ethics. The former will not see the problem. The latter will not believe it can be solved. *The Foundations of Bioethics* speaks to both audiences. It takes seriously the limitations of secular moral reasoning while seeking through it to provide moral guidance that is not just one more content-full secular morality hopelessly in search of a general secular moral justification.

Many will not recognize the challenges facing bioethics, not so much because they do not acknowledge the weakness of secular reasoning, but because they deny a real diversity among moral perspectives. Such cosmopolitan ecumenists hold that men and women share enough in common so that a concrete and authoritative moral consensus can be discovered in societal undertakings that will allow them to justify a particular bioethics and to direct health care policy with moral authority. One can see why many are tempted to endorse this view. Many have goals that are primarily instrumental and immanent. For such persons, intractable moral disagreements may appear to be the result of fanaticism or ignorance. In addition, cosmopolitans often live their lives far from the substantive moral convictions that guide committed Orthodox Jews, Orthodox Catholics, Roman Catholics, Protestants, Moslems, and others who understand themselves within enduring and concrete moral traditions. It is difficult for cosmopolitan ecumenists to understand life within the embrace of traditional communities framed by transcendent commitments or to fathom the gulfs that separate different communities of the ideologically committed. One reviewer of my work even argued that he had refuted claims regarding real differences in moral visions by holding that he and I share a common concrete moral vision. He is wrong.

The account offered in *Foundations* does not provide a content-full ethics by which men and women can live their concrete moral lives. Rather, it justifies a moral framework by which individuals who belong to diverse moral communities, who do not share a content-full moral vision, can still regard themselves bound by a common moral fabric and can appeal to a common bioethics. It offers a moral perspective that can reach across the diversity of moral visions and provide a moral lingua franca. By not endorsing a particular moral vision, it seeks to avoid the difficulties that beset secular accounts that do: they beg the question, arbitrarily affirm a particular point of departure, or invoke an infinite regress. If the project of fashioning a general secular morality without commitment to a particular moral vision fails, then the modern philosophical project of justifying a general secular bioethics fails as well. Those who sought moral guidance from secular morality would then indeed be left with nihilism and unqualified relativism. If this project succeeds, even if individuals cannot discover a common, canonical, concrete ethics, there will be a procedure by which moral strangers can create webs of morally authorized undertakings, including endeavors in health care. Not all can be secured that one would wish. The alternative would be worse—the failure to secure any shred of a general secular morality.

The challenge for secular bioethics is substantial: attempts to bridge moral diversity concretely through a canonical, content-full secular morality fail in principle. The difficulty is that all concrete, secular moral accounts presuppose what they seek to prove. Perhaps here the reader wonders whether the author himself can avoid this same difficulty with his account. My response is twofold. First, this is not a book about the concrete moral views of the author. It is an account of the common morality that can bind moral strangers. Second, this book does not carry with it a concrete moral perspective. Many have regarded *The Foundations of Bioethics* as a defense of the value of individualism and of the worth of freedom or liberty. If it were, the criticism would hold. What would be offered would be yet just one more particular secular ethics. Again, neither the first nor the second edition claims a value for individual choice, freedom, or liberty. The book acknowledges that, when individuals attempt to resolve controversies and do not hear God (or do not hear him clearly) and cannot find sound rational arguments to resolve their moral controversies, they are left with the device of peaceably agreeing how and how far they will collaborate.

In this circumstance, individuals have priority because moral authority cannot be derived from a canonical concrete moral vision. If in secular circumstances one cannot derive moral authority from God or reason, authority can only be derived from the concurrence of individuals. Because the only morally authorized social structures under such circumstances are those established with the permission of the individuals involved, the morality that binds moral strangers has by default an unavoidably libertarian character. However, this is not out of any value attributed to freedom or individual choice. The plausible scope of societal moral authority is limited because of plausible limits of the consent to be governed by others. One need only apply the same requirements for consent in health care to the consent needed to authorize government and particular societal undertakings in order to recognize the limits of secular moral authority that limit limited democracies and the content of secular morality.

This libertarian character of a defensible general secular morality is not antagonistic to the moralities of concrete moral communities whose peaceable commitments may be far from libertarian (e.g., the communism of monasteries). In actual communities framed around content-full moralities, liberty is usually far from the most important good (sectarian Texans to the contrary notwithstanding). The arguments in *The Foundations of Bioethics* are not opposed to such sentiments within particular, peaceable, moral communities. Strictly, with respect to such sentiments, the arguments are neutral. Still, many have misunderstood

*Foundations* as a libertarian manifesto celebrating the value of freedom, as an attempt to secure a particular concrete morality hostile to the communitarian moralities that bind many, indeed most, particular moral communities.

As a step to dispelling confusion, in this second edition I have rebaptized "the principle of autonomy" with the name "the principle of permission" to indicate better that what is at stake is not some value possessed by autonomy or liberty, but the recognition that secular moral authority is derived from the permission of those involved in a common undertaking. The principle of permission underscores the circumstance that, when God is not heard by all in the same way (or is not heard by some at all), and when all do not belong to one closely-knit, well-defined community, and since reason fails to discover a canonical, concrete morality, then secularly justifiable moral authorization or authority comes not from God, nor from a particular community's moral vision, nor from reason, but from the permission of individuals. In this deafness to God and the failure of reason, moral strangers meet as individuals.

If one wants more than secular reason can disclose—and one should want more—then one should join a religion and be careful to choose the right one. Canonical moral content will not be found outside of a particular moral narrative, a view from somewhere. Here the reader deserves to know that I indeed experience and acknowledge the immense cleft between what secular philosophical reasoning can provide and what I know in the fullness of my own narrative to be true. I indeed affirm the canonical, concrete moral narrative, but realize it cannot be given by reason, only by grace. I am, after all, a born-again Texan Orthodox Catholic, a convert by choice and conviction, through grace and in repentance for sins innumerable (including a first edition upon which much improvement was needed). My moral perspective does not lack content. I am of the firm conviction that, save for God's mercy, those who willfully engage in much that a peaceable, fully secular state will permit (e.g., euthanasia and direct abortion on demand) stand in danger of hell's eternal fires. As a Texan, I puzzle whether these are kindled with mesquite, live oak, or trash cedar. Being schooled in theology, I know that this is a question to be answered only on the Last Day by the Almighty. Though I acknowledge that there is no secular moral authority that can be justified in general secular terms to forbid the sale of heroin, the availability of direct abortion, the marketing of for-profit euthanatization services, or the provision of commercial surrogacy, I firmly hold none of these endeavors to be good. These are great moral evils. But their evil cannot be grasped in purely secular terms. To be pro-choice in general secular terms is to understand God's tragic relationship to Eden. To be free is to be free to choose very wrongly.

Because this point has so frequently been misunderstood or ignored, it bears restatement. This book is not a presentation of my concrete moral ideals, my concrete morality, or my concrete bioethics. Quite to the contrary, I regard this book as exploring the possibility for morally authorized collaboration with moral strangers in the ruins of the Enlightenment project. It examines the failure of moral philosophy to deliver a canonical, concrete morality. It explores the implications of this failure for bioethics. It gives justification for the hope of salvaging something from the wreckage of the project of establishing a secular morality that can bind all. It does not provide a concrete moral vision.

Because of the need to address these various misunderstandings, as well as to take account of the substantial debate regarding health care reform that emerged in the United States, this second edition is in great measure a new book. The arguments in each chapter of the new edition have been further developed. All chapters, save for chapter 5, have been significantly recast, not only to avoid previous misunderstandings, but to give greater attention to key philosophical considerations. For those who were unclear that I, while recognizing the sparse morality that binds moral strangers, am also committed to a particular moral community, this second edition should be an enlightenment. The contrast between the morality of moral friends and the morality of moral strangers is further elaborated in order unambiguously to present important moral contrasts. Finally, although arguments throughout the book have been reshaped in terms of the shifting texture of bioethical and health care policy debates, this is nowhere more salient than in chapter 8, which speaks to issues of the allocation of health care resources, including recent reflections on health care reform. The debacle of President Clinton's health care proposals receives special attention in order to illustrate an ideological failure to address candidly the moral issues at stake in health care policy. Much can be clarified even within the sparse morality that binds moral strangers. Despite philosophy's modest capacities, it can make essential contributions to dispelling unwarranted claims and to directing energies to the challenge of creating morally justifiable health care policy for large-scale secular pluralist societies.

*Houston*                                                                       H. T. E.
*May 1995*

# Acknowledgments

This edition and the one that preceded it consumed a total of nearly two decades in the writing. Over this period I benefited from numerous discussions concerning various ancestral manuscripts. I am in the debt of many for their criticisms, suggestions, and support. In particular, the development of this volume benefited significantly from my conversations with my colleagues at the Institute for the Medical Humanities in Galveston, the Kennedy Institute of Ethics of Georgetown University, and the Center for Ethics, Medicine, and Public Issues in Houston. Colleagues and students at Baylor College of Medicine, Rice University, and the Institute of Religion helped me to see many important issues anew. In this regard, I must also mention those who sponsored conferences on the first edition, thus helping me to recognize the need for revision and further development: the Society for Health and Human Values, Liberty Fund, the Institute for Humane Studies (George Mason University), and the Societé pour la Philosophie de la Technique (Paris) with the Centre de Recherches Interdisciplinaires en Bioethique (Université Libre de Bruxelles). Indispensable in beginning these revisions was my stay as a Fellow at the Institute for Advanced Study in Berlin, 1988–89.

Many have read the manuscripts of the first and second editions in various stages, in whole or in part. Their insightful and vigorous responses often brought me to recast large elements of this project. Through forgetfulness and the multitude of names I have surely not recalled them all. Here I can only mention a few among those who have been so generous in time and energies: Baruch A. Brody, Thomas J. Bole III, Xavier de Callatay, James F. Childress, Mary Ann Gardell Cutter, Christina Engelhardt, Dorothea Engelhardt, the Reverend George Eber,

Lee Friedman, Stanley Hauerwas, Corinna Delkeskamp-Hayes, Benjamin
Hippen, Brid Hollywood, Ross W. I. Kessel, B. Andrew Lustig, Laurence B.
McCullough, Mary Rawlinson, James Reagan, Michael A. Rie, Hans-Martin
Sass, Earl E. Shelp, Stuart F. Spicker, Lawrence T. Ulrich, Stephen Wear, and
the Reverend Kevin Wm. Wildes, S.J. I have a particular debt to four individuals
for their especially thorough reading and criticism of the final version of the
manuscript of the second edition: S. G. M. Engelhardt, Mark Cherry, Rui-Ping
Fan, and George Khushf.

Having acknowledged all of this good guidance and advice, I must acknowledge as well that I have not always followed it. Where the volume succeeds, this
can be attributed in no small measure to the various individuals who commented
on the various manuscripts as the two editions went through manifold rewritings.
The shortcomings, missteps, and mistakes are all my own.

# Contents

# The Foundations of Bioethics

Χαῖρε φιλοσόφους ἀσόφους δεικνύουσα·
Χαῖρε,τεχνολόγους ἀλόγους ἐλέγχουσα.
Ο ΑΚΑΘΙΣΤΟΣ ΥΜΝΟΣ

# 1

## Introduction: Bioethics as a Plural Noun

### Bioethics in the face of moral pluralism

Moral diversity is real. It is real in fact and in principle. Bioethics and health care policy have yet to take this diversity seriously. Those who teach bioethics, those who engage in bioethics consultations in the clinical arena, those who serve on ethics committees, even those who produce textbooks of bioethics tend to discount the diversity of understandings regarding the morality of particular health care choices (e.g., regarding abortion, commercial surrogacy, euthanasia, germline genetic engineering, inequalities in access to health care, infanticide, organ sales) or the nature of morality (e.g., teleological, deontological, virtue-based). It is as if one needed only to lay out the canonical account of justice[1] and of the proper physician–patient relationship.[2] The expectation persists of simply disclosing how resources ought to be distributed and how patients and physicians ought concretely to regard each other. All this is supposed to be possible outside of any particular moral narrative or perspective, at least outside of any narrative or perspective with the idiosyncrasies of a particular ideology or religion.[3] After all, this is what the project of secular morality and bioethics has promised: an account in general of what individuals owe each other and ought to do.

This failure to recognize the depth of the moral diversity that characterizes our context is understandable. The presumption that there is a concrete morality available to all through rational reflection has deep roots in Western history. It was the West that first aspired in a systematic fashion to see reality from the anonymous perspective of reason, of *logos*, of any person—to articulate a norma-

3

tive view from nowhere and outside of any particular history.[4] One finds already in the Pre-Socratics the notion of a canonical viewpoint transcending cultures and open to all. Heraclitus (fl. 504 B.C.) held, for example, that "Thought is common to all. Men must speak with understanding and hold fast to that which is common to all, as a city holds fast to its law, and much more strongly still. For all human laws are nourished by the one divine law. For it prevails as far as it wills, suffices for all, and there is something to spare."[5] The aspiration to articulate *the* rational account of being and morality was further shaped by Plato, Aristotle, and the Stoics. These pagan understandings were then developed and strengthened by Western Christianity.

The Western Christian synthesis marginalized the skepticism that existed in the ancient world alongside strong defenses of reason, replacing a polytheistic multicultural world with the monocultural monotheism of Latin Christianity. All reality, value, and social structure were to be understood from the perspective and judgment of the one true God. All history was to be retold within the context of the Christian narrative of salvation and given a unique, canonical context and direction. As a metaphysical account, the Judeo-Christian vision offered a coincidence in the foundations of being of the origin and justification of morality, as well as of the motivation to be moral. Western Christianity involved, in particular, a presumption that its morality could to a great extent be known and understood through reason without faith.[6] Even as the faith of the West shattered, these convictions remained. The West entered modernity with robust expectations from reason.[7]

Contemporary bioethical questions arise against the backdrop of a fragmentation of moral perspective and vision that is closely tied to a series of losses of faith and changes in Western ethical and ontological conviction. When Martin Luther nailed his ninety-five theses to All Saints' Church in Wittenberg on Halloween in 1517, he marked a new era for the West and signaled the crumbling of the presumed possibility of a uniformity of religious moral viewpoint. One could no longer hope to live in a society that could aspire to a single moral viewpoint grounded in faith, governed by a single supreme religious moral authority. In little over a century this rupture led to the Thirty Years' War and the British Civil War. The Pax Westphalica that followed in 1648 heralded the unlikelihood of ever cementing western Europe in one Christian vision.

While the religious roots of ethical and metaphysical consensus were fragmenting, progress in the sciences undermined established understandings of man's place in the world, indeed in the cosmos. This progress also strengthened the expectations from secular rationality. In 1492 Columbus discovered America in the radical sense of disclosing, along with Magellan who would follow, the geography of our world and the vast expanse of world cultures. When the first copy of Nicolaus Copernicus's *De revolutionibus orbium coelestium* was placed on his deathbed in East Prussia on May 24, 1543, a bequest was made to a shift in ideas that was to become the metaphor for dramatic and extensive changes in world views. The Copernican revolution was one of the many changes in ideas and understandings that would leave our secular vision devoid of a sense of absolute or final perspective: man ceased to be at the center of the universe. Matters were made even worse in 1859 by Darwin's *On the Origin of Species,* which deprived that vision of a canonical human environment, Eden. The human species seemed no longer privileged in the development of life, nor was there a regnant secular understanding of human nature as having a univocal, much less a divine design.

As the Western Christian religious synthesis weakened, Enlightenment and progressivist hopes grew that reason (through philosophy or rational reflection generally) could disclose the character of the good life and the general canons of moral probity outside of any particular moral narrative. This hope arose against the background of the Thirty Years' War and the Civil War in England. The aspiration was to discover by reason a common morality that should bind all and provide the foundations for perpetual peace.[8] This has been the modern philosophical moral project: to secure the moral substance and authority that had been promised by the Western Middle Ages through a synergy of grace and reason, but now through rational argument. This hope has proved false.[9] Rather than philosophy being able to fill the void left by the collapse of the hegemony of Christian thought in the West, philosophy has shown itself to be many competing philosophies and philosophical ethics. The attempt to sustain a secular equivalent of Western Christian monotheism through the disclosure of a unique moral and metaphysical account of reality has fragmented into a polytheism of perspectives with its chaos of moral diversity and its cacophony of numerous competing moral narratives. This circumstance as a sociological condition, reflecting our epistemological limitations, defines postmodernity. Secular rationality appears triumphant. But it has become many rationalities. It is not clear whether it can give moral or metaphysical orientation.

Still, some have aspired to translate particular secular philosophies into governmentally imposed secular mass movements. These attempts have failed as well. The once most widely established world philosophy, Marxism, has in great measure collapsed, as if in one night faith failed. The major established churches of the West have for their part seen significant losses of belief, despite attempts to reclaim a social centrality. The Roman Catholic Church convened Vatican II and vigorously engaged energies in what many of its members regarded as a renewal that would usher in a Second Pentecost of commitment and the flowering of faith. Hierarchs attempted to accommodate to the conditions of contemporaneity and to be relevant to the needs of the day. This *aggiornamento* was greeted, especially in Western Europe, by empty pews and departing priests.[10] Rather than unity in the Spirit, there was dissidence and discord. Rather than a harmony of conviction, there was a legion of disputatious diversity. Established and mainline Protestant churches have experienced similar losses of attendance and cultural salience. With the exception of a dramatic Moslem revival and the development of some other fundamentalist religious movements, established religious belief, especially that which has attempted to accommodate to modernity, has in general waned. Pope John Paul II thus laments: ''Dechristianization, which weighs heavily upon entire peoples and communities once rich in faith and Christian life, involves not only the loss of faith or in any event its becoming irrelevant for everyday life, but also, and of necessity, *a decline or obscuring of the moral sense.*''[11] Contemporary bioethics is thus set against a background of considerable skepticism, lost belief, persisting convictions, a plurality of moral visions, and mounting public policy challenges. It is within such a moral chaos that health care policy must be framed.

Contemporary Western societies are now secular as the result of historical forces that have dissociated the major institutions of most democracies from any established church, even where vestiges may remain. Societies are pluralistic, encompassing communities with a diversity of moral sentiments and beliefs. Such diversity has always been present, however hidden. Western Europe of the Middle Ages, though nominally Roman Catholic, included significant populations of Jews, in addition to heretics, agnostics, and atheists. Pluralism was suppressed through the force of the dominant culture. Outside of such dominance, it is difficult to fashion a society that is not pluralist. One must quite likely settle for a society on a very small scale, probably not exceeding the compass of a Greek city-state. This is the case, at least if one wants a geographically located society on the model of most contemporary states. One must remember that the vision of Aristotle's polis, which so influenced the West and indirectly the world, was of a small city unreceptive to immigrants and others who might fragment its cultural unity.[12] The exemplar moral community was one of considerable uniformity.

The modern philosophical hope, despite such difficulties, has been to discover a general communality of persons. This communality has been sought through discovering a canonical, content-full morality that is more than procedural, one that should bind moral strangers, members of different and diverse moral communities. We should be able to discover a content-full secular morality (including the content-full foundation for a bioethics) that can reach across diverse communities of religious and ideological belief. Such has been a goal of the modern philosophical project. Many have thought that one can dispel religious beliefs as remnants of an irrational past and live in the light of the content-full morality that rationality can disclose. There has been the hope to establish an understanding of justice and right action as expressing the requirements of rationality and humanity, and not as simply the expression of a particular world view or ideology.

This last paragraph introduces two terms that have a technical significance throughout this volume: *content-full morality* and *moral strangers*. A content-full morality is to be contrasted with a purely procedural morality in which persons convey to common endeavors the moral authority of their consent. Moral strangers are persons who do not share sufficient moral premises or rules of evidence and inference to resolve moral controversies by sound rational argument, or who do not have a common commitment to individuals or institutions in authority to resolve moral controversies. A content-full morality provides substantive guidance regarding what is right or wrong, good or bad, beyond the very sparse requirement that one may not use persons without their authorization. *Moral friends* are those who share enough of a content-full morality so that they can resolve moral controversies by sound moral argument or by an appeal to a jointly recognized moral authority whose jurisdiction they acknowledge as derived from a source other than common agreement. Moral strangers must resolve moral agreements by common agreement, for they do not share enough of a moral vision so as to be able to discover content-full resolutions to their moral controversies, either by an appeal to commonly held moral premises (along with rules of evidence and inference) and/or to individuals or institutions commonly recognized to be in authority to resolve moral controversies and to give content-full moral guidance. Still, moral strangers need not be alien to each other. They can recognize each other's moral commitments and understand them to be misguided or disordered. A different ranking of fundamental values will render individuals moral strangers, but not incomprehensible to each other. Moreover, given the complexity of human circumstances and inclinations, moral strangers can be the best of affective friends.

The distinction between moral friends and moral strangers can often be captured in a stipulative distinction between communities and societies. In the arguments that follow in this book, *community* is often contrasted with *society*. In such contrasts, *community* is used to identify a body of men and women bound together by common moral traditions and/or practices around a shared vision of the good life, which allows them to collaborate as moral friends. The moral practices and traditions that bind individuals within a community may be more or less thick or thin. Members of a monastery will be very thickly or tightly bound together with overarching and robust moral traditions and practices. Other communities may not be as tightly joined. *Society* is used to identify an association that compasses individuals who find themselves in diverse moral communities. Though they can collaborate in a common association, they find their substantive moral location within those communities they share with moral friends. The Amish, the Hassidim, devout Orthodox Christians, or the members of an ideologically unified commune may understand themselves as citizens and therefore members of a larger American society, but their primary moral place and identification will be in a particular community. Others who commit themselves less robustly to any particular moral community will find themselves in overlapping communities to which they give different allegiances and differing levels of moral commitment. Even these individuals, if they look at the larger society, will discover that there are many associates or citizens who are members of moral communities with which they have significant disagreement, but yet with whom they can still collaborate as limited associates or citizens, albeit moral strangers.[13]

## Bioethics and postmodernity

A canonical, content-full secular morality cannot be discovered, as we will see in the next chapter. The recognition of this failure marks the postmodern philosophical predicament. It is a circumstance difficult to accept, given our intellectual history and its exaggerated expectations for reason. The failure of the modern philosophical project to discover a canonical content-full morality constitutes the fundamental catastrophe of contemporary secular culture and frames the context of contemporary bioethics. One encounters moral strangers, people with whom one does not share sufficient moral principles or enough of a common moral vision to be able to resolve moral controversies through sound rational argument or an appeal to moral authority. When one attempts rationally to resolve such controversies, the discussions go on and on without a final conclusion. Rational argument does not quiet moral controversies when one encounters moral strangers, people of different moral visions.

The stridency of the abortion debate marks the strength of such disagreements. Some regard abortion as profoundly morally evil (e.g., the same as or equivalent to murder, as does the author of this volume), while others see it as at most a physical evil. The abortion debate is only one of a number of issues where the controversies are both impassioned and reflect well-entrenched and conflicting moral visions. Limiting access to high-cost medical interventions, fetal experimentation, and organ sales are among the many issues regarding which there is little concurrence, but instead lively dispute. Still, over the past decade there has been an increasing acceptance by many of medical practices that would have been for many unthinkable only a half century ago (e.g., abortion on demand and active euthanasia as in Holland). A widespread, well-articulated coalition of diverse permissive bioethics has developed. Yet, this apparent concurrence reveals deep disagreements when issues are raised such as commercial surrogacy and euthanasia services, or the development of an explicitly two-tier health care system (i.e., one tier accessible to all and the second only to those who can obtain the means to purchase the additional benefits).

There are disagreements intertwined with disagreements. There are fundamental differences separating many of the secular visions and between secular understandings of bioethics and traditional religious moralities. The latter then disagree with each other as well. There is a foundational tension between achieving the good of persons and respecting them as free and responsible moral agents. There are foundational disagreements as to who should define the good of persons, how, and with respect to what standards. Issues in bioethics are regarded as important, though they remain divisive. We could never do more in medicine. Yet we remain in deep disagreement about what we may or may not do.

Many who work in applied ethics or bioethics seem to disregard these difficulties that lie at the very roots of modern thought. Many proceed with the task of applying ethics as if it were obvious which secular ethic ought to be applied. Many provide bioethics consultations or advice as if there were one content-full bioethics, one canonical content-full bioethical orthodoxy, that should guide all secular moral decisions and justify all health care policy. Such consultations and advice can then lead to imposing a particular moral vision, ideology, or moral orthodoxy as if it were required by reason itself. Such consultants work somewhat as priests, rabbis, or ministers do within a religious context, but without acknowledging their sectarian position. Each has a view of a proper physician–patient relationship,[14] often with a very content-full understanding of free and informed consent. They speak for reason as such, without acknowledging the particular moral commitments that guide their choices. They advance content-full accounts of justice and fairness in health care distributions. They claim to know *the* content-full secular moral vision, which is canonical for all persons. The only difficulty is that such does not exist. There is no content-full morality without a particular moral commitment.[15] There is no content-full bioethics outside of a particular moral perspective. Moreover, there are diverse and profoundly different moral understandings: bioethics is in the plural. This book explores the consequences of this state of affairs: the irremedial plurality of postmodernity.

For those who live outside a traditional community and without transcendent or ideological convictions, differences in belief will often be presumed to mask a more fundamental communality of immanent concerns.[16] The ever-present pleasures and opportunities of this life are seen to have first claim and ground final judgments. A foundation is sought in that which is material and common. But history separates, and belief gives transforming meaning to the ordinary. There are even differences in perspective and tradition that separate cosmopolitans. There is more than one vision of the cosmopolis and of the cosmopolitan (e.g., the liberal democratic cosmopolitan versus the defender of a quasi-dictatorial capitalism a la Singapore).[17] Substantial differences in belief and moral vision remain and define action, character, and virtue. These differences shape living communities of diverse moral understanding, cosmopolitans to the contrary notwithstanding. This volume endeavors to take this real moral diversity and pluralism seriously and explore its consequences for bioethics and health care policy.

Morality is available on two levels: the content-full morality of moral friends, and the procedural morality binding moral strangers. As a consequence, much must be allowed in large-scale secular states that many, including the author, know to be grievously wrong and morally disordered. This circumstance will disappoint those who hoped that the general society or a large-scale state would constitute *the* moral community, which could be guided by *the* content-full secular bioethics. Their hope is sociologically ungrounded and, in terms of the possibility of a secular morality, unjustifiable. Large-scale states compass numerous peaceable moral communities, a diversity that states have no secular moral right to suppress. The great murderous endeavors of this century from Stalin and Hitler to the Gang of Four and Pol Pot have been born of attempts by force to make states single moral communities. Despite brutal repression, diversity remains.

This is not to say that diversity is good in itself. When Jesus asked the devil whom He drove out of the man in Gerasenes, "What is your name?" the devil answered, "My name is Legion" (Mark 5:9). The orthodox Judeo-Christian understanding of being is that at its source there is One Person, One Unbegotten, One Father, and that evil is centrifugal, dispersing, sundering, and personal. Against this diversity, the state is not the hand of God. At least in general secular terms, the state cannot be shown to be the hand of God, however, in fact, Providence may act or God may dispose. The secular state thus appears by default unavoidably polytheistic.[18] One finds numerous visions, a chaos of voices, a legion of beckoning goods, alternative lifestyles, and diverse communities. As a whole, without God, there is nothing ultimately good in all of this. The author recognizes in the landscape of secular bioethics a diversity that is often perverse, but which the secular state cannot find warrant to set aside. This volume does not celebrate the chaos, or even much of the diversity, and surely not the moral perversity and vacuity of this landscape. Instead, this volume offers secular means for coming to terms with the chaos and diversity of postmodernity. The means are meager and offer no transcendent fulfillment. But they are all that is available in general secular terms.

Many yearn for the Western Middle Ages, while at the same time wanting to avoid belief in its God. They aspire to discover a content-full secular bioethics that can warrant a particular health care policy. They seek by secular reason to discover a content-full morality and the moral authority for government to impose it. Many imagine that philosophers and bioethicists can provide the kind of moral guidance once received from ministers, priests, or rabbis. They seek concrete instruction about the meaning of life, or at least a content-full account of justice, fairness, and morally acceptable health care policy. They hope to find content-full moral answers in reason. They seek from the state something like the community they may have once known as members of a church or synagogue. They yearn after a secularly normative consensus in a large-scale state and hope that a large-scale society can be the same as a concrete moral community. They seek a secular religion without belief. These hopes are vain.

This was, after all, the modern moral philosophical project: to secure by reason alone the core of the moral vision and authority that the Western medieval era promised to deliver through its faith in reason and its particular Faith. The modern hope has been to secure morality and political authority without the medieval commitment to a particular revelation and a particular history. The failure of the modern moral philosophical project returns us to the polytheism and skepticism of ancient times with a remembrance of the philosophical monotheism and Faith that fashioned the West. There is a feeling of loss. Against the recollection of a unity and community sought, if never achieved, there is a diversity of moral visions and content-full bioethics that will not submit to a single content-full understanding. This is the price of postmodernity and the multiperspectival and multicultural vision it imposes. Bioethics remains in the plural.

## Politics, morality, and bioethics

This book provides not simply a political theory, but an account of the morality that should guide individuals when they meet as moral strangers to fashion health care policy. It is the case that, when they so meet, they tend to collaborate in the realm of politics, through a *res publica,* a common thing that moral strangers of diverse moral communities can share. Within that perspective, nothing can contentfully be shared by all. The picture is in this respect a disappointing one. But it is all that can be justified in general secular terms. The reader may then retort, "this justification is not enough to motivate moral behavior." Or, "religious and ideological zealots will not be convinced—they will use force to impose their views." To this the author will respond, "That may be the case; still, the moral account justified in this volume provides a secular moral warrant to authorize coercive force to protect persons when acting peaceably, whether individually or in communities, including the establishment of social institutions, within which, albeit in limited ways, common goods can be pursued and health care policy framed." Philosophical arguments may not move the masses, but, if successful, good arguments can show when force may with moral justification be used to motivate and the extent to which welfare entitlements can be created. In addition, there is sufficient room for the market impelled by greed to create goods and services, which will enrich many, if not all. There is space for charity to respond to those in need independently of social interventions and the contributions of the market. To which the reader may respond again, Is all this in the end good? Is this what God wants? Is this the transcendent truth? Is this all one can get for and from bioethics?

Within a project in secular philosophical reasoning, ultimate questions cannot be answered. Even the project of secular philosophical reason cannot itself be valued or endorsed, at least in general secular terms. It is rather a possibility within which morally authoritative collaboration may take place while the various participants bring to it various views of its value and importance.

Perhaps the reader hungers after the unification of the genesis and justification of morality, as well as of the motivation to be moral, that can only be found with reference to the Deity.[19] In terms of what the Deity is and wills, one can find an ultimate genesis of what it is to be right and what it is to be good and virtuous. The standpoint of the Deity also offers an account of why morality is rational in terms of an ultimate grounding of morality in God, the ultimate ground of rationality. Finally, the standpoint of the Deity provides ultimate sanctions against misconduct. This coincidence of the grounds of knowledge and of being, of the genesis and justification of morality, as well as of the motivation for being moral, all of which are so often sought in the philosopher's God, cannot be found in a generally justifiable secular account.[20] Secular moral reflection cannot provide such a deep account of why it is rational and prudent to be moral. Indeed, rationality and prudence fracture into numerous understandings so that one must always specify to which prudence, justice, or moral rationality one is making appeal.

One is left with a polytheism of moral perspectives, none with the capacities sought from the univocal perspective of God. Still, secular moral reflection can offer the possibility of a secularly authoritative moral discourse as well as collaboration among moral strangers, despite the collapse of the modern philosophical project. If individuals are interested in resolving issues peaceably (i.e., without a basic reliance on force itself as authority), and even if the individuals do not hear God in the same way, and despite the fact that secular sound rational argument cannot establish as canonical a particular content-full moral vision, what is offered will still function to secure a general secular bioethics. Meager and content-less as it is, it is all that can be justified in general secular terms. In general secular terms, one cannot even show that it is good.

This means that there is little in general secular terms that one can say about proper physician–patient relationships, or the allocation of scarce resources. For example, there will be no secular content-full moral guidance, whether it is good or bad, to promote or prohibit commercial surrogacy and for-profit euthanatization services. There will simply be limits on what coercive restrictions can be justified in general secular moral terms. There will be no specific secular moral content that one can give to the notion of a virtuous physician. One may know that one ought to do the good, but there will be no common understanding of the goods and goals of medicine, or even of the meaning of beneficence. For example, is it beneficent or maleficent to pay the poor to be sterilized or to buy organs from them? Should one condemn or praise the reasonable person test for informed consent? Or may physicians band together and announce that they will provide information only according to a professional standard? Outside of an already taken-for-granted moral perspective, people will meet as moral strangers who, in secular terms, will be bound only by their own agreements both explicit and implicit. There will be a fabric of common secular moral authority, but it will be empty.

Outside of a particular moral community, there is no canonical content-full moral guidance, or content-full bioethics. One can show that informed consent, market transfers, and the decisions of limited democracies can create structures with moral authority. But they will provide no substantive, nonprocedural moral instruction. For example, one will not be able to discover whether it is wrong as such to experiment on human embryos. One will only learn that one must acquire the consent of those who own the embryos and that one may not act to harm future persons. Of course, there is much more that ought in fact to be said. But a general secular bioethics cannot say it. Still, outside of such concrete communalities of belief, there is a procedural morality that can bind us and ground a procedural bioethics. Secular morality and bioethics do not disappear into a language of emotive persuasion or discourse in the service of wills to power. Despite the logical positivists and against Nietzsche, and while heeding the heralds of post-modernity, it is still possible to save a shred of the modern moral philosophical project, though most (including the author) may find that this salvageable shred is very much less than they had wanted or expected.

### Bioethics in the ruins

Between conflicting moral visions, amid the ruins of once powerful orthodoxies, and in the context of peaceable secularity, how can one understand the virtues? How is one to understand the virtue of courage? Are physicians courageous when they employ heroic measures? One must first know what goals justify what risks and from whose standpoint. How can one understand the virtue of modesty? About what ought a patient to feel shame? Outside of a content-full vision of human flourishing, it is impossible to answer such questions. In a general secular moral context, the virtues are evacuated of moral content. What were once substantial matters of moral character become matters of taste. The moral world of secularity provides at best procedures for negotiation and agreement. Contractual rights and obligations displace what were once rich languages of character and virtue.

Little of traditional concerns about virtue and character can be understood in general, secular terms outside of the context and content provided within particular moral communities. These observations concur with those of Alasdair MacIntyre and others: we live amid the shattered remnants of once vibrant and integrated moral visions and understandings that could have sustained content-full accounts of proper contemporary health care policy.[21] The residue of those collapsed understandings provides the denizens of the contemporary world with often contradictory and in the end, in general secular terms, unjustifiable moral visions. Moral intuitions, severed from the moral visions that sustained them and gave them sense and meaning, persist as prejudices, unsecured sentiments, taboos, and isolated moral intuitions. Those who believe, those who live within intact moral communities and possess content-full moral visions, will have no trouble discerning the meaning of character and virtue. However, they will feel the immense gulf between their vision of human flourishing and what little can be secured in general, secular terms.

Traditional moralities and their communities remain. Their adherents accept grace and submit to a history. They know concretely about virtue and character. Some even strive for sanctity and holiness. They know what is worth dying for, when, and why. They know that morality commands, that its content is not chosen. In the contemporary world, they are both a curiosity and a challenge. They have content-full views of the good death, of shameful uses of health care technology, and of courage in the face of suffering. They provide numerous vivid presentations of human meaning, dedication, and community. They offer a range of bioethics with often diverse views of human obligations. Thus, one finds Roman Catholics stopping lifesaving treatment they see to be unduly burdensome,[22] whereas Orthodox Jews find themselves obliged to treat until the patient is in the process of dying.[23] From the outside, particular moral communities can be regarded as providing engaging varieties of moral taste. Their views can be heuristic, even for the ecumenist cosmopolitan, who may wonder about how to strike an appropriate balance between costs and benefits in the project of postponing death.

### Toleration in the face of moral diversity

Diversity is not only engaging. Diversity with substance offends. To have particular beliefs over against others is to invite judgment. A canonical content-full vision has teeth. Thus, Orthodox Judaism and Orthodox Catholicism both condemn abortion for convenience, as well as consensual euthanasia. These religions regard such activities as wrong, not just for their own adherents, but for persons as such.[24] Even if these religions are tolerant in the sense of not using coercive force to constrain those who persist in their errors, they are not tolerant in the sense of viewing these matters as mere issues of personal choice or preference. They allow in the sense of not coercing, but they do not accept.

It is here that cosmopolitan ecumenists are often offended most deeply. They are offended as well by lifestyles and moral visions that violate accepted contemporary understandings of social roles, as when Orthodox Jews, because of a fundamental proscription against a woman having more than one husband, but not against a man having more than one wife, may be able to allow donation of gametes for in vitro fertilization, but only from unmarried women, never from men.[25] This, however, is one of the morally unavoidable costs of postmodernity.

The moral vision that binds moral strangers forbids unconsented-to force, but not the moral affront that arises from the knowledge that others condemn moral diversity (e.g., as heresy, perversion) or act within consensual communities in ways that give moral offense.

So, too, a secular bioethics cannot develop conclusive secular arguments for forbidding many actions that Christian societies have taken to be seriously morally disordered, such as suicide or the active euthanasia of severely defective newborns. As this volume will show, it is not possible to demonstrate in general secular terms the grave moral evil of direct abortion (again, the author of this volume knows on religious grounds and firmly states that *direct* abortion is gravely wrong, not to mention suicide and euthanasia). A secular bioethics will not justify coercively realizing egalitarian visions or content-full understandings of political correctness. Particular ideologies will be no better advantaged in general secular terms than particular religions. In addition, secular bioethics will usually qualify its answers, leaving vexing areas of uncertainty. This will not be out of a pursuit of a minimalist ethics, such as Daniel Callahan has criticized,[26] but rather out of a recognition of the limitations of secular reasoning. These conclusions about the capacities of bioethics require changes in secular public policy, insofar as such policy is to be justified in general secular terms. If there are no general rational arguments to show that certain actions are wrong, then the secular moral authority to prohibit such actions by force is at best undermined. But at the same time, particular communities should be at liberty to fashion substantive moral understandings with their own members. The more one lives within the embrace of a particular community and a particular moral vision, the more one will appreciate the starkness of the contrast between the ethics (and bioethics) that can bind moral strangers and that which can bind moral friends.

We live in a century in which more people have been slaughtered in the cause of secular visions of justice, human dignity, ideological rectitude, historical progress, and purity than have ever been killed in religious wars. Countries that professed commitments to the working class and to peasants have killed workers and peasants in the millions because they failed to conform to the regnant political correctness. These atrocities were the actions of regimes that aspired to secularity and professed humane sentiments but failed to tolerate the de facto diversity and plurality of moral visions that characterize the human condition. Tolerance of wrong choices has not been commonplace. Indeed, Thomas Aquinas recommends that the stubborn or relapsing heretic be exterminated from the world by death.[27] We will need to learn to be tolerant, even about issues less important than salvation. We will need to eschew contemporary secular versions of the *writ de haeretico comburendo*. Perpetual peace in the absence of repression will likely come, if ever, when we are willing to endure the choices persons make with themselves, their private resources, consenting others, and in their communities however deviant, even when those choices are profoundly wrong.

In the past decade much has changed beyond expectation. Perhaps the political structures born of this age will give way to arrangements in which we can peaceably accept the flourishing of concrete differences. An ideology that aspired to world domination collapsed largely from its own failure of conviction (not just from its abject failure as an economic system). Perhaps in the ruins of old social and political structures we will learn to live peaceably and frame secularly justifiable health care policy in the face of limited secular moral authority, a vacuous secular morality, and real moral differences. This will require a toleration of discordant and diverse moral differences, and an acceptance of the limits of secular morality. But should the grace of such peaceable collaboration in diversity not be ours, still, in purely secular terms, it is all that can be justified.

Toleration does not mean that we will need to forgo moral condemnation of those acts we find reprehensible (e.g., "those who provide direct abortion do a great evil"). After all, toleration only makes sense in terms of that which one holds to be wrong or improper. One does not tolerate the good; one tolerates that which is evil. It is just that there are many evils against which one cannot secularly justify the coercive intervention of the state. In all of this, religious and ideological believers should recognize that a secular bioethics provides the peaceable neutral framework through which they can reach out to others and convert or recruit through witness and example, even if not through force.[28] Those of orthodox religious belief should know that prayer makes plain what secular reason cannot discern. The grace of conversion is not the force of coercion, but rather the attraction of the Divine.

The distinction drawn in this volume between a general secular morality and the moralities of particular moral communities is related to the traditional Western Christian distinction between what unaided reason can establish and what revelation can teach.[29] Unsupplemented by some special source of content, our understandings of morality and of the ultimate purpose of our lives remain impoverished.[30] Most of the traditional questions of Western metaphysics concerning the significance of human existence will in general secular terms go largely unanswered.[31] The general differences between the conclusions in this volume and those offered by traditional natural law theory, as for instance one finds drawn from the reflections of Thomas Aquinas, lie in the limitations of secular reason that this volume acknowledges.[32] Or to put matters more precisely, this volume sketches what reason can disclose when it turns forthrightly neither toward nor away from grace, but instead attempts to exercise its abilities apart from any of the contributions that grace, tradition, or a particular ideology can bring.[33] In such circumstances, few of the hopes of natural law accounts can be fulfilled.

The impossibility of establishing the concrete vision of the good life, proper deportment, health care policy, or bioethics by an appeal to general rational secular arguments leads to the development of two divergent understandings of bioethics: secular bioethics and the bioethics of content-full moral commitment. The first is the focus of this volume.

## Notes

1. There is a wealth of volumes, not to mention articles, focused on the topic of justice in health care policy, providing a rich range of views of fairness among which to choose. See, for example, Henry J. Aaron and William B. Schwartz, *The Painful Prescription* (Washington, D.C.: Brookings Institution, 1984); Thomas J. Bole III and William B. Bondeson (eds.), *Rights to Health Care* (Dordrecht: Kluwer, 1991); Larry R. Churchill, *Rationing Health Care in America* (Notre Dame, Ind.: University of Notre Dame Press, 1987); Norman Daniels, *Just Health Care* (New York: Cambridge University Press, 1985); Paul T. Menzel, *Strong Medicine* (New York: Oxford University Press, 1990); E. Haavi Morreim, *Balancing Act* (Washington D.C.: Georgetown University Press, 1995) ; Martin A. Strosberg, Joshua M. Wiener, and Robert Baker (eds.), *Rationing America's Medical Care: The Oregon Plan and Beyond* (Washington, D.C.: Brookings Institution, 1992); and Robert M. Veatch, *The Foundations of Justice* (New York: Oxford University Press, 1986).

2. An engaging contemporary attempt to reexamine the physician–patient relationship is provided by Edmund Pellegrino and David Thomasma, who criticize current understandings and call for a restoration of the relationship to its proper character. See *A Philosophical Basis of Medical Practice* (New York: Oxford University Press, 1981), and *For the Patient's Good* (New York: Oxford University Press, 1988). See also Edmund Pellegrino and David Thomasma, *The Virtues in Medical Practice* (New York: Oxford University Press, 1993).

3. The term *ideology* has carried a bad connotation since Napoleon used ''idéologues'' in ridicule and Karl Marx employed ''Ideologie'' to identify a collective illusion, a false consciousness regarding reality, primarily social and economic reality. ''Idéologie'' was coined by Antoine Louis Claude Destutt, Comte de Tracy (1754–1836), in 1796 to name his materialistic account of ideas, and his psychology generally, which he took to be a part of zoology. Against the background of Étienne Bonnot de Condillac's (1715–80) development of John Locke's theory of ideas into an empirical sensationalism (a theory that all ideas are to be understood in terms of their derivation from sensations), and in accord with the materialism of Pierre Jean George Cabanis (1757–1808), Tracy offered a reductive account of ideas. In this fashion, Tracy advanced his science, ideology, as a theory of human ''ideological'' or psychological activities. Along with Condillac, Cabanis, and others, Tracy sought, in light of his understanding of ideology, to effect radical social reforms, including reforms in education. The ''idéologistes'' were opposed by Napoleon and scorned under the title of ''idéologues.'' In the nineteenth century, ideology came to be used to compass a particular genre of the philosophy of mind, the science of ideas, speculation, visionary reflection, impractical theorizing, and unrealistic revolutionary enthusiasms.

   Karl Marx (1818–83) and Friedrich Engels (1820–95) in *Die deutsche Ideologie* give ideology a special set of meanings as a part of their account of how systems of ideas reflect economic arrangements, due to the division of labor, which alienates workers from the ruling social structures as well as from the value of their labor. An ideology is then a superstructure of ideas and beliefs, which makes a particular social organization (e.g., bourgeois capitalism) both plausible and effective. An ideology represents "the ruling ideas of the epoch. . . . The ruling ideas are nothing more than the ideal expression of the dominant material relationships, the dominant material relationships grasped as ideas; hence of the relationships which make the one class the ruling one, therefore the ideas of its dominance." Marx and Engels, *The German Ideology* (New York: International Publishers, 1967), p. 39. An ideology is a false consciousness that is false in canonizing a particular historically conditioned set of political, social, and economic arrangements, and in rationalizing the alienation of labor from workers. In this context, thinkers become employed to develop and sustain the ideology that protects the interests of the ruling class. These are "conceptive ideologists, who make the perfecting of the illusion of the class about itself their chief source of livelihood" (ibid., p. 40). However, since history in Marxist accounts leads to the triumph of the proletariat, there is as a consequence a conflict between bad ideologies and the good ideology, the communist ideology. In this last case, Marxist-Leninism is the ideology of the revolutionary working class in its struggle against the bourgeois ideology of the capitalists. Thus, Gorbachev in attempting to justify perestroika could speak of turning to Lenin as an ideological source of perestroika. Mikhail Gorbachev, *Perestroika* (London: Collins, 1987), for example, pp. 25–26. Socialist ideology in this case is regarded as a new type of ideology.

As a result, ideology in Marxist circles has also taken on a neutral meaning, in that it compasses ideologies on both sides of the "ideological struggle." "All ideologies stem from one root, viz., the *psychology* of the given age, characteristic of this particular age, the totality of its manners, customs, morals, feelings, views, aspirations and ideals." B. M. Boguslavsky et al., *ABC of Dialectical and Historical Materialism* (Moscow: Progress, 1978), p. 451. So, too, ideology is defined as a "System von Anschauungen, Ideen und Theorien über die soziale Wirklichkeit als Ganzes bzw. über einzelne ihrer Seiten, Prozesse und Probleme, in denen die jeweiligen Klasseninteressen konzentrierten Ausdruck finden sowie dementsprechende Stellungnahmen, Entscheidungen, Bewertungen, Regeln und Normen für soziale Verhaltensweisen." Georg Assmann et al. (eds.), *Wörterbuch der Marxistisch-Leninistischen Soziologie* (Berlin: Dietz, 1977), p. 261. See, also, F. W. Konstantinow et al., *Grundlagen der marxistischen Philosophie,* trans. from Russian by Otto Finger et al. (Berlin: Dietz, 1966), especially pp. 193–651; and Wolfgang Eichhorn et al., *Marxistisch-leninistische Philosophie* (Berlin: Dietz, 1979), especially pp. 661–674. For examples of ideology, including understandings of science and the physical world, see G. Domin and H.-H. Laufmann (eds.), *Imperialismus und Wissenschaft* (Berlin: Akademie-Verlag, 1977); Herbert Hörz, *Marxistische Philosophie und Naturwissenschaften* (Berlin: Akademie-Verlag, 1974); and Alexander Wernecke, *Biologismus und ideologischer Klassenkampf* (Berlin: Dietz, 1976). For a brief critique of the zealous attempts to account for social structures and beliefs in terms of ideological analyses, see Jon Elster, *An Introduction to Karl Marx* (New York: Cambridge University Press, 1986), especially pp. 168–85. For an excellent overview of many of these issues, see Klaus Hartmann, *Die marxsche Theorie*

(Berlin: de Gruyter, 1970), pp. 196–204, 554–66.

In this book, *ideology* is used to identify, grosso modo, a concatenation of ideas, images, values, metaphysical assumptions, and epistemological presuppositions that provide a group of people with understandings of morality, justice, proper social structures, as well as of legitimate political authority. The term is used to identify the secular equivalent of the nexus of moral, axiological, political, epistemological, and metaphysical understandings such as are provided by a religion. This use is in stipulation because, inter alia, according to Marxist accounts religious beliefs are an element of an ideology. Moreover, there is in my use a recognition that ideas play a role in a world view other than to direct action. Thus, Copleston's definition is too narrow. "The word 'ideology' is here understood as a system of ideas oriented to the realization of a social or political goal through concerted human action, the action of a group." Frederick Copleston, *Philosophy in Russia* (Notre Dame, Ind.: University of Notre Dame Press, 1986), p. 4.

4. Because the West has through its scientific, technological, imperialistic, and commercial successes exported its religions, laws, cultures, and languages throughout the world, much is said in this volume about Western philosophical arguments and the development of Western culture and thought. First, the West exported its traditional cultures to the world and then, second, its self-critical, antitraditional view of culture, which has fashioned the posttraditional culture of the contemporary world. The West, by and large, has created the contemporary world culture.

As a consequence, it is Western philosophical reflections and expectations, as well as Western bioethics, that have immediate salience in bioethical discussions, whether one is in Tokyo, Bei-jing, Sydney, Jerusalem, Mexico City, Manila, Buenos Aires, or Austin, Texas. For an overview of contemporary approaches to bioethics, see, for example, B. A. Lustig et al. (ed.), *Regional Developments in Bioethics: 1989–1991* (Dordrecht: Kluwer, 1992). Attempts to articulate indigenous bioethics are endeavors to preserve something of local traditional culture against the critical forces of Western modernity and are thus defined over against Western bioethics. A substantial attempt to give an account of bioethics from the perspective of the developing world is found in a book under preparation by Angeles Tan Alora and her colleagues from the Southeast Asian Center for Bioethics, Manila, namely: *Bioethics: Readings and Cases from the Developing World.* See also Rosemarie Tong, *Feminist Thought: A Comprehensive Introduction* (Boulder, Colo.: Westview Press, 1989).

5. Heraclitus, *On the Universe,* in *Hippocrates,* trans. W. H. S. Jones (Cambridge, Mass.: Harvard University Press, 1959), xci, vol. 4, p. 499. The Stoics saw Heraclitus's account as an anticipation of their theory of the *koinos logos.*

6. Western Christianity's rationalistic account of faith took form through various stages. It included the view that one could by reason show the existence of God, either by ontological proof, as with Anselm of Canterbury (A.D. 1033–1109), by the *quinque viae,* as with Thomas Aquinas (A.D. 1225–74), or at least by some form of rational considerations. *Constitutio dogmatica de fide catholica, Canones,* II. *De revelatione,* 1, from the Fourth Session of the Vatican Council, April 24,1870. This marriage of philosophy and theology followed an earlier incorporation of rationalism that developed out of the Frankish court and was expressed in its endorsement of the

novel doctrine of the filioque. John S. Romanides, *Franks, Romans, Feudalism, and Doctrine* (Boston: Holy Cross Orthodox Press, 1981). These rationalistic commitments and aspirations were as well bound to a legalistic understanding of morality. Christos Yannaras, *The Freedom of Morality* (Crestwood, N.Y.: St. Vladimir's Seminary Press, 1984). For a brief account of the period of transition as Western Christianity separated from the tradition and gave itself its own form, see Chrysostom Frank, "St. Bernard of Clairvaux and the Eastern Christian Tradition," *St. Vladimir's Theological Quarterly* 36 (1992): 315–28.

7.  In this book I refer to the ancient, middle, modern, and postmodern worlds, eras, or ages. By the ancient world I identify that great circum-Mediterranean pagan cultural synthesis framed primarily from Greek and Roman sources, which came to an end some time after the Edict of Toleration (A.D. 313) and before the middle of the sixth century. Alaric's sack of Rome (A.D. 410), the abdication of Romulus Augustus (476), the closing of the pagan academies (529), and finally the great four-year plague that began in 542 marked the collapse of an up until then regnant cultural understanding and the beginning of a new world. For reflections on the character of the circum-Mediterranean world after the plague, see, for example, John E. Sandys, *A History of Classical Scholarship* (New York: Hafner, 1958), vol. 1, pp. 269–71, 383. After this period, the Western world had changed decidedly in character and tone. Already in a letter written in 494–95, Pope Gelasius (492–96) of Rome distinguished between *antiquus* and *modernus*. Walter Freund, *Modernus und andere Zeitbegriffe des Mittelalters* (Cologne: Böhlau, 1957), p. 4. By the sixth century the terms were used in a developed way by the Roman senator and commentator on the Psalms, Magnus Aurelius Cassiodorus (480–575), to identify the ancient world, much as we would today.

The notion of the Middle Ages as the millennium extending from the fall of old Rome to around the fall of new Rome, Constantinople (May 29, 1453) appears in part shaped by a monumental history by Flavio Biondo, *Historiarum ab inclinatione Romanorum imperii decades,* written between 1439 and 1453, which compassed the period from the sack of Rome (A.D. 410) by Alaric to A.D. 1442. See, for example, Alfred Masius, *Flavio Biondo, Sein Leben und seine Werke* (Leipzig: B. G. Teubner, 1879), and Denys Hay, "Flavio Biondo and the Middle Ages," *Proceedings of the British Academy* (London: Oxford, 1960), pp. 97–125. Terms such as *media tempestas* (1469), *media aetas* (1518), and *medium aevum* (1604) came to be used. Otto Brunner, Werner Conze, Reinhart Koselleck (eds.), *Geschichtliche Grundbegriffe* (Stuttgart: Klett-Cotta, 1978), vol. 4, p. 98. See also Christoph Cellarius, *Historia Universalis, breviter ac perspicue exposita,* in *Antiquam et Medii Aevi ac Novam divisa* (1685). One finds individuals speaking of "auncient, middle-aged, or moderne writers." Nathan Edelman, "The Early Uses of Medium Aevum, Moyen âge, Middle Ages," *Romanic Review* 29 (Feb. 1938): 7; see also "Other Early Uses of *Moyen âge* and *Moyen temps,*" *Romanic Review* 30 (Dec. 1939): 327–30. From the vantage point of the Renaissance, this period was regarded as an epoch of darkness separating modern times from the ancient world, thus establishing a threefold division of history with modernity identifying Europe shaped by the Renaissance and Reformation.

Modernity incorporated a critical relation to the literature, culture, and knowledge of the past. One of the first expressions of this sense of modernity is found in the so-called *querelle* or quarrel whether the literature and culture of the moderns were better than those of the ancients. "As early as the eighteenth century, the word 'modern' acquired something of the ring of a war cry, but then only as an antithesis of 'ancient'—implying contrast with classical antiquity." Carl E. Schorske, *Fin-de Siècle Vienna* (New York: Alfred Knopf, 1985), p. xvii. See, also, Hans Baron, "The *Querelle* of the Ancients and the Moderns as a Problem for Renaissance Scholarship," *Journal of the History of Ideas* 20 (Jan. 1959): 3–22; and J. W. Lorimer, "A Neglected Aspect of the 'Querelle des anciens et des modernes,' " *Modern Language Review* 51 (Apr. 1956): 179–85. With the French Revolution (1789) and its subsequent attempt on November 9, 1793, to establish a cult of Reason, modernity took on a distinctly anticlerical, anti-Roman Catholic, if not anti-Christian, character. André Latreille, *L'Église catholique et la révolution française* (Paris: Hachette, 1948), 2 vols. Sentiments against established religion were supported by the secularization in Germany that followed the *Reichsdeputationshauptschluß* on August 24, 1803, which transferred Roman Catholic holdings to secular hands, destroying a system of eleemosynary care dating from the Middle Ages and unleashing a *Bildersturz* or iconoclasm that destroyed both rare books and precious art. "Der Reichsdeputationshauptschluß," in H. H. Hofmann (ed.), *Quellen zum Verfassungsorganismus des heiligen römischen Reiches deutscher Nation,* (Darmstadt: Wissenschaftliche Buchgesellschaft, 1976), pp. 329–58. As Octavio Paz observes, the modern age can be characterized as a "breaking away from Christian society." Octavio Paz, *Children of the Mire,* trans. Rachel Phillips (Cambridge, Mass.: Harvard University Press, 1974), p. 27. Indeed, after World War I and the collapse of progressivist hopes, modernity took on the sense of being an adversary culture. Lionel Trilling, *Beyond Culture* (London: Secker & Warburg, 1966). It opposes not just Christianity, but much of traditional Western culture. The modernity of the nineteenth century and early 20th century had been full of hope and confidence in scientific and social progress. See, for example, J. Howard Moore, *The Universal Kinship* (London: George Bell, 1906). The modernity that followed was not only critical of the past but self-critical and self-doubting. Modernity became "an unending permanent revolution against the totality of modern existence." Marshall Berman, *All That Is Solid Melts into Air* (New York: Simon & Schuster, 1982), p. 30.

Within religion, modernity took on the sense of accommodating to the science and circumstances of the contemporary world. In Roman Catholicism, this included the heresy of modernism condemned by Pope Pius X in his encyclical *Lamentabili,* July 3, 1907; see Joseph Schnitzer, *Der katholische Modernismus* (Berlin: Protestantischer Schriftenvertrieb, 1912). See also Gabriel Motzkin, *Time and Transcendence* (Dordrecht: Kluwer, 1992). Modernity came later to have special meanings in art and literature. A prominent element of modern art has been its disengagement from the past and classical art. "Modern architecture, modern music, modern philosophy, modern science—all these define themselves not out of the past, indeed scarcely against the past, but in independence of the past." Schorske, *Fin-de-Siècle Vienna,* p. xvii. See also Matei Calinescu, *Faces of Modernity: Avant-Garde, Decadence, Kitsch* (Bloomington: Indiana University Press, 1977).

The term *postmodernity* may first have been used by Arnold Toynbee to indicate the historical period when reflection takes place concerning the modern age. Harry Levin, *Refractions* (New York: Oxford University Press, 1966), p. 277. The term also initially was used to identify the massive social, industrial, and technological changes that became salient after World War II. To capture the changes, authors spoke of a postbourgeoise society. George Lichtheim, *The New Europe: Today and Tomorrow* (New York: Praeger, 1963). This society was "postindustrial." Daniel Bell, *The Coming of Post-Industrial Society* (New York: Basic Books, 1973). "The advent of the post-modern period has been marked by the rapid rise of a new technology of knowledge, which serves data collection and analysis, simulation, and systems analysis. It has been said that the computer is to the production of knowledge what the steam engine was to production of materials." Amitai Etzioni, *The Active Society* (New York: Free Press, 1968), p. 9. Postmodernity also came to identify both a sociological and epistemological condition: the loss of a universal narrative in terms of which to interpret human experience, along with the loss of the capacity to justify or to disclose in general secular terms the content of such a narrative. Jean-François Lyotard, *The Postmodern Condition,* trans. G. Bennington and B. Massumi (Manchester: Manchester University Press, 1984). This last sense of postmodernity, the absence as a matter of fact and in principle of a universal secular moral narrative, is cardinal for this work on bioethics. As the reader will note, though I take Lyotard's observation on the fracturing of the universal moral narrative as heuristic, there are many points of disagreement with Lyotard regarding our condition. Though I agree that one "destroys narrative monopolies" in recognizing the lack of secular moral authority for any particular secular moral account or narrative, I recognize considerable limits to the authority "to will the power to play out, listen to, and tell stories." The "non-centrism, non-finality, non-truth" that Lyotard underscores is that of any content-full secular narrative. Andrew Benjamin (ed.), *The Lyotard Reader* (London: Blackwell, 1989), pp. 153, 120. As a consequence, *pace* UNESCO and other organizations forwarding content-full understandings of positive human rights and rights to forbearance beyond those grounded in the principle of permission, the articulation of universalist positive rights is an impossible undertaking. See, for example, Eugene B. Brody, *Biomedical Technology and Human Rights* (Paris: UNESCO, 1993).

In summary, when speaking of the ancient world, era, or age, I wish to identify that polytheistic, multicultural period of the circum-Mediterranean world in which there were at best modest expectations from reason qualified by robust traditions of skepticism. The Middle Ages is used to identify the Western European Christian synthesis, the period during which the Roman Catholic religion was fashioned and against which, later, the Protestant Reformation reacted. The Western Middle Ages provided a monotheistic, monocultural moral vision with not only a strong commitment to faith in a Revelation, but a robust faith that reason could disclose much of the moral content and moral authority that faith secured. Within this context, a strong skepticism did in fact count as a form of heresy. See, for example, the Holy See's condemnation of fideism on November 25, 1347.

Modernity, as the foregoing indicates, is an ambiguous term. First, it identifies a period after the Middle Ages, most clearly after the Renaissance and Reformation when, in the spirit of the *querelle,* Western European culture confidently asserts its powers over the ancient world with a self-confidence born of its successes in exploration, astronomy, anatomy, physics, chemistry, and art. It attempts in its philosophy to span the divisions created by the Reformation and to set behind it the religious wars of the first part of the sixteenth century. Modernity in this sense has its culmination in the Enlightenment, which proclaims the centrality of reason. It does so looking to the past as constraining and to the future as liberating. Immanuel Kant's (1724–1804) 1784 manifesto on the Enlightenment is an epiphany of this viewpoint. "Enlightenment is man's release from his self-incurred tutelage. Tutelage is man's inability to make use of his understanding without direction from another. Self-incurred is this tutelage when its cause lies not in lack of reason but in lack of resolution and courage to use it without direction from another. *Sapere aude!* 'Have courage to use your own reason!'—that is the motto of enlightenment. . . . By the public use of one's reason I understand the use which a person makes of it as a scholar before the reading public." "What Is Enlightenment?" in *Foundations of the Metaphysics of Morals,* trans. L. W. Beck (Indianapolis: Bobbs-Merrill, 1976), pp. 85, 87, Akademie Textausgabe, vol. 8, 35, 37. AK citations are to the standard German text of Kant's writings: *Kants gesammelte Schriften* (Berlin: de Gruyter). After the French Revolution and until World War I, there remained a strong confidence in progress and in reason. But from Friedrich Nietzsche to the present, modernity came to identify a strongly adversarial culture, which was not merely anti-Christian but which, as with Dada, brought reason itself into question. This second sense of modernity is the beginning of postmodernity's loss of the unifying focus of reason. In talking of modernity I will use it in the first sense and regard the second as the anticipation of the fragmentation of traditional Western culture into the self-doubt, loss of faith in reason, and cultural diversity of postmodernity. With postmodernity the West becomes posttraditional—it abandons central elements of some fifteen hundred years of its culture.

In this first sense, modernity (as well as terms such as *the modern period*) is characterized by the project of securing by reason the substance of the Judeo-Christian morality, along with an account of moral authority not by faith, but by sound rational argument. It is the attempt to have what is taken to be the core of the Judeo-Christian moral vision without the necessity of confessing the Judeo-Christian God. The attempt to secure this core of the Judeo-Christian account of moral authority and of morality, albeit now in secular terms, I shall often refer to as the modern philosophical project or the modern moral philosophical project (or simply as the moral philosophical project), using the former to include the hope of giving not just moral but also metaphysical or ontological orientation. Although the modern philosophical project antedates the Enlightenment and indeed was brought into question by Enlightenment figures such as David Hume (1711–76), it can generally be seen as continuing in the Enlightenment and in the nineteenth- and early twentieth-century progressivist aspirations to justify and frame a universal secular moral narrative. The term *Enlightenment project* (and related terms) is used to identify the endeavor to establish a canonical, content-full morality in secular terms justifiable to persons generally. Postmodernity is the recognition that this project is vain.

8. Kant at the end of the Enlightenment and six years after the French Revolution writes
   in favor of establishing a league of nations to frame the condition for world peace.
   *Zum ewigen Frieden: ein philosophischer Entwurf* (1795).
9. The justification for this claim is advanced in chapter 2. For an account of its historical
   and philosophical roots, see Alasdair MacIntyre, *After Virtue* (Notre Dame, Ind.:
   University of Notre Dame Press, 1981); *Whose Justice? Which Rationality?* (Notre
   Dame, Ind.: Notre Dame University Press, 1988).
10. In the seven years following Roman Catholicism's introduction of its Novus Ordo
    Mass (1969), along with its severely limiting the use of its "traditional" Tridentine
    Mass, the number of Roman Catholic priests in the world declined from circa
    410,000 to about 245,000. In many areas of the world, there was also a dramatic drop
    in Sunday Mass attendance. For instance, while between 1965 and 1974 Protestant
    church attendance in Canada decreased only 19 percent, Catholic attendance dropped
    29 percent. *Index to International Public Opinion, 1978–1979* (Westport, Conn.:
    Greenwood Press, 1980). In some places in Europe, the decline has been even more
    dramatic. In the sixteen years prior to 1989, the number of churchgoers in Amsterdam
    declined from 45,000 to 10,000, and the number of open churches declined from 65
    to 45, with the likelihood that half of the remaining would close by the end of the
    century. Siggi Weidemann, "Altäre unter dem Hammer," *Süddeutsche Zeitung*
    (Apr. 18, 1989). The accommodation to modernity does not appear to have been a
    success. Unlike Trent, the Second Vatican Council was the herald of much catastro-
    phe.
11. John Paul II, *Veritatis Splendor* (Vatican City: Libreria Editrice Vaticana, 1993),
    p. 158.
12. Aristotle, *Nicomachean Ethics* 9.10; *Politics* 7.4.
13. In all of this, it is important to underscore that moral strangers do not find each other
    morally inscrutable. Moral strangers may share the same values, but only have
    different orderings of those values. They will understand each other only too well.
    They will see each other as mistaken but not as mysterious or alien. There can be
    mutual understanding across divergent moral communities, even when different
    values are at stake. Southern Baptists can understand committed Moslems. Devout
    Moslems can understand committed atheist socialists. In understanding each other,
    they can both disagree with each other and yet still in some areas be partners (i.e.,
    *socii*) in certain public undertakings.
       Also, it is important to recognize that persons who do not live their lives fully
    embedded within a very thickly joined community, such as a monastery or some other
    committed religious community, or a group of ideologically dedicated, will find that
    they are both moral friends and moral strangers in different areas with the same
    people—which is to say that, in some areas of discussion, they will be able to resolve
    disputes by sound rational argument or by commonly acknowledged moral authori-
    ties. In other areas, resolution will be possible only by agreement. The distinction
    between moral friends and moral controversies, between societies and communities,
    is directed to the way in which controversies can be resolved with commonly recog-
    nized moral authority.
       The contrast of community with society becomes less helpful as one deals with

individuals whose moral lives are so vacuous and whose moral commitments are so tenuous that their association in a large-scale society appears to them plausibly the same as membership in a moral community with substantial traditions and practices. The conflation of community and society is further abetted by the commitment of governments to creating identities for citizens around constitutions, patriotic traditions, and social customs. Yet for most polities, their heterogeneity makes such attempts at large-scale community building unsuccessful. The seeming communality of such societies trades on moral ambiguities grounded in shards and pieces of once cohesive communities and once firmly shared moral visions.

In any event, no sharp line is presupposed between moral friends and moral strangers, communities and societies. Also, moral friends can become moral strangers overnight through heresy or schism. Instead, what is at stake is the difference between those moral contexts in which individuals can discover how they ought to act as well as how they should resolve moral controversies and those in which they must create by moral agreement how they should act together or resolve moral controversies. In the latter case, common moral authority is derived from permission.

Even with this qualification, it must be acknowledged that moral friends in community may possess morally authoritative procedures for creating answers. One might think of the dispute in the Talmud between Rabbi Joshua and Rabbi Eliezer regarding whether a particular oven was clean or unclean. Despite miracles invoked by Rabbi Eliezer, Rabbi Joshua prevailed, buttressed by Rabbi Jeremiah, who argued "that the Torah had already been given at Mount Sinai; we pay no attention to a Heavenly Voice because Thou hast long since written in the Torah at Mount Sinai, *After the majority must one incline.*" Baba Mezia 59b (Soncino edition). Unlike procedures accepted by associations, the foregoing procedure reflects an authoritative Lawgiver (Who among His laws authorizes a procedure), rather than being grounded in authority derived merely from the participants who create the procedure and endow it with authority. It is derived from a common accepted moral vision of true authority. One should note that, after the decision, Rabbi Eliezer was excommunicated. "On that day all objects which R. Eliezer had declared clean were brought and burnt in fire. Then they took a vote and excommunicated him" (ibid.). He had become in an important sense a moral stranger.

14. In this volume, the term *patient* is used in preference to the term *client*. A patient is a person who undergoes, suffers, or endures a problem, with respect to which health professionals can provide preventive, curative, comforting, caring, and diagnostic interventions. *Client,* on the other hand, derives from the Latin *cliens,* which can identify one who is a retainer, a follower, or a dependent, and may have unnecessarily demeaning connotations.

15. A very helpful account of the need to assume a particular moral viewpoint in order to gain moral content is found in Hegel's *Philosophy of Right.* The dialectical necessity of moving from Abstract Right and Morality to the Ethical Life (*Sittlichkeit*) lies in the failure of either of the first two to provide the content necessary to understand what contracts ought to be made or what the good is that ought to be pursued. Such can be made out in a content-full fashion only within a view from somewhere, within the context of a particular moral community. As Hegel puts it in the beginning of

"Sittlichkeit," "In an *ethical* community, it is easy to say what man must do, what are the duties he has to fulfill in order to be virtuous: he has simply to follow the well-known and explicit rules of his own situation." *Hegel's Philosophy of Right*, trans. T. M. Knox (London: Oxford University Press, 1965), sec. 150, p. 107. An exploration of Hegel's arguments for the necessity of the contingency of moral content, is found in Allen Wood, "Does Hegel Have an Ethics?" *Monist* 74 (July 1991): 358–85.

16. An interesting defense of the perspective of cosmopolitan ecumenism is provided by Francis Fukuyama's popular study, in which he argues that history will culminate in the universal recognition of the moral propriety of capitalist liberal democracy. He contends that the conjunction of capitalism's ability to satisfy desires, liberal democracy's capacity to provide peaceable mutual recognition, and modern science's contribution to the alleviation of life's difficulties have transformed history. History has changed from being directed to duties and projects that transcend this world or that involve conquest, to duties and projects directed to satisfying desires and concerns realizable in this world through consumption and without conquest. "The modern liberal project attempted to shift the basis of human societies from thymos to the more secure ground of desires. . . . Liberalism also made possible the modern economic world by liberating desire from all constraints on acquisitiveness, and allying it to reason in the form of modern natural science" (p. 333). Under such circumstances, the content-full language of particular moral communities, so Fukuyama argues, will evaporate. "For the apparent differences between peoples' 'languages of good and evil' will appear to be an artifact of their particular stage of historical development" (p. 338). *The End of History and the Last Man* (New York: Free Press, 1992). Philip Grier provides a powerful critique of Fukuyama and the peculiar dependence in his arguments on Alexander Kojève ("The End of History, and the Return of History," *Owl of Minerva* 21 [Spring 1990]: 131–44). Kojève argues that the Americans of the late 1940s and 1950s were the true realization of Russian and Chinese Communist aspirations. Kojève, for example, observes that

Now, several voyages of comparison made [between 1948 and 1958] to the United States and the U.S.S.R. gave me the impression that if the Americans give the appearance of rich Sino-Soviets, it is because the Russians and the Chinese are only Americans who are still poor but are rapidly proceeding to get richer. I was led to conclude from this that the "American way of life" was the type of life specific to the post-historical period, the actual presence of the United States in the World prefiguring the 'eternal present' future of all of humanity. Thus, Man's return to animality appeared no longer as a possibility that was yet to come, but as a certainty that was already present.

To be animal, to have fallen out of history, is to have become a good consuming cosmopolitan ecumenist who eschews further confrontations directed toward recognition or satisfaction of thymos. In Kojève's account, the only humans not to become animals at the end of history are the Japanese because they are saved by snobbery.

"Post-historical" Japanese civilization undertook ways diametrically opposed to the "American way." No doubt, there were no longer in Japan any Religion, Morals, or Politics in the "European" or "historical" sense of these words. But Snobbery in its pure form created disciplines negating the "natural" or "animal" given which in effectiveness far surpassed those that arise, in Japan or elsewhere, from "historical" Action—that is, from warlike and revolutionary Fights or from forced Work. To be sure, the peaks (equalled nowhere else) of specifically Japanese snobbery—the Noh Theater, the ceremony of tea, and the art of bouquets of flowers—were and still remain the exclusive prerogative of the nobles and the rich. . . . Now, since no animal can be a snob, every "Japanized" post-historical period would be specifically human.

*Introduction to the Reading of Hegel* (Ithaca, N.Y.: Cornell University Press, 1969), pp. 161–62. One way to understand these claims is that the American consumerist way of life is beyond history and transcendent concerns, sustaining a set of bioethics whose concerns are all and only immanent.

The Canadian film, *The Decline of the American Empire* (1986), directed by Denys Arcand, provides a cinematic portrayal of postmodern, posthistorical North America.

17. By cosmopolitans I identify those individuals who regard themselves as possessing the canonical, content-full, secular morality (and bioethics) and see it as being justifiable outside of a particular moral history and tradition. I use the term *cosmopolitan ecumenist* to identify those individuals who hold that, given sufficient discussion, individuals will come to see that they share a common content-full morality, however sparse. For reflections on allied themes, see MacIntyre, *Whose Justice? Which Rationality?* See also H. T. Engelhardt, Jr., *Bioethics and Secular Humanism: The Search for a Common Morality* (Philadelphia: Trinity Press International, 1991), pp. 33–40.

18. Here I regard polytheism metaphorically as the personalized presentation of the diverse possibilities for human flourishing. The possibilities are incarnate in contrary and competing biographies of human excellence, none of which has priority and which cannot be fully integrated in a single moral standpoint. In secular terms and building on the polytheistic metaphor, the last would be a monotheistic moral vision. The contemporary secular pluralist state is polytheist. One may choose among contrary moral communities as the ancients chose to whom among the pagan gods they would give special devotion. In this regard, one might consider Severus Alexander's (emperor A.D. 222–35) piety with regard to the gods. "His manner of living was as follows: First of all, if it were permissible, that is to say, if he had not lain with his wife, in the early morning hours he would worship in the sanctuary of his Lares, in which he kept statues of the deified emperors—of whom, however, only the best had been selected—and also of certain holy souls, among them Apollonius, and according to a contemporary writer, Christ, Abraham, Orpheus, and others of this same character and, besides, the portraits of his ancestors." Aelius Lampridius, "Severus Alexander," in *Scriptores Historiae Augustae,* trans. David Magie (Cambridge, Mass.: Harvard University Press, 1967), 29.2, p. 235. There is no sense of the singularity of the moral claims made by Abraham and Christ. They are regarded as providing partial, attractive, yet still competing visions of truth, somewhat like competing bioethics.

19. With special qualifications anent Kant's account of motivation, Kant makes reference to God's standpoint in order coherently to account for a secular philosophical ethic that possesses content. In order rationally to understand the duty to promote the highest good, Kant is compelled to assume the existence of God.

Now it was our duty to promote the highest good; and it is not merely our privilege but a necessity connected with duty as a requisite to presuppose the possibility of this highest good.

This presupposition is made only under the condition of the existence of God, and this condition inseparably connects this supposition with duty. Therefore, it is morally necessary to assume the existence of God. . . . In this manner, through the concept of the highest good as the object and final end of pure practical reason, the moral law leads to religion. . . . Therefore, morals is not really the doctrine of how to make ourselves happy but of how we are to be worthy of happiness. Only if religion is added to it can the hope arise of someday participating in happiness in proportion as we endeavored not to be unworthy of it.

*Critique of Practical Reason,* trans. L. W. Beck (Indianapolis: Library of Liberal Arts, 1956), pp. 130, 134, AK V, 125, 129–30. Here, in general outline, Kant is correct. The Divine perspective unifies the ground of being, the justification of morality, and the basis for a motivation to be moral.

20. This portrayal of the Deity and of the philosophers' God reflects Greco-Judeo-Christian understanding of Deity. It sought to justify a single coherent view of values and of reality in terms of a God who is the ground of being, value, and knowledge.

21. MacIntyre, *After Virtue.*

22. For a discussion of the limits on the obligations to save life within Roman Catholic moral theology, see Russell E. Smith (ed.), *Conserving Human Life* (Braintree, Mass.: Pope John Center, 1989).

23. As soon as the patient is *goses,* there is an obligation not to begin the use of stimulants that will prolong dying. See Immanuel Jakobovits, *Jewish Medical Ethics* (New York: Bloch, 1962). Also, Fred Rosner, "The Jewish Attitude toward Euthanasia," in Fred Rosner and J. D. Bleich (eds.), *Jewish Bioethics* (New York: Sanhedrin, 1979), pp. 260–64.

24. Orthodox Judaism appears to hold that the moral constraints against abortion are more severe for gentiles than Jews. A study in this regard is provided by Baruch A. Brody, who notes that abortion for a bnai Noah is a capital offense. "The Use of Halakhic Material in Discussions of Medical Ethics," *Journal of Medicine and Philosophy* 8 (August 1983): 317–28.

25. The reason is that the Torah does not forbid a man from having more than one wife, though a woman is forbidden from having more than one husband. Therefore, it is easier to regard the donation of ova from an unmarried woman as not raising the issue of adultery than it is so to regard the donation of sperm for artificial insemination. For discussion of some of these complex issues, see Avraham Steinberg, "Jewish Medical Ethics," in B. A. Brody et al. (eds.), *Theological Developments in Bioethics: 1988–90* (Dordrecht: Kluwer, 1991), p. 184. See also David M. Feldman, *Health and Medicine in the Jewish Tradition* (New York: Crossroads, 1986), p. 71. The matters are complicated by the decree of Gershom ben Joseph (960–1028/40) forbidding European Jews to have more than one wife, and by the question of how long this decree binds and whom.

26. Daniel Callahan, "Minimalist Ethics," *Hastings Center Report* 11 (Oct. 1981): 19–25.

27. As the Angelic Doctor puts it, "I answer that with regard to heretics . . . on their own side there is the sin, whereby they deserve not only to be separated from the Church by excommunication, but also to be severed from the world by death. For it is a much graver matter to corrupt the faith which quickens the soul, than to forge money, which supports temporal life. Wherefore if forgers of money and other

evildoers are forthwith condemned to death by the secular authority, much more reason is there for heretics, as soon as they are convicted of heresy, to be not only excommunicated but even put to death." *Summa Theologica of St. Thomas Aquinas* (Westminster, Md.: Christian Classics, 1948), vol. 3, p. 1220; 2-2, Q. 11, art. 3. See also 2-2, Q. 10, art. 8. In this regard, Aquinas was reflecting the general ethos of Western Christianity. The Fourth Lateran Council, for instance, granted the same indulgences to those who exterminated heretics at home as to those who went to the Holy Land. "Catholici vero qui, crucis assumpto charactere, ad haereticorum exterminium se accinxerint, illa gaudeant indulgentia, illoque sancto privilegio sint muniti, quod accedentibus in Terrae sanctae subsidium conceditur." "Concilium Lateranese IV" [1215], *Conciliorum Oecumenicorum Decreta* (Basil: Herder, 1962), *Constitutiones* 3, p. 210. In this respect, one might note, Thomas Aquinas and the council departed from the traditional teachings of the Catholic church. A canon (variously numbered 27 or 28) of the eighty-five Apostolic Canons states: "We command that a bishop, or presbyter, or deacon who strikes the faithful that offend, or the unbelievers who do wickedly, and thinks to terrify them by such means, be deprived, for our Lord has nowhere taught us such things. On the contrary, 'when Himself was stricken, He did not strike again; when He was reviled, He reviled not again; when He suffered, He threatened not.'" Alexander Roberts and James Donaldson (eds.), The *Ante-Nicene Fathers* (Grand Rapids, Mich.: Wm. B. Eerdmans, 1989), vol. 7, p. 501. This opposition to coercive conversion was underscored by the Council of Carthage (A.D. 418 or 419), whose canons were later accepted by the Quinisext (or Quinisextine) Council (commonly known as the Trullan Council, A.D. 692). "Canon CXIX. There has been given a law whereby each and every person may by free choice undertake the exercise of Christianhood." Sts. Nicodemus and Agapius (eds.), *The Rudder of the Orthodox Catholic Church,* trans. D. Cummings (1957; repr. New York: Luna Printing, 1983), p. 673. It is because of the violation of these canons, as well as other offenses, that Orthodox Catholicism traditionally held the pope of Rome to have been deposed and removed from every Church office. "After stigmatizing the transgressions and innovations of the Popes [of Rome] many times the Orthodox Church has decreed their deposition and has divested them of every grace required for the celebration of Mass or of any other divine service. . . . It is an admitted fact . . . that the Pope [of Rome] not only strikes faithful followers and infidels, but even murders many like a blood thirsty man, who is one abominated by the Lord. So, how can a bishop subscribing his name to capital penalties, and acting as the instigator and cause of wars and murders and so many other nefarious deeds, possess any title to holy orders?" *The Rudder,* p. 788.

28. Christianity traditionally did not regard itself as a religion to be imposed by state force, but as a faith embraced freely and learned as one advanced in commitment. It even has an esoteric character. Cyril of Jerusalem (A.D. 315–86) warns, for example: "If after the class a catechumen asks you what the instructors have said, tell outsiders nothing. For it is a divine secret that we deliver to you, even the hope of the life to come. Keep the secret for the Rewarder. If someone says, 'What harm is done if I know about it too?,' don't listen to him. So the sick man asks for wine, but, given to him at the wrong time, it only produces brain-fever, and two evils ensue: the effect on

the sick man is disastrous, and the doctor is maligned.'' St. Cyril of Jerusalem, Procatechesis 12, in *The Works of Saint Cyril of Jerusalem,* trans. L. P. McCauley and A. A. Stephenson (Washington, D.C.: Catholic University of America Press, 1969), vol. 1, p. 79. Indeed, one must note the great reluctance of Christianity to reveal even its liturgy to unbelievers. One still finds before the first prayer of the faithful in the Orthodox liturgy the injunction, ''Depart, all ye Catechumens, depart. Depart, all ye Catechumens: let no Catechumen remain: but let us who are in the faith again, yet again, in peace pray unto the Lord.'' *Service Book of the Holy Orthodox-Catholic Apostolic Church,* 6th ed., trans. Isabel Hapgood (Englewood, N.J.: Antiochian Orthodox Christian Archdiocese, 1983), p. 92.

29. In the West, there was a distinction made between what can be known by natural reason, by reason unaided by grace and revelation, and what can be known through revelation. As Thomas Aquinas states, ''I answer that, It was necessary for man's salvation that there should be a knowledge revealed by God, besides philosophical science built up by human reason.'' *Summa Theologica* 1, Q. 1, art. 1, vol. 1, p. 1.

30. The impoverished character of secular bioethics can be understood within the traditional Western distinction between nature and grace. Or it can be seen in the more traditional Christian account. Understanding ''without grace'' can be interpreted as a fictive stage prior to the mind being drawn toward the law of God, toward the creation of a well-formed conscience. This account finds a classical articulation by John of Damascus (676–750). ''The law of God, then, acts upon our mind by drawing it to Him and spurring on our conscience. . . . Hence, it is impossible to observe the commandments of the Lord except by patience and prayer.'' St. John of Damascus, ''The Orthodox Faith,'' in *Saint John of Damascus Writings,* trans. F. H. Chase, Jr. (Washington, D.C.: Catholic University of America Press, 1981), pp. 388–89. Thus, one can understand the prayer at Great Vespers as a petition that one be given a well-formed conscience: ''Blessed art Thou, O Lord; teach me Thy statutes. Blessed art Thou, O Master; make me to understand Thy commandments. Blessed art Thou, O Holy One; enlighten me with Thy precepts.'' Hapgood, *Service Book,* p. 10. Rational argument will not establish a content-full morality. Rather, it is through being embedded in a content-full morality that one comes to understand reality. ''We may study as much as we will but we shall still not come to know the Lord unless we live according to His commandments, for the Lord is not made known through learning but by the Holy Spirit.'' Archimandrite Sophrony, *Wisdom from Mount Athos: The Writings of Staretz Silouan 1866–1938,* trans. R. Edmonds (Crestwood, N.Y.: St. Vladimir's Seminary Press, 1974).

31. Metaphysics in the West traditionally includes natural theology and explorations concerning the immortality of the soul. One might think here of the three questions of Kant: ''1. What can I know? 2. What ought I to do? 3. What may I hope?'' *Critique of Pure Reason* A805 = B833, in Norman Kemp Smith (trans.), *Immanuel Kant's Critique of Pure Reason* (London: Macmillan, 1964), p. 635. The last question has traditionally been addressed through considerations regarding the existence of God and the immortality of the soul. Following Kant, I consider the limits of our ability to answer such questions through secular rationality. My focus is on the second question.

32. The Roman Catholic Church contends that on the basis of natural reason one can

demonstrate a range of truths from the existence of God to the immorality of contra-ception. For example, the First Vatican Council held as an article of faith that the existence of God can be proved by natural reason alone. *Constitutio dogmatica de fide catholica, Canones,* II. *De revelatione,* 1, from the Fourth Session of the Vatican Council, April 24, 1870. *Conciliorum Oecumenicorum Decreta* (Basel: Herder, 1962), p. 786. So, too, Roman Catholicism came to hold that contraception can be evil as a matter of natural law. "The artificial limitation or prevention of births is immoral because it is contrary to the natural law." John P. Kenny, *Principles of Medical Ethics,* 2d ed. (Westminster, Md.: Newman Press, 1962), p. 102. As a matter of natural law, contraception becomes an action that persons should recognize as immoral, independently of any religious commitments. "All men, then, are called upon to obey the natural law. Hence it matters not whether one be a Roman Catholic, a Protestant, a Jew, a pagan, or a person who has no religious affiliations whatsoever; he is nevertheless obliged to become acquainted with and to observe the teachings of the law of nature." Edwin F. Healy, *Medical Ethics* (Chicago: Loyola University Press, 1956), p. 7.

Given this understanding of natural law, Roman Catholic moral theologians in general, and Roman Catholic medical ethicists in particular, came to regard them-selves as having a special scientific purchase on a body of morality accessible in principle to persons as such.

But the [Roman] Catholic moralists do have a just claim to special competence in the *science of ethics,* the science of moral right and wrong, the science of applying the moral law to the problems of human living. They are highly trained and experienced men in this particular field. Their preparation for this professional capacity is intense and comprehensive; they usually teach the science of morality over a number of years; and they are constantly dealing with practical applications of this science. Aside from any question of religion, the [Roman] Catholic moral-ists represent by far the world's largest group of specialists in the science of ethics. And they have a tradition of scientific study that extends over centuries.

Gerald Kelly, *Medico-Moral Problems* (St. Louis, Mo.: Catholic Hospital Associa-tion, 1958), p. 34. So, too, Marxist ethics in the late Soviet Union similarly regarded itself as providing objective scientific conclusions. Loren R. Graham, "How History and Politics Affect Closure in Biomedical Discussions: The Example of the Soviet Union," in H. T. Engelhardt, Jr., and A. L. Caplan (eds.), *Scientific Controversies* (New York: Cambridge University Press, 1987), pp. 249–64. Thomas Aquinas was less sanguine about the capacity to know natural law by reason. Though he held that the first principles of natural law are discoverable by all, he acknowledged that culture and context can limit the ability to perceive the secondary principles accu-rately. Aquinas, *Summa Theologica,* 1-2, Q. 94, art. 6.

33.  The realm of secular reason is, to mix metaphors, a kind of limbo. Here the Orthodox, not the Western, understanding of grace and nature cuts to the issue. It is not as if there ever were nature without grace. Grace is not a *donum superadditum.* To appre-ciate the secular world is not to see the world as it is without grace, without the energies of God. It is rather to use the moral language that must be employed with those who live ignoring grace, ignoring those energies. Natural law can only be seen truly within the moral perspective, vision, and endeavor of the community bound in correct worship and belief. Natural law is not accessible by reason alone.

# 2

## The Intellectual Bases of Bioethics

Moral controversies appear irresolvable. Some moral controversies can surely be shown to have been conceptual confusions or misunderstandings of crucial facts about the world. Such can be dispelled by conceptual clarification and analysis or the provision of more accurate information. Established orthodoxies and norms of political correctness may suppress evidence of some controversies. But the old questions seem perennial. This is nowhere more true than in bioethics where the issues at stake bear on matters of life and death. Plato[1] and Aristotle[2] discussed the morality of abortion and infanticide. Plato explored the issue of the allocation of resources to health care and informed consent.[3] We are left with similar questions, if not the same questions. Is it morally correct to limit the public funding of high-cost, low-yield health care in order to control costs? May a policy be established not to provide treatment for very low birthweight babies because of the high costs, low chance of survival, and the often low quality of life of those who survive? Or should one attempt to save life at all costs? Does it make any moral difference if the monies involved are governmental and the funds saved will be used to fund higher per-diem rates for scientists consulting on governmentally funded projects? Or to build formal gardens? Or to lower taxes? Is it wrong if the rich can privately purchase for their newborns care not available through public sources? How can one know which policy is the one that should be endorsed?

## Varieties of ethics

There are numerous ambiguities at the very roots of ethics. There is not even one sense of ethics, but a family of senses. To answer moral questions, one must first be clear about the meaning of morality and about the kind of morality at stake. One might construe morality as an account of how agents ought to act to be praiseworthy, not blameworthy. In such accounts, moral agents will take center stage, for it is only they who can be the subject of justified blame and praise. Or is morality an account of how to maximize happiness or satisfaction? Or perhaps morality is best understood independently of a focus on what agents should accomplish, and is instead concerned with achieving the good. It is not just that the border between moral and aesthetic concerns is fuzzy. There are also concerns about defilement, purity and impurity, being clean or unclean, that elide into moral interests in acting rightly, achieving the good, or being worthy of praise. Contemporary moral philosophical reflection in the academy addresses only a small portion of the issues that have captured the interest of individuals considering what should count as proper conduct. Even within academic reflections, there are differences between those moral theories that provide (1) accounts of when moral agents are blameworthy and praiseworthy (e.g., Immanuel Kant), (2) accounts of what it means to achieve happiness (e.g., John Stuart Mill), and (3) accounts of what it is to realize the good (e.g., Thomas Aquinas).

The term ethics is itself ambiguous. First, as its etymology suggests, ethics can mean that which is customary. As that which is habitual to a people, ethics is similar in meaning to the root of the word morals, *mos* (pl. *mores*), the customs of a people, a sense that is close to the meaning of the English word mores. In medical ethics, these senses are found in many of the Hippocratic works portraying the Greek physician.[4] In such cases, one is dealing with taken-for-granted webs of moral values and expectations that constitute the character of the everyday lifeworlds of medical practice. It is in terms of ethics as ethos that many live most of their lives, and in terms of which most health care is usually provided. From within an assumed matrix of values, we derive many of our moral intuitions and have our consciences formed before we become self-conscious moral reasoners. When physicians speak of having learned proper medical practice from the example of an excellent teacher, they are often referring to the initiation into a lifeworld of virtue and dedication that such distinguished "role models" provide.

If the community within which one lives is cohesive and not subject to forces that encourage social change, or if the community has successfully maintained the fabric and social structure of its moral commitments, despite sociotechnological pressures (e.g., the Hassidim and the Amish), this taken-for-granted sense of moral propriety is likely not only to be largely unquestioned, but also to appear largely unquestionable. The more one lives within the secular pluralist embrace of a cosmopolitan society, the more the fabric of taken-for-granted morality will be a cento woven haphazardly out of pieces of diverse moral visions. Taken-for-granted moral sensibilities, even if they are only regnant norms of political correctness, provide a point of departure for ethical reflections and decisions. But postmodernity fragments moral understandings and brings taken-for-granted moral sensibilities under scrutiny. Moreover, the recognition of multicultural diversity discloses important differences in ethos. Ethics as ethos exists in the plural.

Ethics is also used to identify the rules of conduct used by professional groups, such as lawyers, accountants, or physicians and nurses. When these rules are articulated as canons of probity for professional conduct, and when the focus is primarily on issues of professional decorum, ethics is best understood as etiquette. Indeed, this is how codes of medical ethics were often styled[5] prior to the American Medical Association's first code of medical ethics in May 1847.[6] A major portion of the issues addressed in such codes of etiquette concern not moral issues in an immediate and direct sense, but questions of fee schedules, advertisement, and the relation of physicians with nonorthodox practitioners. Yet the concerns of etiquette blend into those of governing ethos. Such rules are not trivial. Such codes of etiquette help formulate and give formal expression to an important dimension of the mores of health professionals. They are like laws. They are explicit enactments or precedents reflecting moral principles and political agreements. Unlike laws, they usually possess only the sanctions of professional disapproval or ostracism. Professional etiquette possesses a more restricted scope and source of authority than law.[7] In addition, there is the foundational question of the authority of such codes and of what shape such etiquette should take.

Laws are often regarded as if they were equivalent to canons of ethics. However, one speaks not only of good laws and bad laws, but of laws that ought to be disobeyed. As a creature born of political forces and compromise, the law is likely only in part to reflect the mores of a society or settled moral judgments. This is more the case the more a legal framework compasses communities with divergent views of the good life and of content-full moral obligations. Also, the more such communities differ in their accepted canons of moral probity, the more explicit laws and bureaucratic rules will need to be.[8] In such cases, explicit laws and rules will be relied on as the social cement binding communities that do not share a content-full matrix of values. The price of providing health care in a society spanning numerous moral communities may be a body of bureaucratic rules and regulations.[9] Still, one needs to know which laws should be written and which should be obeyed.

For guidance one might turn to a particular ideology, moral vision, or religion. This, though, will not resolve disputes across communities of ideological conviction or religious belief. The same can be said about theories of justice that depend on particular thin theories of the good or moral rationality. Consider the view that self-respect is tied to security and wealth rather than to personal liberties. Such a thin theory of the good, if properly framed, would lead to principles of justice justifying an authoritarian capitalist system rather than a liberal democracy. Those who live in Cambridge, Massachusetts, may find it morally bizarre for one to establish principles of justice on the basis of such a thin theory, since they would in many areas be hostile to the civil liberties of a liberal democracy. Those who live in successful authoritarian capitalist systems may find it incomprehensible that one would rank liberty higher than security and prosperity. Because not all are favored by the grace of true belief or proper ideological insight, the world is explained by prophets of competing moral and metaphysical accounts, and the cacophony of their contradictory claims can be heard in any large society in its debates concerning health care policy. There appears to be no greater uniformity among philosophers or theories of morality and justice than among religious leaders and the various religions.

Until a general conversion to the Faith or to a particular ideology, or to a generally imposed orthodoxy, one will need to search for common grounds to bind rational peaceable individuals and to direct health care decisions. Canons of proper action that can be peaceably established on grounds disclosable or acknowledgeable by moral strangers would constitute the core of a secular ethics, as introduced in chapter 1. It is an ethics that aspires to provide a logic or grammar for speaking across a plurality of ideologies, beliefs, and bioethics. If one is a patient or a health care professional in a society that includes patients, physicians, and nurses of different communities of moral belief, one reaches for this sense of ethics precisely because one needs to justify a viewpoint that can span divergent communities of moral conviction.

In resolving moral controversies in a secular pluralist context, the appeal to ethics as ethos, etiquette, law, or ideology (including particular forms of moral conviction and religious belief) will not suffice. The hope is to find a moral fabric, understanding, or vision that can be shared by moral strangers, by rational persons as such. This has been the modern moral philosophical or Enlightenment hope.

## The problem of objectivity in morals

To find answers to moral questions, one must know how moral disputes can in principle be resolved. The procedures for answering a question disclose both the meaning of the question and the significance of the answer. To decide which choice is better requires deciding better for whom and by what criteria.

The search for a flawless answer can be understood as an attempt to achieve the position of the perfect knower. Ideally and traditionally, this has been the viewpoint of the Creator, God. The Deity (a perfectly advantaged, totally unbiased Knower) would be able to provide the best of answers. The Deity's answers are taken to be impeccable, because there is no better-placed knower. No one could rebut the answers of the Deity by claiming a more advantaged position. Furthermore, since the Deity created things, the Deity knows them from the inside out. After all, the Deity created even their hidden essences. One could attempt, therefore, to portray reality as known by the Deity. In comparison with this perspective, all other portrayals of reality, all other understandings of things, would be deficient cases. What the Deity holds to be the nature of reality *is* the nature of reality, for it is the Deity's will, informed by His understanding of reality, that shapes the structure of reality. Thus, the Deity cannot be wrong. It is not simply that the Deity's view of reality cannot fail to accord with things in themselves. The Deity's account is the paradigm of an all-encompassing coherent account of reality. In the Deity's case, criteria for truth based on the agreement between the knowledge claim and the object to be known and criteria for truth based on ideal conditions for intersubjective agreement coincide. The Deity satisfies both correspondence and coherence conditions for truth.

This privilege of the Deity is usually held to obtain for issues of both fact and value. The Deity knows the structure of reality because He can best examine reality and because reality is His own creation. Similarly, in the case of values, the Deity can best judge the consequences of various possible choices, and can therefore offer the most exhaustive evaluation of their comparative merits in this regard. Even if values, as well as rules of logic, were beyond the Deity's control, still the Deity is uniquely placed to judge and compare them. In this sense, the Deity is the existing realization of the philosophical device of the ideal observer who judges moral choices, uninfluenced by improper prejudice and supported by an exhaustive knowledge of the relevant facts. The Deity can provide the perfect answers to the perfect questions.

However, all do not listen to the Deity, or listen in the same way. As a consequence, there is general disagreement about the perfect questions and their perfect answers. Nonetheless, some have attempted to employ a notion of the Deity's viewpoint as an intellectual focus against which to measure particular attempts to assess reality and to judge conduct. One might think here of the importance of the divine perspective for the philosophical accounts offered by René Descartes (1596–1650), Benedict Spinoza (1632–77), and Gottfried Wilhelm Leibniz (1646–1716), where the Deity possesses the paradigm case of clear and distinct ideas, of clear and distinct perceptions. Such viewpoints presume that the world of facts, and often the world of values, has a unique pattern of rational coherence.

This *monotheistic presumption* (i.e., that there is one unique vantage point in terms of which a concrete account of knowledge and ethics can be given), when transferred from the context of a religious understanding to the aspirations of secular reason, becomes the keystone of the modern philosophical project: the presumption that philosophy can disclose the canonical view of reality and morality. If, however, there is no satisfactory secular access to that singular viewpoint, then it will not be clear in general secular terms whether such a viewpoint exists. It will by default in secular transactions be as if there were many gods and goddesses, many competing viewpoints. Put poetically, insofar as one abandons the presumption of the possibility of a single, authoritative, concrete account of knowledge and ethics, one embraces a *polytheistic presumption*.[10] The contemporary world is polytheist by default.

The more one moves from a secular monotheistic presumption (that there is a unique moral perspective available to secular reason) toward the secular polytheistic presumption (that there are a number of equally defensible, but quite different, moral perspectives), the more one moves from modernity to postmodernity and the recognition of irradicable secular moral diversity. The more one can hope for access to a unique authoritative viewpoint, the more one can hope to give a generally satisfactory answer regarding the proper compass of a public health care system (e.g., whether it should provide funds for the treatment of very low weight neonates). Insofar as a unique, authoritative viewpoint appears unobtainable secularly, content-full moral answers in bioethics and elsewhere will turn more on matters of particular inclination and of common decision, rather than on points open to general resolution through the discovery of correct answers via sound rational argument. This book argues that the polytheistic presumption in matters of secular morality and bioethics is unavoidable. The polytheism of postmodernity is the recognition of the radical plurality of moral and metaphysical visions.

*Problems in justifying a particular moral viewpoint*

What can one in principle establish, and with what certainty, in the area of secular morals and bioethics? One will need to know what bases exist even for taken-for-granted rules such as "It is immoral to torture or kill the unconsenting innocent for sport."[11] Such an approach does not carry a prejudice against traditional morality, nor is it designed to place the rights of persons or cherished human values in jeopardy. Rather, it involves the honest realization that much of what structures the concrete fabric of the everyday moral lifeworld, when explored for its secular justification, has the character of the arbitrary and conventional. This is often most clearly seen in the encounter of different cultures.

For example, Captain Cook and his men were shocked because Hawaiians thought it quite natural and proper for men and women in certain circumstances to have carnal conversations without the benefit of marriage and to engage in immodest speech. However, the Hawaiians were disquieted by the fact that the Europeans found it proper for the sexes to eat together—this the Hawaiians knew to be taboo:

The women never upon any account eat with the men, but always by themselves. What can be the reason of so unusual a custom, it is hard to say; especially as they are a people in every other instance, fond of Society and much so of their Women. They were often asked the reason, but they never gave no other Answer, but that they did it because it was right, and expressed much dislike at the custom of Men and Women eating together of the same Victuals . . . more than one-half of the better sort of the inhabitants have entered into a resolution of enjoying free liberty in Love, without being troubled or disturbed by its consequences . . . both sexes express the most indecent ideas in conversation without the least emotion, and they delight in such conversation beyond any other. Chastity, indeed, is but little valued.[12]

Since nearly all would now see no moral difficulty in allowing men and women to eat together, and many would take no exception to fornication, this example may not be seen to constitute a serious challenge to the fundamentals of traditional morality. It may lack the heuristic force of more extreme examples.

Or one might consider the Ik, who live in the mountains separating Uganda, the Sudan, and Kenya. They live according to a moral system in which little if any altruism is supported, and where the good is equivalent to a full stomach. Taking food from the starving could thus be termed a good act.

The very word for "good," *marang,* is defined in terms of food. "Goodness," *marangik,* is defined simply as "food," or, if you press, this will be clarified as "the possession of food," and still further clarified as "*individual* possession of food." Then if you try the word as an adjective and attempt to discover what their concept is of a "good man," *iakw anamarang,* hoping that the answer will be that a good man is a man who helps you fill your own stomach, you get the truly Ikien answer: a good man is one who has a full stomach. There is goodness in being, but none in doing, at least not in doing to others.[13]

Is the viewpoint of the Iks immoral, and, if so, why?

Such case examples of divergent moral viewpoints bring home the central question regarding the justification of moral claims: how can one establish *anything* as morally binding? How can one show that morality in general and bioethics in particular are any more than matters of taste? To begin with, one will need to distinguish among three issues: (1) the genesis of a moral viewpoint, (2) the justification of a moral viewpoint, and (3) the grounds for being rationally motivated to act morally. Actual moral viewpoints are fashioned under the force of various sociohistorical influences. This condition of morality is shared with the sciences. The world has the science and technology it possesses today in great measure because of the West and its sociohistorical circumstances. This genesis in the West of much of contemporary science and technology does not thereby render it parochial, nonobjective, or *merely* Western. The issue of the scope of its cardinal significance turns on its justification, its merits, its claim to the acknowledgment of others. In the case of both science and morality, in seeking a justification one is asking for the claim of the activity or practice on the concurrence of persons as such.

As soon as one attempts to justify particular customs or opinions as those rational individuals ought to acknowledge, one has entered into an attempt to free oneself from merely accepted viewpoints. One has moved from taking for granted that children with very low birthweights should be aggressively treated, to attempting to seek the justification for such practices. In the face of moral pluralism, one will hope to find an understanding of knowing and valuing that will show that some criteria for knowing or valuing correctly are better, that is, more defensible, more justifiable to persons as such. Even if the final, absolute, or divine perspective is not accessible in secular terms, one can still ask what should rationally resolve controversies regarding facts and values.

In conflicts among rival scientific accounts, one has the advantage of being able to compare their predictive power, given a sufficiently common understanding of what is at stake. One can determine how one could decide what the etiologic infectious agent for yellow fever is. Disputants can test competing accounts with reality and thus falsify some competitors and strengthen the claims of others. Some accounts will stand out as preferable in being simpler accounts of the facts with fewer anomalies and with fewer ad hoc assumptions. The "facts" can cause difficulties for many conjectures concerning empirical reality. Thus, for example, given the recent exploration of the planets (e.g., Venus and Mars), Ptolemy's account of the solar system is shown to be false—Flat Earthers, Cardinal Bellarmine, and Pope Urban VIII to the contrary notwithstanding. Of course, in many cases such crisp choices between competitive scientific accounts are not available. One must then also consider the varying explanatory powers of competing theoretical accounts and their ability to encompass different ranges of data in ways that variously promise to be fruitful for further exploration. One must recognize that attempts to test predictions require interpretations of data that are always made within theoretical and factual expectations. Inquiry is guided by antecedent theoretical value commitments[14] and *ceteris paribus* clauses (i.e., this will obtain, all else being equal). These all involve decisions made with the guidance of generally accepted scientific paradigms, historically conditioned by the thought styles of the particular scientific communities of the investigators.[15] Finally, and most significantly, rival communities of empirical scientific investigators do not usually claim scientific authority coercively to close down laboratories and stop scientists from engaging in empirically "bad" science. Moral controversies are closely tied to disputes regarding the proper use of force.

In short, even science is not an ahistorical deliverance of the gods. Scientific truth, as all human truth, is historically and culturally shaped. However, the empirical sciences benefit from a discipline imposed by an external reality, even when that reality always appears dressed in the expectations of particular times, societies, and persons. In the case of conflicts regarding morals, such appeals to "facts" do not appear to be as decisive, since what is at stake are not simply the "facts," but evaluations of the "facts." The constraints on ethics would appear to be first and foremost logical. If one asserts contradictions, one need not be taken as attempting to offer a rational answer to a rational question about what one ought to do. Indeed, in secular ethics and bioethics one wants, as in a scientific explanation, to give as encompassing and systematic an account of the moral life, with as few ad hoc explanations and contradictions as possible. Yet, without the constraints of empirical reality, ethicists, including bioethicists, enjoy considerable latitude in the development of their accounts of the moral life. Under such circumstances, how can one tell who is a moral authority and in what sense? In answering this question, one must again bear in mind that it might seem proper to ask for a greater level of certainty from ethics than science, since ethics, unlike science, directly authorizes coercive interventions in the activities of persons.

With regard to secular moral claims in bioethics, the question is the extent to which one can secure a similar toehold on intersubjectivity analogous to what is available in empirical science. Are there ways in which one can approach the intersubjectivity available in determinations about matters of fact, when answering questions in bioethics or ethics generally?[16] Here it should be stressed that morality must be a potentially intersubjective endeavor if it is to provide a secular basis for moral agents being held to have acted wrongly or in a blameworthy fashion. It is surely the case that individuals have various strongly held views about right actions. Many disagree regarding the morality of abortion, artificial insemination, and the rights of patients to free health care. The question is whether any of these views is correct such that other moral agents ought rationally to concur. Can one provide for morality and bioethics more than (1) the formal rational constraints of avoiding contradictions and (2) the conditional constraints of embracing the means to the ends one holds to be obligatory insofar as one holds them to be conditionally or overridingly obligatory?

*Attempts to justify a content-full secular ethics: why they all fail*

There is a fundamental difficulty in establishing the objectivity of claims regarding content-full moral obligations, content-full moral rights, any moral preferences, or evaluations generally. In particular, to resolve moral controversies by sound rational argument, one must share fundamental moral premises, rules of moral evidence, and rules of moral inference and/or of who is in moral authority to resolve moral controversies. In the presence of different understandings of moral premises, rules of moral evidence, etc., moral controversies will not be able to be resolved by sound rational argument. One needs a standard by which to judge, order, or compare what is morally at stake. How does one compare the interests of a group of patients who could be treated in a protocol that offers them a considerable amount of noxious side effects and only limited chances of cure, with the interests of future patients who in a decade will very likely be the real beneficiaries of such protocols through the advances to which they may eventually lead? How does one balance interests in treating a pregnant woman with a drug to control a nonfatal but serious disease, with the risk of damaging the fetus she is carrying? To provide answers one must judge or rank some outcomes or considerations as more important than others. But where can a standard basis or point of reference for comparison be found?

The modern philosophical or Enlightenment hope was that one could by reason discover a communality binding persons and disclosing common moral standards. Focus was turned away from an encounter with God and with grace to a rational secular encounter with a reality all persons could share. In its various expressions, this hope concentrated efforts on the examination of reason itself, human sympathies, human nature, or other elements of our condition, so as to disclose what binds us in one community and in one common moral understanding. In the various national and cultural contexts within which this intellectual project was undertaken, there were various accents given to the role of reason or to common sympathies, sensibilities, and sentiments. As we shall see, the difficulty is to determine which reason should guide or which sympathy should be canonical. For example, if one seeks the communality that should bind persons in sympathies and sensibilities, one quickly encounters a diversity of human sympathies and sensibilities and a plurality of visions regarding concrete moral obligations. The problem is then which sympathies or obligations should be canonical and why. Moreover, how can particular de facto sympathies or sensibilities or inclinations to recognize an obligation achieve a de jure moral status? How does one show that particular sympathies, sensibilities, sensitivities, or inclinations to recognize particular obligations or rights are canonical? One must already possess a moral criterion independent of the sympathies, sensibilities, and sensitivities, obligations, or rights in question.

The need is for a standard. Standards in ethics and bioethics can be sought (1) in the very content of ethical claims themselves, in intuitions, in what appears to declare itself to be self-evidently right or wrong, or at least (2) in a study of exemplar cases; (3) in the consequences of moral choices; (4) in a notion of unbiased choice, the ideal of an impartial observer, or a group of unbiased contractors; (5) in rational moral choice or discourse itself; (6) in a game theoretical (or prisoner dilemma) account of the problems of social interaction; (7) in the character of reality or nature; (8) in an appeal to middle-level principles; or (9) to some moral reference point that can canonically direct moral choice. More broadly, a standard can be sought in the content of moral thought (e.g., in intuitions), in the form of moral reasoning (e.g., in the idea of impartiality or rationality), or in some external objective reality (e.g., consequences of actions or the structure of reality).

As we shall see, there are insuperable problems with each of these approaches because (1) an appeal to any particular moral content begs the question of the standards by which the content is selected, (2) an appeal to a formal structure provides no moral content and therefore no content-full moral guidance, and (3) an appeal to an external reality will show what is, not what ought to be or how what is should be judged. Somewhat procrusteanly, these alternatives, all of which are unsatisfactory, can be displayed under the eight headings just noted (the ninth listed being a marker for the attempt to remedy the failures of the first eight approaches). In what follows, intuitionist accounts, casuistic accounts, consequentialist accounts, hypothetical-choice theoretic accounts (including hypothetical contractor theories), rational choice and discourse theoretic accounts, game-theoretical accounts (including prisoner dilemma–based accounts), natural law accounts, and middle-level principle-based accounts will all be briefly reviewed to show that they suffer from quite common problems. Each presupposes exactly what it seeks to justify: a particular moral content. Rather than possessing the means for discovering or justifying the canonical, content-full secular morality, understanding of the good or content-full account of fairness, each is rather at best an expository device disclosing the implications of a particular moral vision. These particular alternative attempts to establish a canonical moral understanding are not meant to be exhaustive of all species of attempts to justify by rational argument a concrete morality which all should endorse. They are rather illustrations of how and why all such attempts always fail in presupposing what they set out to establish: canonical moral guidance. They illustrate why any attempt to justify a particular content-full moral understanding as canonical will either beg the question at issue by presupposing what is at stake (i.e., the existence of a content-full oral standard) or involve an infinite regress. Content-full moral controversies cannot be resolved by sound rational argument in the absence of common basic moral premises, rules of evidence and inference, and view of who is in moral authority.

First, one might attempt to settle moral controversies by an appeal to intuition. One might even endeavor, constrained by certain disciplines, to intuit moral standards as well as content-full moral claims, obligations, or rights. Perhaps to be intuitively grounded, a moral precept, obligation, etc., would need to be clearly and precisely formulated, appear self-evident in careful reflection, be consistent with other intuitively known moral propositions, and be of the kind to be recognized by other moral experts to be correct.[17] Such a discipline may incorporate an appeal to a reflective equilibrium among intuitions. Holding some intuitions to be true may have implications that violate other more deeply established moral intuitions. Thus, if one holds that one is obligated to save life at *all* costs, there will be no resources left over for any enjoyment of life. Which is then more important, saving life or enjoying life? How can one tell? How can one determine how to balance these concerns? Is there a rationally conclusive way to determine the correct answer or correct balance of concerns?[18]

Or to put the matter somewhat more starkly, consider the choice between two possible worlds, each with ten persons. World *A* has 1 person with 12 utiles (hedon units, units of preference satisfaction or units of goodness), while each of the remaining 9 persons has only 1 unit each, giving the world a sum total of 21 units. In world *B* each person has 2 units, but the world thus has only 20 units. Which is the better world? World *A* has more of whatever units of excellence one measures than does world *B*, though world *B* has greater equality. Should one have second thoughts and want to say that world *B* is better than *A*, it must be because one has decided to recalculate matters on the basis of a special value now given to average utility or to equality. On the other hand, one might reconsider the virtue or excellence of having a person with 12 units of goodness. The achievement of such perfection may itself merit special extra weighting somewhat like a very rare flower can give special merit to a garden.

One might also consider a choice between world *C*, in which all individuals have 5 utiles (hedon units, units of preference satisfaction, units of goodness, etc.), and world *D* in which all individuals have 5 utiles, save for 1 person who enjoys 10 utiles. The enjoyment of the 10 utiles has no other effect but to make people unequal. Is world *D* better or worse than *C*? In world *D* there are more utiles, but there is also inequality. Answers to such questions turn on judgments regarding equality and have implications for the allocation of health care resources. How can an appeal to intuition resolve the matter? Choices between worlds *A* and *B* and between worlds *C* and *D* depend on starkly different views of what is morally to be endorsed. The appeal to such case examples indicates the impossibility of an appeal to intuition resolving deeply rooted moral controversies. One's judgment of the cases depends on one's intuitions, and that is what is at stake. An appeal to cases may clarify or display differences, but it will not resolve them.

Depending on which intuitions one holds to be better established, one will revise one's intuitions regarding such matters as the propriety of saving life at all costs versus enjoying life, tolerating inequalities, or obliterating them. But how can one determine which intuitions ought to be held to be better established? One could appeal to a further intuition, perhaps to the intuition that it is best to concur with the preponderance of one's intuitions. But how would one know that this is the tack to take? One will need to appeal to increasingly higher order intuitions, intuitions regarding methodology, or simply arbitrarily embrace one intuition, or set of intuitions, as final. An appeal to intuitions is not able to offer a satisfactory solution to the problem of resolving moral controversies, because any one intuition can be countered with a contrary intuition. There is no conclusive way to mediate among conflicting intuitions by appealing to intuitions.

Second, the problem with appeals to intuitions will not be circumvented by reference to exemplar cases or to casuistic analyses.[19] For casuistry not simply to involve an appeal to intuitions (i.e., intuitionally to choose to be guided by particular cases selected by intuition as exemplar), the guiding cases must be understood within a framing context. This is, in fact, how Roman Catholic casuistry functioned. Individual cases were understood within both a dogmatic framework that offered authoritative content and confessors who were in authority to interpret cases and guide penitents. One cannot discursively know how, and under what circumstances, particular cases should direct ethical decisions without a framing context, narrative, or set of rules. Casuistry or the case method of ethical controversy resolution depends on a guiding framework beyond the cases themselves.

This difficulty is not apparent if one discusses the resolution of moral controversies with moral friends. Under such circumstances exemplar cases can be straightforwardly recognized as exemplary and as giving guidance. Indeed, in such contexts it is hard to imagine that all persons will not simply *see* certain exemplar cases as governing. When one meets moral strangers, such expectations are broken. Imagine a discussion between Dominican friars and well-bred samurai regarding the exemplar bushido shown by the forty-seven samurai, the forty-seven ronin, who decapitated Kira Yoshinaka in order to avenge their master, Asano Nagononi, Lord of Ako, and then in 1703 committed seppuku (ritual suicide), were buried in the cemetery of the Senga Kuji Zen Buddhist Temple (Tokyo), and immortalized in the Kabuki play, *Chushingura*. They are to this day the object of moral and religious devotion, revered for their loyalty to their Daimyo. How will the Dominicans succeed in explaining to the samurai that this exemplar act of courage and devotion in fact involves the perversion of important moral values? The Dominicans will need to convert the samurai to being Christians. True conversion, as the Orthodox Church reminds us, involves a metanoia, a fundamental changing of one's mind. After conversion, as in a gestalt shift, one can see matters anew. But beforehand there will simply be a conflict of minds. The discussants are in different lifeworlds with different taken-for-granted moralities. They do not share common moral premises or rules of moral evidence.

The matter is the same in bioethics. One need only imagine the discussion between a devout Southern Baptist who opposes nontherapeutic abortions and the atheist director of an abortion clinic who sees no significant moral evil in abortion. The Southern Baptist may regard those who chose to have an abortion in order to avoid an unwanted child as paradigm examples of those whose values are deformed. In contrast, the director may see such choices as paradigmatic presentations of a proper freedom of women to control their own bodies, thus regarding such choices as not just to be secularly protected but as, in a way, praiseworthy.

Similar conflicts will occur when adherents of different ideologies meet. Imagine the discussion between an egalitarian and an impassioned devotee of the free market regarding whether it is good or bad that the rich can purchase more and better health care than the poor. The devotee of the market will hold that the good of free choice in the market outweighs any evils associated with inequalities. And of course, the egalitarian's view will be the very opposite, as will be his interpretation of cases. Each will have different understandings of what is shown by particular cases of equality, inequality, free choice, or constrained choice. The problem is how such and similar controversies can be resolved by sound rational argument.

It will not be possible to circumvent these difficulties faced by intuitionist and casuist accounts by acknowledging the existence of different forms of major ethical appeals such as appeals to consequences, rights, respect of persons, virtues, cost-effectiveness, and justice. A model that acknowledges the variety and conflicting character of moral appeals, and that then requires a proper sensitivity to all appeals so as to determine how to apply them in resolving controversies regarding particular cases, will still need to determine which sensitivity is proper or improper. To assess properly the success of competing appeals requires an antecedent notion of proper assessment. One can retreat to higher-level considerations or appeals regarding proper sensitivity and proper assessment, but this will effectively beg the question. In such accounts, which acknowledge the pluralism of moral appeals and attempt to assess them, there can be a notion of the education of the moral sense so as to choose rightly: a notion of the development of discernment, phronesis, or prudence. Outside of any particular tradition of discernment, phronesis, or prudence, how will one be able to determine who is descerning and who is imprudent? This criticism invokes a moral epistemological skepticism, not a metaphysical skepticism. It does not require holding that there is no moral truth or moral sense to discern. It is just that no general secular account can determine which moral sense has discerned rightly or wrongly without begging the question.

Consider the attempt to address the difficulties of appeals to intuition by asserting that humans possess a faculty by which they can know what is moral.

To a large degree, our fundamental moral intuitions about particular actions, agents, and institutions are forced upon us by our moral cognitive faculties. To the extent that this is so, there are constraints on our intuitive judgments and it is not the case that "anything goes." However unsatisfactory our understandings of these notions and however much that means that we have no rules for evaluating choices, the individual, in making these choices, finds many forced upon him by his cognitive makeup.[20]

The difficulty is to know when this faculty is functioning rightly, as well as why. Given the pleomorphic character of all species, including humans, such a faculty should be uniform across humans and always produce the same judgments.

Third, given the failure of intuitionist and casuistic accounts, one may attempt to resolve moral controversies by comparing the consequences of different systems of moral choices. But how can one assay the comparative virtues of competing systems without appealing to a background moral understanding that will allow one to assess the relative merits of the competing systems? The possibility of establishing such an understanding is exactly what is at issue. Imagine a utilitarian attempting to assess the comparative merits of two major methods of distributing health care, one that provides acute and chronic care and some preventive care versus a system that concentrates resources on preventive medicine and short-term acute care, but with only a small amount of resources given to long-term acute care and to chronic health care. Each will have different costs and benefits, including moral costs and benefits. In the first system, because the prime focus is on acute and chronic care, the claims of individuals seeking such treatment will be better met than in the second, where they may be denied treatment with the remark that in the end the greatest good will be achieved through research in, and application of, preventive medicine. Of course, those in the second system will have their interests in preventive medicine addressed more adequately than they would be in the first. If those are held to be very important interests by the proponents of the second system, they too can consistently claim that their system will lead to the greatest good for the greatest number. Apart from empirical claims that may be at stake, and focusing only on how to compare different interests, who is right, and why? To what extent may one discount the need of those seeking health care now in favor of those whose interests may in the future be secured against the evils of preventable diseases? How does one compare the preferences of those who seek health care now with those seeking better prevention now? One would need to appeal to a particular moral sense, a particular way of comparing present and future interests in order to decide. One cannot simply decide on the basis of an appeal to consequences, for that would beg the question. One needs to know how to rank or compare consequences, including present versus future consequences.

To answer such questions, one must know which outcomes are more important and to which preferences priority ought to be given. However, consequentialist accounts (including utilitarian accounts), which compare outcomes, are no better advantaged than intuitionist accounts with regard to demonstrating which ranking or comparing of benefits and banes is to be preferred, since both presuppose an antecedent, indeed authoritative means of judging, ranking, or comparing benefits and harms. If one agrees, for example, that one must be concerned about liberty, equality, security, and prosperity consequences, depending on how one ranks these consequences one will be living in Texas, Massachusetts, Singapore, Japan, North Korea, or the Vatican. One must already have a vision of the good in order to rank consequences. One cannot appeal to consequences to determine the correct ranking of consequences. One must already have a correct ordering of consequences or a normative vision of human flourishing or of the good. Indeed, the choice between maximizing total utility versus average utility (or the total aggregate of the good) depends on different understandings of what it means to maximize utility or achieve the good. The same is the case in deciding how to compare the significance of the good, pleasure, utiles, preferences realized, or hedon units experienced by persons versus higher and lower animals.

One possibility for answering such questions might be by showing the consequences of particular actions. One might argue that if one does not seek free and informed consent from patients, the fabric of mutual respect will be weakened. But other advantages may be gained. Such goal-oriented teleological approaches presuppose that one already knows what goals ought to be pursued, when, and how to compare them. In order to choose among competing moral practices on the basis of the consequences, one must already know which consequences are better or worse than others. Consequentialist ethics presupposes a nonconsequentialist ethics. For example, does one know which is preferable for a society— Spartan virtues in the framing of health care policy or those of an indulgent latter-day Athens? Is it better to organize society around the virtues of a Texas Ranger or a samurai warrior? Is it better for a society, and consequently its bioethics, to be founded on the moral sentiments of the Ik or on those of the Mennonites? How does one know which choice is better? To answer any of these questions, one will need to know the answer to two questions in advance. Better for whom? Better with respect to which values? To assess consequences one needs independent moral criteria.

These difficulties exist prior to considering the problem of utility or consequence monsters. Such large-scale good realizers or pleasure experiencers can lead to conclusions unacceptable to many who already hold a particular content-full moral vision, if they attempt to resolve moral controversies by an appeal to consequences. Consider, for example, a world in which 20 percent of the population realizes great good, advantage, pleasure, preference satisfaction, or a balance of benefits over harms by subjecting 1 percent of the population (an identifiable minority) to painful experiments, while the remaining 79 percent is indifferent (i.e., feels a balance in moral sympathies, pleasures, or preferences between disturbance from the torture and the vicarious pleasure or satisfaction given the pleasure and advantage that redounds to the 20 percent). If this world maximizes both the greatest total and average amount of good, pleasure, preference satisfaction, utiles, or hedon units in comparison to any other materially possible world, it must be affirmed by consequentialists as the materially best possible world.

The calculation of the best choice depends on how one compares goods, consequences, preferences, and the like. Those who would want to object may forward, for example, a revised approach to calculating benefits, harms, pleasures, utiles, and preferences. Which is to say, they will implicitly reveal that they possessed a vision of the good prior to their appeal to a consequentialist or utilitarian account. The appeal to a detailed account of consequences helps to direct particular choices and can serve as a heuristic or expository device that may aid in making clearer or systematizing the character of one's initial moral vision. But it cannot justify that vision. Further, the content of the vision that identifies utility monsters as monsters is prior to the appeal to consequences or utility insofar as this understanding leads to revisions of weighting of outcomes, consequences, preferences, and the like, in order to avoid certain "morally unacceptable," "morally outrageous," or "morally counterintuitive" conclusions. In order to know that one ought to correct preferences and how, one must already possess a background moral vision and be able to show that it is binding. In addition, one must be able to show that it is the canonical background moral vision, not just one more parochial moral understanding. To make such definitive moral judgments, one needs a standard of the preferences to be satisfied, of the consequences to be realized, the utiles to be secured, the pleasures to be experienced, or the hedon units to be had. Any particular calculation of the achievement of the good, utiles, pleasure, preferences, or hedon units requires choices among different weightings and comparisons of good, consequences, pleasures, utiles, and hedon units.

Without a standard, how does one compare interests? How does one compare, for example, $X$'s interest in not being taxed with $X$'s interest in not being drafted, with $X$'s interest in not being the subject of experiments without consent, with $X$'s interest in not being raped, with $X$'s interest in not being killed, with $Y$'s interest in taxing $X$, with $Y$'s interest in drafting $X$, with $Y$'s interest in experimenting on $X$ without $X$'s permission, with $Y$'s interest in raping $X$, with $Y$'s interest in killing $X$. Does one appeal to the intensity or the quality of the interests? One will need a God's-eye perspective to compare intensities of interest (i.e., to produce an interpersonal comparison of utiles), if one could decide the antecedent question about how one should take into account the qualities and kinds of interests. A calculation will require comparing interests not only between individuals, but within individuals over time. When such calculations are done over time, the question will not simply be that of the discount rate of time for interests, preferences, and the like, but also whether and why one should maintain a stable method of comparing kinds and qualities of interest over time. Such choices presuppose an antecedent view or moral theory of consequences.

In comparing interests, preferences, and the like, one will as well need to know whether all interest holders count equally. If different species are able to generate different qualities and intensities of interests or preferences, will they count differently? If intelligent individuals with proper schooling in interests and preferences are able to enhance the intensity and quality of their interests and preferences, will they count more than the ignorant or untutored because they have more intense, better-quality interests or preferences? To answer such questions, one will need to know how and why one compares intensity and quality of interests and preferences. One will need already to possess a particular moral vision of interests and preferences that judges, ranks, or compares interests and preferences and assesses their value.

These difficulties are not escaped if one attempts to focus only on maximizing preferences. In order to determine which actions, choices, rules, policies, or practices lead either to the greatest total maximization of preferences or the

THE INTELLECTUAL BASES OF BIOETHICS

greatest average maximization of preferences, one must know how to compare present and future preferences and their satisfaction. One must know how God discounts time. One must know whether all preferences and their satisfaction count equally. Do rationally considered preferences, brute preferences, and impulsive preferences count the same? Does the preference to help the members of some despised group count the same as (or more or less than) the preference to torture the members of that group to the glee (and preference satisfaction) of the many?

Any attempt to distinguish between manifest and rational preferences in order to provide an account of properly corrected preferences requires choosing a particular set of inclinations to satisfy. One can distinguish morally wholesome from morally pathological preferences only with reference to a particular moral sense or norm. In order to deliver a content-full account of secular morality, one must have already made a prior choice regarding the proper character of moral rationality.

Fourth, one might attempt to remedy this circumstance by constructing a hypothetical-choice theory. Such a theory might invoke the notion of a disinterested observer, as have Roderick Firth[21] and Richard B. Brandt,[22] in order to specify what rational individuals would choose, and therefore what one ought to choose if one is seeking a rational outcome. But any such observer must be specified in some detail. The observer must be informed (fully or partially through a veil of ignorance) concerning the consequences of various possible choices and be able to imagine how such consequences will affect those concerned (here the similarities to the Deity are considerable). The observer must also be impartial in weighing everyone's interests and siding with none.

If the observer is totally morally disinterested, how will it be able to perform the task of identifying morally right or preferable outcomes? The observer cannot be so impartial as not to favor certain consequences over others. If it is not partial to certain choices, the observer could not serve as a guide to moral choices, much less health care policy. That is, one must impute to the impartial observer a particular moral sense (a set of moral intuitions, an understanding of moral rationality, etc.). The observer or hypothetical chooser must be a partisan of a particular moral view or moral sense. But what is at stake is how to establish the preferability of a particular moral view or moral sense, and the ordering of goods it can secure, over alternative moral senses and their orderings of moral goods. Without a solution to this difficulty, one will not be able to appeal to a disinterested observer in order to decide, for example, whether it is right or preferable to provide high-cost neonatal intensive care for very low birthweight babies who have only a low chance of survival, or to let them die and suggest that the parents try to secure a healthy baby through another pregnancy. A disinterested observer can choose between these alternatives only if the observer has a particular moral vision with particular moral implications.

It will not help here to multiply the number of impartial observers as Rawls has done in his hypothetical-contractor theory.[23] John Rawls, in attempting to determine the grounds for identifying just social institutions, appeals to an intellectual device in which one is invited to imagine oneself establishing the basic principles of justice that will govern the constitution and laws of the society into which one will be born.[24] Rawls suggests that one would want to increase one's share of the primary social goods (e.g., powers and opportunities, income and wealth) as long as this would not be at the expense of one's share in equal liberty.[25] In addition, one would not want to risk losing an acceptable amount of the primary social goods in order to secure the possibility of acquiring an even greater amount of these goods.[26] He therefore invites us to picture a number of rational contractors who are equally ignorant with respect to what their future places in society will be, what their natural assets or abilities will be, what conception of the good they will have, the special features of their psychology, the particular circumstances of the society, or even the generation into which they will be born.[27] Such strategically ignorant contractors, not knowing what their position will be, should agree, so Rawls contends, on an unequal distribution of the primary social goods (other than liberty) when such a distribution is to "the greatest benefit of the least advantaged, consistent with the just savings principle," given that such primary social goods are "attached to offices and positions open to all under conditions of fair equality of opportunity."[28] In addition, Rawls holds that such rational contractors would value liberty more highly than other primary social goods, such that they would not see it to be appropriate to trade basic liberties for increased prosperity. Rawls also holds that the contractors would not be egalitarians, if unequal distributions would advantage all.[29] Which is to say, he does not assign a significant independent value to equality for its own sake.[30] However, the contractors are to regard fortunate outcomes, if not the result of principled social planning under just institutions, as arbitrary and therefore open to be set aside. This approach has been widely applied in discussions of what should count as a just distribution of medical resources, though Rawls himself has not made such an application.[31]

Rawls's account makes a number of crucial presuppositions about rational contractors. They must (1) rank liberty more highly than other societal goods,[32] (2) be risk aversive,[33] (3) not be moved by envy,[34] (4) be heads of family (or be concerned about at least some members of the next generation),[35] and (5) not assign a very high ranking to such goods as living peaceful lives in a state of nature. They must have a very particular moral sense.

On the last point, consider the BaMbuti, pygmies who inhabit the forests of Zaire. They move about the forest in small bands, living in very small groupings in relative harmony and free from warfare. They do not invest energies in accumulating goods that could save severely defective children born into their groups or the elderly in need of special health care.[36] Thus, though they live in near-

Rousseauean, idyllic circumstances (at least at the time of the study), they violate the just-savings principle of Rawls. Would they, under the principles of Rawls, be morally compelled to abandon their traditional ways of life? Ought one to hold their society to be unjust, if they could now join the larger society of Zaire and provide health care for their defective children and needy elderly, though such interventions are likely to disturb the cultural integrity of the BaMbuti living in the forests? May the BaMbuti legitimately reject such help because they value their own way of life more highly? The answer will turn on the moral sense of the rational contractors to whom one appeals in order to resolve this and similar controversies. It will depend on how one ranks particular harms and benefits. In short, Rawls presupposes the legitimacy of a particular moral sense. He is best understood as having engaged in a limited, but still important, goal of providing a rational reconstruction of the moral world of a liberal member of the Cambridge, Massachusetts, community.[37]

The difficulty is that appeals to hypothetical-choice theories (including hypothetical contractors) will not disclose a canonical secular content-full morality or give canonical content-full guidance in the framing of health care policy. In order for such an appeal to vindicate a particular moral understanding of the right or the good and to direct some choices over others, some approaches to health care policy over others, one must already have answered foundational questions by choosing a particular moral sense, cluster of intuitions, or variety of moral rationality for the hypothetical observer, chooser, or group of hypothetical contractors. One only derives from a hypothetical-choice theory those choices which one has foreordained or predestined by an antecedent choice of a particular thin theory of the good, moral sense, cluster of moral intuitions, or notion of moral rationality. Matters are complicated beyond a dependence on a particular moral sense, vision, or understanding. Hypothetical-choice theories, as indeed any moral theory with implications for public policy, must trade on assumptions regarding other key notions. Consider two different notions of freedom and which is the more important: freedom to use unhindered the fruits of one's labor for investment and for the purchase of the goods and services one desires or freedom to speak one's mind openly on whatever political issues touch one's fancy.[38] The first focuses on freedom from state intervention through taxation. The second focuses on freedom from state interventions through state censorship. Which is worse and why: state taxation or state censorship? The ordering of these two senses of freedom involves ranking political liberties versus economic liberties (as well as economic prosperity), which ranking is tied to a choice of political structures along a spectrum that may lead from an oligarchically controlled democratic capitalism (one might imagine Singapore or South Korea in periods of their history) to a majoritarianly dominated democratic socialism (something like Sweden in periods of its history). Different choices will lead to different levels of toleration for the coercive state restriction of political and economic liberties (e.g., free speech regarding the morality of abortion versus the freedom to purchase better basic health care). There is no single concept of freedom, equality, or democracy to be delivered or reconstructed by the appeal to such expository devices as hypothetical contractors and original positions without already begging the question by incorporating in advance particular moral content.

So, too, one must select among concepts of equality such as equality in protection of one's forbearance rights (e.g., the right not to be interfered with in contracting with others, including the right to use one's resources with consenting others unhindered) versus equality of outcome (e.g., equality in wealth and position).[39] The choice will have significant implications for how one may fashion a health care system. Also, if the focus is on moral agency or moral agents, then those entities that have experience and interests but cannot act as moral agents (e.g., fetuses), will not count equally with moral agents. If the focus is on those who can achieve happiness, then interests in equality will be directed to the equality of happiness realizers. If the focus is on the realization of the good, the focus may be on entities insofar as they can realize the good. Concerns of equality will be quite different depending whether the account of morality is focused primarily on concerns regarding worthiness of blame and praise, the achievement of happiness, or the realization of some other more complex good. Concerns about equality will gain their meaning from the moral account within which they are considered.

Since there are numerous competing understandings or senses of liberty and equality, a hypothetical-choice theory must incorporate into the chooser a particular disposition toward such understandings or senses. In addition, hypothetical-contractor accounts such as Rawls's must address what it is to choose regarding a biography. Should such contractors regard themselves as guaranteed a life, they will have grounds to support prenatal diagnoses and selective abortion in order to maximize their future health and abilities. If they have a risk of not having a life, not being born, they will oppose contraception and abortion in order to maximize their chances. Different initial assumptions deliver quite different conclusions. However, even if these theoretical challenges can be met without appealing to a particular intuition or moral sense, there will still be the insoluble difficulty of choosing the correct moral sense, vision, understanding, or thin theory of or disposition to the good in order to have any hypothetical-choice theory (or any other account) produce particular outcomes.

Fifth, attempts to discover a concrete view of the good life, content-full moral obligations, a content-full understanding of right conduct, or justice through an analysis of rationality, neutrality, or impartiality suffer from the same difficulties as hypothetical-choice theories (e.g., impartial-observer theories and rational-contractor theories). One must not only know beforehand which sense of rationality, neutrality, or impartiality one ought to choose. One must in addition incorporate a particular moral vision, moral sense, or thin theory of the good.

Which is more rational, to invest in health care to treat the pains of the young or the pains of the old? How many resources should be invested in health care when it only marginally postpones death or diminishes suffering? Appeals to reason alone will provide only logical constraints, not moral content and concrete directives. To direct moral choices, a notion of rationality, neutrality, or impartiality must include a particular disposition toward comparing liberty, prosperity, security, and the like. One might think of Bruce Ackerman, who imports concepts of entitlement into his neutrality principle in order to impeach privileges due to success in the natural lottery (e.g., being born healthy) and social lottery (e.g., being born rich), even when those privileges do not involve trespasses against others.[40] Ackerman attempts, by embracing a particular interpretation of neutrality, to disallow libertarian outcomes such as those endorsed by Robert Nozick,[41] who accepts the results of the natural and social lotteries. Just as with Rawls's *Theory of Justice,* an account of rational neutrality must give particular guidance in deciding how to be neutral toward competing interests—for example, economic liberties versus economic needs. Further, in order to produce one pattern of outcomes rather than another, the choice of a notion of moral rationality must include a particular view toward risk taking and toward the manner in which equalities matter—again, all central issues in framing health care policy.

The same occurs if one attempts to give an account of society and morality in terms of a theory of discourse such as Jürgen Habermas's *Theory of Communicative Action.* Habermas offers an analysis of what he takes to be the character and consequences of rational discourse. The discourse that Habermas takes to bind individuals requires a therapeutic critique in which the participants have freed themselves from illusions, in particular, self-deceptions about their own subjective experiences. "Thus the critique of value standards presupposes a shared pre-understanding among participants in the argument, a pre-understanding that is not at their disposal but constitutes and at the same time circumscribes the domain of the thematized validity claims. Only the truth of propositions and the rightness of moral norms and the comprehensibility or well-formedness of symbolic expressions are, by their very meaning, universal validity claims that can be tested in discourse."[42] But it is the general specification and testability of moral norms that is impossible. Either such secular norms do not exist or they cannot be tested without presupposing what is at issue: a particular moral sense or notion of moral rationality. It is for this reason that the Enlightenment's hope for a universal moral narrative, account of the moral life, or content-full moral community is not realizable. Habermas, however, both in *The Theory of Communicative Action* and elsewhere, requires the assumption that sound rational arguments can in principle be regarded as able to resolve moral controversies.

I shall speak of 'discourse' only when the meaning of the problematic validity claim conceptually forces participants to suppose that a rationally motivated agreement could in principle be achieved, whereby the phrase 'in principle' expresses the idealizing proviso: if

only the argumentation could be conducted openly enough and continued long enough
. . . [and] thus every valid norm has to fulfill the following condition: (U) All affected
can accept the consequences and the side effects its general observance can be anticipated
to have for the satisfaction of everyone's interests (and these consequences are preferred to
those of known alternative possibilities for regulation.[43]

Given different understandings of the significance of consequences and the
proper ordering of interests, there can be no such rationally principled acceptance. The only acceptance possible under such circumstances will be the kind of
volitional acceptance that occurs in the market.

Habermas wishes to escape a foundationalism by drawing on a process that
critically takes regard of psychological and social theories and facts. He also
hopes to be able to show that some ways of regarding reality and morality are
preferable simply by reference to the character of reciprocal reason giving in
discourse.

For agreement and disagreement, insofar as they are judged in the light of reciprocally
raised validity claims and not merely caused by external factors, are based on reasons that
participants supposedly or actually have at their disposal. These (most often implicit)
reasons form the axis around which processes of reaching understanding revolve. But if, in
order to understand an expression, the interpreter must *bring to mind the reasons* with
which a speaker would if necessary and under suitable conditions defend its validity, he is
*himself* drawn into the process of assessing validity claims. For reasons are of such a nature
that they cannot be described in the attitude of a third person, that is, without reactions of
affirmation or negation or abstention.[44]

For such contentions to be convincing, one must already concur with Habermas's
bold Enlightenment assumption that reason giving will be sufficient to bring into
mutual criticism differing moral senses.

Habermas's philosophical account, as opposed to his historical and empirical
reflections on social and psychological theories, is offered as a kind of high-level
empirical generalization guided by norms of rational discourse. "A philosophy
that opens its results to indirect testing in this way is guided by the fallibilistic
consciousness that the theory of rationality it once wanted to develop on its own
can now be sought only in the felicitous coherence of different theoretical fragments."[45] If this theory is meant as a causal or genetic one, it may in fact provide
a nonmoral, empirical account of how conversion and convergence are effected
by dialogue. But unless the concept of reason employed itself possesses a normative status, Habermas will not be able to show why there may not simply be
repeated abstentions. Given certain views of the facts of the matter (e.g., a
heterogeneity of moral inclinations), one would indeed expect divergent dialogues. For his account to have morally normative weight (i.e., to be more than
an account of what is likely to happen when discourse occurs within a certain
understanding of rationality), he will need to have already made a choice among

different content-full notions of rationality. Somewhat like Kant (as we will see in the next chapter), Habermas smuggles considerable content into his notion of discourse.

One might consider a sixth approach to the problem of establishing a concrete content-full secular ethics as a basis for bioethics and health care policy, namely, that of game theory. One can explore what societal or political constraints are required in order for others as well as oneself to act in coordination so that mutual harms can be avoided and goods achieved. Framing a society, including establishing health care policy, is seen to be like a game in which the participants may engage in various moves and countermoves so that it behooves the participants (i.e., members of the society) to decide which rules will allow them to cooperate so as to achieve their individual and common goals.[46] The focus is on how rationally to cooperate and coordinate actions.

Imagine that Bubba Joe and Billy Bob have participated in a bank robbery for which they have been arrested. Yet there is insufficient evidence to convict either if neither gives evidence. Yet Bubba Joe and Billy Bob may each be motivated to turn state's evidence at once in order to be immune from prosecution before the other confesses. They will both be advantaged if they can coordinate their actions (i.e., so that neither confesses, neither is known to be a criminal, and neither is convicted). The usual sense of what should count as a correct solution is threatened if one of the participants has transcendent commitments or immanent goals that make outcomes that others hold to be unacceptable either acceptable or desirable. If Bubba considers his robbery of a New York–based bank located in Texas a virtuous act of patriotism against the Damnyankee, then the glory of conviction may be a goal worth pursuing. This attraction may be enhanced if Bubba is convinced that his act as a freedom fighter is pleasing to God. Or, perhaps, he holds there is an independent moral good in confessing.

In more general terms, the more individuals value personal freedom and autonomy over other goods, the more they will regard as unacceptable the costs to freedom and liberty that come from coordination that does not increase the amount of freedom or liberty. On the other hand, as the value of nonliberty interests (e.g., prosperity) increases, the more constraints on freedom and liberty will be acceptable if the result is greater prosperity. Different views of the value of freedom, caprice, prosperity, etc., will give different game-theoretical solutions. The same will be the case with regard to other values, goals, and harms. One will also need to discover the correct discount rate for future benefits and harms. One will also need to avoid absolute right- or wrong-making conditions. Imagine the difficulty of discovering a game-theoretical solution to the task of framing abortion policy when some hold that the recognition of abortion rights is an essential element of respecting women, and others that abortion is an act of murder that can lead to eternal damnation. A game-theoretical justification requires at least some common ranking of values and harms as well as some common understanding of moral rationality, if it is to be more than an analysis of market mechanisms.

Seventh, one will also not be able to resolve moral controversies in ethics, bioethics, and health care policy by an appeal to the structure of reality or to so-called natural law without again begging the question. In order for the character of reality to serve as a criterion for resolving moral disputes, it must be shown to be morally normative. For example, if one could show that the general tendencies of nature were established by God, not as a challenge for humans to overcome, but as a guide for humans in their conduct, then appeals to reality or nature could provide a guide to conduct. But establishing the first proposition requires special religious or metaphysical premises not open to a general secular defense. To know whether the general tendencies of nature or the structures of reality are to be acknowledged as morally instructive, or as obstacles to be set aside, as for example through contraception, one must have standards by which to judge which states of affairs or structures of nature ought to be accepted, as being that to which one ought to submit. But the availability of such standards is what is at issue. One must have standards by which to judge whether what is is normatively natural or good in order to derive moral implications from nature. Nature, and the laws of nature, are not by themselves morally normative (a point we will examine further in chapter 5). They simply are.

A similar difficulty besets those who appeal to moral facts. How does one know whether the failure of two people to recognize the same moral facts or objective moral truths comes not from the failure of one to see correctly, but from each of the two imposing different interpretive moral visions or senses on reality? The attempt to look out to reality in order to determine for moral strangers what should be binding confronts the same difficulty as the attempt to look inward to one's intuitions. One requires for guidance an antecedent criterion to resolve controversies. One must already have accepted a particular moral vision by which to interpret reality and to know who is and who is not blind to values.

Eighth, one cannot avoid these difficulties by appealing to middle-level principles as suggested by Beauchamp and Childress.[47] Beauchamp and Childress contend that middle-level principles can be used by individuals with different theoretical and moral perspectives, thus allowing both consequentialists and deontologists to employ the middle-level principles in order to resolve bioethical controversies. This tactic, if successful, would provide a nonfoundationalist approach to bioethics. Such appeals may indeed be feasible when individuals with the same or very similar moral visions or thin theories of the good and justice have reconstructed their moral sentiments within divergent theoretical approaches. One might imagine individuals starting with very similar moral sentiments and dispositions, but then some giving rule-deontological and some rule-teleological accounts of these original sentiments and dispositions. The con-

sequentialists will analyze a particular bioethical case by considering the consequences that make it appropriate or inappropriate to embrace a particular decision. The consequentialists may also contend that their own theoretical approach
best portrays what is morally at stake. The deontologists will consider the right-
and wrong-making characteristics of the actions involved in order to endorse the
same decision. The deontologists may as well contend that their theoretical
approach best portrays what is morally at stake.

Consider the issue of whether a health care system should allow a second
luxury tier for the rich. Those who belong to a community dominated by certain
varieties of an egalitarian moral vision may ''justify'' their prior egalitarian
sentiments by arguing (1) by an appeal to consequences that a two-tier system
will disadvantage the poor, because the rich, having their own system, will not be
concerned about the quality of the health care for the poor, causing more harm
than benefit when compared with a one-tier system (this calculation will depend
on a particular weighting given to health care consequences versus certain kinds
of liberty consequences), or (2) by an appeal to right- and wrong-making conditions that a two-tier system incorporates the significant wrong-making characteristic of treating people differently in the matter of life and death decisions. If
such teleologists and deontologists lived in the same moral lifeworld before their
theoretical reconstruction of their morality, it is not at all amazing that their
different theoretical apparatuses generally justify the same choices.[48] Though the
individuals use different theoretical languages and frameworks, they in fact live
in the same or similar moral lifeworlds. It is not that remarkable, then, that they
are able to produce middle-level principles that can help them resolve controversies within their common moral perspective. It is not remarkable that they are
able to come to similar practical choices using middle-level principles, since they
began with similar moral commitments or prejudices.

Such success will not be available when there is not only a theoretical difference, but also one of moral perspective. In such circumstances, the appeal to
middle-level principles will not resolve controversies, but instead highlight their
depth. For example, in determining whether and to what extent high-cost, low-
yield medical intervention should be provided by the government to the poor,
how will an appeal to the principle of justice provide a resolution when the
disputants include individuals who are both Rawlsians and Nozickians (i.e.,
individuals who hold that justice involves providing all with the material conditions for equality of opportunity versus those who hold that justice involves not
interfering with the property rights of others)? The differences depend not just on
different reconstructions of the same moral understandings, but grow out of
foundationally different moral visions. Nor will an appeal to the principle of
autonomy resolve disputes concerning the appropriateness of a twenty-eight-
year-old quadriplegic committing suicide. Those who understand the principle of
autonomy as expressing an overriding right of people to be in authority over

themselves will recognize the right of competent individuals to exit this life whenever they want, with whosoever help they may be able to obtain. Those who understand the principle of autonomy as underscoring values associated with liberty may argue that an early death is a loss of many years of enjoying liberty and therefore find such choices not only wrong, but meriting coercive restraint. Nor will it help to appeal to principles of beneficence to determine whether it is morally good or bad for people to sell their organs unless one already has a common understanding of exploitation, the importance of free choice, the importance of financial advantage, and so on. The advocates of organ sales and the opponents of organ sales often constitute their moral lives within radically different, taken-for-granted moral assumptions. Advocates may see no moral difference between selling their organs and selling their labor, if the risks and returns are comparable. Moreover, advocates may see a nobility in individuals having the freedom and responsibility to make such choices over their own lives. In addition, they may be hostile to appeals to power differentials (i.e., as impeaching the capacity to consent) because such appeals set at jeopardy one vision of a truly free society. The opponents for their part may regard these views as perverse.

An appeal to the middle-level principles of autonomy, beneficence, nonmaleficence, and justice may be a helpful device: (1) to resolve moral controversies between individuals with similar moral sentiments but different theoretical approaches, (2) to explore and compare the ways in which different theories reconstruct the same set or similar sets of moral sentiments and intuitions, (3) to determine the differences among moral views and their implications for bioethics and health care policy, but not (4) to resolve controversies between individuals who do not share the same moral vision or moral sense. The appeal to middle-level principles may succeed in bridging the gulf between those who share a moral vision, but who are separated by their theoretical reconstruction of that vision. But it will not bridge the substantive gulf between those separated by different moral visions or different moral senses.[49]

Theoretical approaches cannot deliver content-full moral guidance unless one already fits them out with a particular moral substance. As a result, each theoretical approach recapitulates the challenge of postmodernity: a moral theoretical account must either beg the question with regard to moral content (i.e., incorporate particular moral content without justification) or give no substantive guidance. Each attempt to justify a particular moral vision presupposes exactly what it seeks to establish so that moral theoretical arguments are at best expository, not justificatory. Even if one attempts a defense of secular ethics or bioethics on the basis of arguments that are not reducible to intuitionist, consequentialist, hypothetical-choice, or hypothetical-contractor arguments, or analyses of the nature of rational choices or game theoretic rationality or natural law arguments or middle-level principles analyses, the arguments will fail as well. All concrete moral choices presuppose particular moral guidance. Moral content is achieved at the price of particularity. To have moral content, one must endorse particular moral premises or rules of moral evidence as a point of departure, thus endorsing one from among the class of available moralities. On the other hand, universality is approached at the price of content. For a morality to have content, it must be particular. But which particularity, which moral content, should be endorsed and on what basis? Again, to answer such questions, one either begs the question or submits to an infinite regress. In the face of these difficulties, no particular moral vision or bioethics, in general secular terms, can be shown to be better than any other.

This problem is in fact recognized by Rawls (especially the later Rawls), who acknowledges the difficulty of giving a general secular justification for a universally applicable account of justice or fairness. His theory of justice is advanced for a society that is a modern constitutional democracy. His theory of justice is not necessarily the basis for claims across societies, for humans as such, for the world as such. "I shall be satisfied if it is possible to formulate a reasonable conception of justice for the basic structure of society conceived for the time being as a closed system isolated from other societies."[50] Indeed, Rawls recognizes that his theory is at root a political expository device.

Since justice as fairness is intended as a political conception of justice for a democratic society, it tries to draw solely upon basic intuitive ideas that are embedded in the political institutions of a constitutional democratic regime and the public traditions of their interpretation. Justice as fairness is a political conception in part because it starts from within a certain political tradition. We hope that this political conception of justice may at least be supported by what we may call an "overlapping consensus," that is, by a consensus that includes all the opposing philosophical and religious doctrines likely to persist and to gain adherents in a more or less just constitutional democratic society.[51]

The theory of justice presupposes a background notion of justice embedded in the idea of a *"just* constitutional democratic society."* Or, as Rawls puts it elsewhere, his conception of justice "presents a way for [citizens] to conceive of their common and guaranteed status as equal citizens and attempts to connect a particular understanding of freedom and equality with a particular conception of the person thought to be congenial to the shared notions and essential convictions implicit in the public culture of a democratic society."[52] This begs the question of what should count as a just or democratic society, in that there are various competing notions of justice and democracy, not to mention freedom and equality.

The contentions the later Rawls makes concerning the existence and significance of an overlapping consensus do not remedy this difficulty. They do not secure an account that should claim the assent of rational persons as such. First, the mere fact of peaceable collaboration among individuals with diverse moral visions does not presuppose or imply a concurrence regarding Rawls's vision of

liberal political values such as equality of oportunity. One need not even presuppose consensus or overlapping consensus regarding notions such as social
equality to justify a constitutional democracy. It is enough that individuals distinguish between moral friends and moral strangers, society and community, while
understanding that a democratic polity has the sparse authority of common consent for a limited sphere of undertakings. Such an understanding will not be
enough to justify Rawls' commitments to social welfare under his rubric of
political liberalism.

Second, instead of seeing an overlapping consensus underlying the de facto
collaboration of citizens in their government, one can take acquiescence in contemporary constitutional democracies as an expediency: it is safer to collaborate
hypocritically than to resort to violence. One may not conclude to an overlapping
moral consensus from the failure of citizens to rise up in arms against taxation for
various welfare programs they take to be immoral, misguided, or unworthy of
their support. When individuals (such as patients, physicians, and hospital officials) in countries with all-encompassing or near all-encompassing health care
systems attempt to circumvent those systems through illicit payments or influence
peddling, they can be regarded as silent freedom-fighters against the purported
overlapping consensus. When in response to all-intrusive governmental regulation and taxation individuals act not only to cheat on taxes, but to create underground, unmonitored businesses (as is common in many countries), they can also
be regarded as silently renouncing the purported overlapping consensus, while
hypocritically giving it lip service by not appealing to overt force. The purported
overlapping consensus to which Rawls appeals is thus amenable to an empirical
reconstruction, so as to reveal not a consensus but an underground overlapping
dis-consensus. In short, Rawls requires a normative account of any overlapping
consensus in order for it to be guiding.

Third, the moral significance of any consensus or dis-consensus is for its part
available for further reconsideration in ways that will not support Rawls's construals. One need only interpret what should count as a reasonable consensus in
terms of a different thin theory of the good, proper moral sense, reasonable moral
understanding, etc. Consider fundamental disagreements regarding key terms
such as fair equality of opportunity. Is appropriate equality of opportunity: (1) the
equal opportunity to act freely on one's ability to collaborate with others unhindered by the intrusion of the state (something of this sort would appear to have
been the sense of equality of opportunity among citizens built into the formal
right foundations underlying the U.S. Constitution of 1787); or (2) the equal
opportunity to act on one's rational plan of life with the provision of the medical,
social, educational, economic, and other welfare support that can help to erase
differential advantages? One need only consider the different views held by
members of the U.S. Congress regarding taxation, welfare, and affirmative action
to doubt that there is an overlapping consensus identifying current institutions as

fair systems of cooperation, rather that as structures in which one will pragmatically acquiesce in the sense of forgoing overt opposing force.

How much diversity is allowable and what falls within the guiding overlapping moral consensus? For Rawls, this is governed by his notion of a *reasonable* pluralism. The guiding overlapping consensus is the one that corresponds to a *reasonable* pluralism. The problem, to recast a phrase from Alasdair MacIntyre, is to determine whose moral reasonableness or which notion of moral rationality should govern. Shifting from an appeal to which political conception of justice is true to an appeal to which conception is reasonable succeeds only in highlighting the diverse understandings of reasonableness in moral and political life. Again, one might consider how Rawls in specifying reasonableness implicitly appeals to a particular view of equality, which is one among many.[53]

What can one then make of the often invoked notion of consensus or overlapping consensus? Does the existence of a significant proportion of citizens in Great Britain who would support the social and political inequality of a hereditary peerage and monarchy disconfirm the existence of an overlapping consensus regarding social and political equality? How much agreement and on what issues constitutes such a normative consensus: 51 percent? two thirds? three fourths? What amount of majority conveys what amount of moral authority? What sense of rationality is required to anoint a majority with moral authority? Since it will be impossible to attribute authority to mere numbers without further moral considerations being engaged, as with Rawls there will be an invocation of what is reasonable and rational. Reasonableness and rationality, to have moral force or content, to be more than merely formal notions, must be partisan to one among a number of competing accounts of reasonableness and rationality in morality and political relations. Perhaps appeals to consensus, other than for reasons of *Realpolitik,* reflect a secular remnant of the Christian appeal to the consent of all holy Christians in order to warrant the authority of ecumenical councils.

At times, claims about the existence of a consensus may trade on the failure to note important differences. Often, one is deceived that there is a considerable concurrence because of the use of similar words or because of features that share some family resemblances.[54] Imagine an ecumenical discussion among Greco-Roman pagans, orthodox Jews, Roman Catholics, and Episcopalians. Those moderating the discussions might point out that all agree to the importance of a priesthood. Yet, the significance and role of priests in Greco-Roman pagan cults is quite different from that within orthodox Judaism, which in turn is quite different from that among either Roman Catholics or Episcopalians. Perhaps after some discussion the ecumenists would think that matters can progress better if they began discussions between the pagans and the Jews, in that both have a notion of a hereditary priesthood. They might also press discussions between the Roman Catholics and Jews, since both require their priests to be male, and between the Episcopalians and Greco-Roman pagans, since both allow priestesses. What amount of agreement and in what areas constitutes a consensus or a normative overlapping consensus?

Or consider controversies regarding the status of private property and its implications for welfare, including the provision of health care for the indigent. Both Nozickians and Rawlsians agree that there is private property; however, the meaning of the practice differs radically. For the Nozickian, entitlements to private property are grounded in principles of just acquisition and just transfer. "From each as they choose, to each as they are chosen."[55] For Rawlsians, private property must be understood in terms of its function within just institutions defined in terms of the two principles of justice. These are quite different notions of ownership. They each imply quite different individual rights to health care. Is there a consensus or overlapping consensus regarding private property in the case of Nozickians and Rawlsians? Does the purported existence of a consensus trade on central ambiguities regarding ownership?

Or consider the issue of abortion. Those who hold that the state should use force to prevent abortions may still conclude in a particular place and time that state interventions would cause more harm than good. Is there a consensus or overlapping consensus with those who hold that it is good to provide abortion on request, since both sides would not support governmental intervention? If the two sides are willing to make compromises to avoid what each holds to be a worse evil, does the outcome then count as a consensus or overlapping consensus? How does one distinguish a consensus from (1) fortuitous concurrence with regard to a particular issue of policy, (2) areas of morally unproblematic limited cooperation and limited agreement, and (3) areas where agreements have been made by parties who consider the outcome the lesser of evils.

Why would so many people hold the view that theories of justice or accounts of bioethics are justified in terms of a societal consensus or a set of overlapping consensuses, if it were so suspect? In part, this may stem from the way in which politicians seek the appearance of widespread concurrence in order to govern. If one is to establish a governmental committee that will endorse a particular policy rather than be riven with dissent, one must structure the process so that there will not in fact be endless debates about fundamental moral or political visions. Thus, one does not appoint persons like William Buckley, Angela Davis, Jesse Jackson, Bella Abzug, Ron Paul, and Mother Teresa to a committee to determine the high school curriculum for safe sex for New York City public schools.[56] If one did, one would quite quickly encounter unbridgeable moral disagreements. Instead, one attempts to appoint individuals who share much in common. One takes control of the agenda for the meetings, so that the discussions do not go aground on issues of deep disagreement. One manages discussion and creates the appearance of consensus as one of the wise strategies of a peaceable *Realpolitik*.

Appeals to consensus and overlapping consensuses function as does an ideology according to Marx. "The ideas of the ruling class are in every epoch the ruling ideas: i.e. the class, which is the ruling material force of society, is at the same time its ruling intellectual force."[57] The consensus to which appeal is made is the cluster of ideas needed to legitimate particular political programs for public policy including health care policy. Against the background of democratic institutions that aspire to impose a particular moral understanding, widespread agreement can be claimed to delegitimate contrary understandings as morally unacceptable and politically incorrect.

Ideology, in short, facilitates domination and exploitation as ongoing social relationships. . . . Socialist thought invites ideological analysis as an instrument in the social struggle among competing groups for access to state power and thereby to the resources the modern interventionist state commands.[58]

As John Gray observes, the circumstance that ideological criticism has not generally been deployed against either communist or socialist ideologies seems to depend on an "undefended assumption that socialist goals stand in need of no ideological demystification."[59] The force of this general point is that even democratic, mildly socialist understandings such as Rawls will count as mere ideologies if they cannot provide a justification to warrant the normativity of their content. An appeal to a consensus without foundational arguments is an appeal to the orthodoxy of a governing elite in order to legitimate its dominance and to make criticism of its basic assumptions appear immoral or irrational. If one seeks to justify moral authority by an appeal to a national consensus, one may mistake Machiavellian strategies and subtle compromises for consensus or even for overlapping consensuses.

After all of this is said and done, the crucial principled question remains: why does the majority possess the true or authoritative vision of fairness or justice, if such a majority exists? Why would a preponderant consensus convey moral authority? Again, how much consensus would be needed for moral authority? Perhaps the force of the appeal to a consensus trades on a strategic ambiguity in the term itself.[60] The word *consensus* in the Latin means both a unanimity as well as an agreement. The same is the case in English. The word consensus can identify both a common feeling, as well as an agreement. But as has just been shown, there can be some agreement even where the basic moral sentiments are in conflict, so that the decision to collaborate in a particular case does not imply a general agreement to collaborate in many, much less most, cases. Moreover, rather than being made out of a concurrence of moral judgments, agreements can be made as a prudent compromise in the face of coercive political pressures where other choices would bring even more harms. Consensus will have a moral force, where it identifies a unanimity of agreement. But when consensus identifies a balance of political power in which individuals with diverse moral sentiments find themselves forced to collaborate and acquiesce in much that they find morally disturbing in order to avoid even worse moral outcomes, much more must be established in order to derive moral authority or legitimacy.[61]

In the ruins of foundationalism, many endorse the contingent commitments to which they find themselves bound by history and chance. Richard Rorty, for example, advances what he takes to be Michael Oakeshott's (1901–90) insight,[62] drawn from Hegel:[63]

We can keep the notion of "morality" just insofar as we can cease to think of morality as the voice of the divine part of ourselves and instead think of it as the voice of ourselves as members of a community, speakers of a common language. We can keep the morality–prudence distinction if we think of it not as the difference between an appeal to the unconditioned and an appeal to the conditioned but as the difference between an appeal to the interests of our community and the appeal to our own, possibly conflicting, private interests. The importance of this shift is that it makes it impossible to ask the question "Is ours a moral society?"[64]

But why remain bound by one's own community's moral prejudices? Why should one in the end endorse the conceits of Rorty's liberalism instead of those of a capitalist authoritarian government, as found in Singapore?

As a liberal of a particular genre, Richard Rorty endorses his variety of liberalism with its particular understanding of freedom, equality, and solidarity as the gift of a particular history. The general view of governance delivered by this moral contingency is taken in its core elements as pragmatically indubitable, because no fundamental doubt can be accepted without setting this moral framework aside and with it our common moral language. Still, those who embrace his morality would at the same time be "people who had a sense of the contingency of their language of moral deliberation, and thus of their consciences, and thus of their community."[65] Yet, contingency cannot guarantee Rorty's ironic balance between remaining a liberal and recognizing its lack of ultimate justification. Doubt is ubiquitous, critical, and corrosive. There is not only the received liberalism of Cambridge, Massachusetts, but the quite different moral presumptions of Singapore, South Korea, and other polities with alternative understandings of the good morality and polity. The contingency of any vision of solidarity can be brought into question by both reason and history. One can always invoke the critical power of universality that Rorty wishes to still and which can always inquire whether the morality one embraces is the morality all should embrace.

Despite this precariousness and in the embrace of contingency, Rorty advances a pragmatic account of philosophy's function that makes it equivalent to that of an ideology in service to the ruling class. Philosophy is not to be viewed as providing a conceptual foundation for democratic political institutions.[66] Philosophy is to be understood in the service of a particular account of democratic political institutions. Philosophy moves from being an intellectual enterprise in its own right to being an ideological tool. If one *believes* firmly enough in the institutions of a particular variety of liberal democracy, then perhaps one can resist the temptation of critically recognizing that the believers are *simply* " 'we twentieth-century liberals' or 'we heirs to the historical contingencies which have created more and more cosmopolitan, more and more democratic political institutions.' "[67] A merely factual, merely contingent moral vision satisfies only as long as one does not give in to the critical doubts that most liberalisms encourage. Doubt opens to other possibilities, including those offered by Nietzsche. Since there is no general secular justification or foundation for the contingent sentiments that frame the various liberal democracies, in general secular terms such societies are, as Rorty admits, no more or less noble, good, beautiful, or inspiring than societies built around a samurai ethic or that of authoritarian capitalism.

Rorty's suggestions work only if one holds that a liberal democracy is preferable, say, to an authoritarian capitalism (i.e., Cambridge, Massachusetts, over Singapore). Any particular choice is plausible, given a particular ranking of liberty, equality, prosperity, and security. Those who can walk safely at night in the security of a prosperous authoritarian capitalism and have (given their value weightings) an apparently much more successful health care system[68] will pity those who live in more dangerous and relatively exiguous circumstances in liberal social democracies. Those who live in developing countries will be able to choose between modeling their country after Cambridge, Massachusetts, or Singapore on the basis of their own rankings of goods and harms.

Who is right? How could one tell? As importantly, how can one justify to moral strangers the imposition of a liberal social democracy versus a laissez-faire capitalist democracy, an authoritarian democracy, a communist dictatorship? Any judgment of outcomes depends on a particular judgment or ranking of harms and benefits, on a particular vision of the good. It is not possible to justify a canonical content-full morality, understanding of right conduct, or bioethics, in general secular terms. Nor will it do simply to canonize the failure to justify moral claims through announcing various nonfoundationalist approaches to morality and bioethics. Unless one can provide some other form of plausible justification for the moral authority of such nonfoundationalist proposals, as through justifying a casuistical or middle-level approach (such tactics appear from the foregoing not to be promising), one will simply be announcing one's moral prejudices. To assert that one has a nonfoundationalist vision that should govern when others do not concur is tantamount to admitting that one has in desperation decided to announce one's moral vision or ideology and then coercively impose it on others.

## At the brink of nihilism

One must appreciate the enormity of the failure of the Enlightenment project of discovering a canonical content-full morality. This failure represents the collapse of the Western philosophical hope to ground the objectivity of morality. This failure bears against theories of justice and accounts of morality generally. It brings all secular bioethics into question. If one cannot justify a particular morality, then one cannot justify claims of immorality. All appears to become a matter of taste. Indeed, if one cannot disclose some lines of conduct as canonically immoral, then the health care provided by Albert Schweitzer and by Nazi death camps will be equally defensible and indefensible. If one cannot discover an objective method to decide when the morally deviant are also the morally wrong, then the action of the morally heinous and the saint will be equally justifiable or lacking in justification, at least in general secular terms. One stands on the brink of nihilism.

The threat of this conclusion is, to say the least, deeply disturbing. Western culture has presumed that there is a fabric of natural law in terms of which one can judge the rightness and wrongness of actions across cultures and times. Such presumptions have guided Western law from the Roman Empire through the Nuremberg trials.[69] Gaius speaks of "the law that natural reason establishes among all mankind [and which] is followed by all people alike, and is called *ius gentium* [law of nations or law of the world] as being the law observed by all mankind."[70] This is a point repeated in the *Institutes of Justinian*[71] and Blackstone's *Commentaries on the Laws of England*.[72] The failure to develop a perspective from which one can rationally choose among competing views of morality brings these moral assumptions into doubt.

The inclination to make bioethics more than an exegesis of a particular moral tradition or vision becomes a temptation of a will to power. To impose a particular bioethics on society generally without moral authority, from a general secular moral perspective, is to use one's will to create a consensus by coercion. It is to conclude that, if God is dead in the secular public area in the sense that not all hear Him, and since a secular substitute is not available in a canonical content-full morality disclosable by reason, there are no general moral constraints. Each may choose a different version of a putative bioethical consensus and then seek to make it de facto, albeit not *de jure morale,* authoritative. Will meets will with no general secular moral constraints.

From the French Revolution to the October Revolution, reason has failed to establish a particular view of the good life and of content-full moral obligations as morally authoritative.[73] The problem is as outlined earlier: to establish a particular concrete understanding of the good life and of content-full moral obligations as morally authoritative, one must appeal to a particular moral sense, vision, or understanding. However, to justify that moral sense one must appeal to a yet higher moral sense, vision, or understanding *ad indefinitum.* Either one undertakes an infinite regress or arbitrarily embraces a particular, content-full moral vision or understanding, thus begging the question regarding which content-full moral vision, understanding, and so forth, should be canonical. To acquire or articulate a particular moral content, one needs particular moral premises, rules of evidence, and the like. As a consequence, the more one attempts to advance a moral vision without appeal to any of the particularities of culture, religion, and history, the more the resulting moral vision lacks content. The more a moral vision, moral understanding, thin theory of the good, account of right conduct, etc., has content, the more it presupposes particular moral premises, rules of evidence, rules of inference, etc. The more it gains content, the more it will appear parochial and partisan to one among numerous particular moral understandings. Universality is purchased at the price of content. Content is purchased at the price of universality. Without a guiding background morality one confronts a babble of competing possibilities. The plurality of content-full moral visions is therefore not simply descriptively the case but a condition of our moral epistemological predicament. To know which secular morality to endorse, we must already know morally. But the question is how to know that one knows morally. If the secular means for establishing the correctness of any particular moral viewpoint fails, then one loses any source of authoritative direction for a secular ethics or bioethics. In addition, without some new approach one will be unable to establish public policy bodies or individuals as having the moral authority to impose any particular policy by force. Public policy, including health care policy, will lack general secular moral authority, and could at best have authority with a bar sinister, an authority based on force.

## *The way out of nihilism: how to save the moral legitimacy of secular bioethics*

Controversies can be resolved on the basis of (1) force, (2) conversion of one party to the other's viewpoint, (3) sound rational argument, and (4) agreement.[74] In particular, one must distinguish between resolutions through *cloture* (main force) and resolutions that have moral authority. An appeal to force will not answer ethical questions, such as intellectual queries as to why a controversy ought to be resolved in a particular fashion, even if the resolution imposes a widespread consensus. Using force, even legally authorized force (e.g., to forbid the private sale of better basic care) will simply be an act of force for any who do not share the moral vision that purports to make such interventions legitimate. Brute force, unless it is justified, remains brute force. Subtle force remains force. A goal of ethics is to determine when force can be justified.

Much can be regained for ethics by remembering what in fact one could hope from it. To ask a secular ethical question is to seek a ground other than force for resolving moral controversies. One seeks authority other than in coercive power. Secular ethics and bioethics are at the very least means for resolving controversies regarding proper conduct on bases other than appeals to force as the fundamental basis for the resolution. Justification for the resolution of moral controversies has often been sought in a commonly held moral viewpoint, a viewpoint to which all in a community have in one sense or another converted. Moral authority is then the moral authority of the moral understanding one holds in common. Rawls and Rorty may provide examples of such appeals to conversion in their appeals to consensus. The appeal to "conversion" involves one of the traditional hopes for the resolution of moral controversies. The Christian West, especially prior to the Reformation, envisaged a single authoritative moral viewpoint, available not only through divine grace, but in great measure through rational argument, and interpreted by the singular authority of the Roman Catholic Church and, in particular, the pope of Rome.[75] This moral vision and authority completed and fulfilled what reason was held to disclose regarding the *ius gentium*.[76]

The fragmentation of Christendom, the secularization of the West,[77] and the failure of such rational arguments have called this ideal into question as a historical possibility. Moreover, the appeal to a transcendent God and His grace cannot resolve controversies in a secular society. By definition, the decisive premises in such a context are available only through divine revelation and grace.[78] Unless the premises and rules of evidence can also be secured by a general rational argument, they will not be accessible to those not so blessed. Force when employed to coerce those not so favored will not be justifiable in general secular terms. Such actions will then be against the possibility of a peaceable, general, secularly defensible morality. Indeed, the Christian states of the Western Middle Ages were without moral authority in much of what they did, as the history of the persecution of Jews and heretics attests.[79]

The Reformation and modernity disclosed the depths of these problems of legitimacy. The fragmentation of moral perspectives called forth the modern philosophical hope of giving morality the authority of reason. The foregoing pages have explored why the various attempts to authorize morality rationally have failed and must fail. This failure marks the collapse of an intellectual project that developed with Western Christianity.[80]

If one cannot establish by sound rational argument a particular concrete moral viewpoint as canonically decisive (and one cannot, because the establishment of such a viewpoint itself presupposes a moral viewpoint, and that is exactly what is at stake), then the only source of general secular authority for moral content and moral direction is agreement. To rephrase the point, because there are no decisive secular arguments to establish that one concrete view of the moral life is better morally than its rivals, and since all have not converted to a single moral viewpoint, secular moral authority is the authority of consent. Authority is not that of coercive power, or of God's will, or of reason, but simply the authority of the agreement of those who decide to collaborate. This basis for morality is available in the notion of ethics as a means of securing moral authority through consent in the face of intractable content-full moral controversies. If one is interested in collaborating with moral authority in the face of moral disagreements without fundamental recourse to force, then one must accept agreement among members of the controversy or peaceable negotiation as the means for resolving concrete moral controversies.

This account of ethics and bioethics requires a minimum of prior assumptions. It requires only a decision to resolve moral disputes in a manner other than fundamentally by force. It commits one to no particular concrete moral view of the good life (e.g., the importance of health care vis-à-vis other human undertakings) or of content-full moral obligations. Any concrete view requires either arguments that cannot be successful (i.e., sound rational arguments establishing a particular view of the good life and of content-full moral obligations as canonical) or special premises available only within particular communities endorsing particular ideological, religious, or metaphysical presuppositions. The appeal to permission as the source of authority involves no particular moral vision or understanding. It gives no value to permission. It simply recognizes that secular moral authority is the authority of permission. This appeal is a minimal condition in relying on what it is to resolve issues among moral strangers with moral authority: consent. It establishes a secularly acknowledgeable authority for its conclusions: agreement. By appealing to ethics as a means for peaceably negotiating moral disputes, one discloses as a necessary and sufficient condition (sufficient when combined with the decision to collaborate) for a general secular ethics the requirement to respect the freedom of the participants in a moral controversy (i.e., in the sense of gaining their permission for using them) as a basis for common moral authority (i.e., from the permission of those collaborating). Since moral controversies can in principle encompass all moral agents (and, as we shall see, *only* moral agents), one has a means of characterizing the secular moral community as the possible intellectual standpoint of persons interested in resolving moral controversies in ways not fundamentally based on force.

Secular moral authority is nothing more or less than the authority of those who agree to collaborate. It does not invoke a moral authority derived from God, reason, or a particular moral tradition or ideology. The secular moral world can be fashioned through free will,[81] even if not on the basis of sound rational arguments with moral content. Even if one does not attain transcendent rationality, one obtains an immanent, transcendental[82] grounding for this decision of the will: a game, a grammatical possibility that cannot be avoided and which comes with inescapable rules but no content. If one resolves moral controversies by mutual agreement, one can account for the moral authority of this common endeavor: mutual consent. If one acts against this one means of resolving secular moral controversies among moral strangers, one loses any general secular moral grounds to protest when visited with defensive or punitive force. Those who endorse the practice find a moral world that can be shared with moral strangers. Those who reject the practice lose recognizable secular grounds for protest when they are punished. In the face of the postmodern plurality of moral perspectives, there is still a generally understandable meaning to acting with moral authority. There is the possibility of intersubjective moral coherence and collaboration without presupposing the objectivity of secular morality in the sense of its corresponding to particular content-full moral truths[83] and without requiring content-full moral agreement.

If an individual refuses to participate in this practice and instead resolves disputes by force, even if supposedly morally justified (e.g., "God tells me that having two tiers of health care is wrong, so therefore we will forbid this by law"), others can retort: "When you use force against the innocent on the basis of moral claims that are not generally justifiable, or agreed to by all parties concerned, you cannot rationally protest when we employ force to protect ourselves from you and reject your supposed authority. What is asserted without proof can as easily be met with a counterassertion. Moreover, rational beings anywhere in the cosmos who are interested in coming to terms with moral controversies with general secular moral authority, and in not using force as the primary basis for the resolution of disputes, should understand you to be an enemy of secular morality, and therefore blameworthy, and hold us to have acted correctly."

On the other hand, when an individual peaceably refuses (which refusal can be protected by defensive force) to participate in a particular agreement, and does not use unconsented-to force against the innocent (e.g., breaking a promise), one has simply discovered a limit to a particular community or area of agreement, and not a warrant to force cooperation. It is here that one also has discovered a fundamental equality among all persons.[84] If no hierarchy of values can be established as canonical, then individuals cannot be subordinated one to the other outside of the wishes or actions of the persons involved (e.g., as a part of just punishment). Moreover, the right of all persons to refuse to participate in any particular community makes all persons equal in their right to be left alone and to seek to fashion a community with willing others.

This view of ethics and bioethics is not grounded in a concern for peaceableness. It is not based on an interest in establishing a peaceable community. This view cannot be shown in general secular terms to be good, praiseworthy, or rationally to be desired. It should, instead, be recognized as a disclosure, to borrow a Kantian notion, of a transcendental condition, a necessary condition for the possibility of a general domain of human life and of the life of persons generally. It is a disclosure of the minimum grammar involved in speaking of blame and praise with moral strangers, and for establishing a particular set of moral commitments with an authority other than through force.[85] This account can be regarded as a transcendental argument to justify a principle of freedom as a side constraint, as a source of authority.[86] The authority of freedom as a side constraint, the principle that one may not use others without permission, derives from this being a necessary condition for the possibility of a major endeavor of persons: a secular moral fabric that can be justified to, and that can bind, moral strangers. Just as certain conditions must be presupposed for the very possibility of scientific reasoning, so here one finds a basic, minimum presupposition of secular ethics.[87]

This analysis has the character of unpacking a tautology. Such circular reasoning (i.e., reasoning from the notion of ethics as the enterprise of resolving moral controversies without a fundamental recourse to force, but rather with moral authority) is acceptable if it discloses the character of a major, unavoidable element of the lives of persons.[88] It provides an intellectual insight. It shows that although one cannot discover content-full moral lineaments of conduct outside of a particular proper concrete view of the good life and of content-full moral obligations, one can still disclose the basis for the fashioning of a secular moral fabric.

These points concerning the resolution of moral controversies with authority may benefit from a summary. Resolution by force carries no intellectual authority either with regard to (1) which viewpoint is correct, or (2) whether the correct viewpoint *may* be imposed by force. Authority in such cases is simply power, the force to compel. Nor will appeals to conversion suffice for a secular pluralist society, though they will suffice for those who form a community of believers or ideologues who experience the grace of common conversion or who are committed to a particular moral sense or set of moral premises. The grace of conversion or special commitment has no general secular moral authority. Sound rational arguments would provide the authority of reason, were they able to justify a particular content-full moral viewpoint. Because sound rational argument fails in principle to establish a canonical content-full moral understanding, one is left with agreement. With the advent of the Reformation (the historical metaphor for the unlikelihood of common conversion) and with the collapse of the Enlightenment hope of delivering a secular, rational justification of the authority of a singular concrete understanding of the good life and of content-full moral obligations, one still possesses a process for peaceably creating common moral authority.

This account of the morality that can bind moral strangers, the one element of the Enlightenment hope that survives, is still sufficient to justify a wide range of human practices and health care policies. Indeed, it can justify all practices that draw their authority from bare consent or from the necessary forbearance from using individuals without their consent, which lies at the foundation of the very possibility of a general secular morality. Thus, a justificatory account can be given of such practices as free and informed consent, the market, and limited democracies. In the acquisition of permission, consent, or agreement, all that will be foreclosed is coercive force on the part of the one seeking agreement. One may take market advantage of those coerced by nature or third parties, insofar as those entering the agreement are not responsible for such coercion. It will not be improper to employ inducements or to engage in peaceable manipulation to garner permission, agreement, or consent. Persuasion, inducements, and market forces are means of making it worthwhile for individuals to agree to join in particular undertakings. Such manipulations form part of the fabric of a secular society of persons acting with common authority, as long as such manipulations are peaceable, as long as they do not involve threats of force or unconsented-to interventions that are undertaken against the possibility of free agreement impossible (in general secular terms, this does not foreclose the possibility of peaceably inducing others to agree to make choice impossible—e.g., the immoral suggestion, "let's get drunk together").

*Moral authority in postmodernity: legitimating health care policy*

Postmodernity discloses the unavailability through sound rational argument of a single, canonical, normative, content-full understanding of morality or bioethics that could provide moral authority for public policy in general and for health care policy in particular. If sound rational argument could have established such content-full moral guidance, then: (1) one could have dismissed all who disagreed as being irrational, (2) one could have visited them with coercive force grounded in the authority of rationality (and they would have no rational grounds for protesting against being visited with such force, as long as it was delivered in accord with the content-full understandings that sound rational argument had been justified), and (3) such coercive force would not be alienating but in fact restorative of individuals to the rational moral conduct proper to them as rational beings. By default, authority is derived not from reason, nor from God, nor from a will to power (i.e., force), but from the bare will to have the one authority moral strangers can share: permission. Secular moral authority is derived from a bare will to morality. Competence to give permission is the ability to so will.

These reflections lead to a reexamination of the moral authority of democracies and of democratic majorities. Unless one has unanimous consent, one must show how much of a majority is normative and why. If one cannot give a sound rational argument to canonize a particular understanding of democracy, or of the authority of democratic majorities, then the secular moral standing of democracy will have been deconstructed and will collapse into contrary and competing ideologies. To avoid the secular delegitimation of all public policy, including health care policy, one must show how much a limited democracy can do, while still deriving its moral authority from its citizens. To illustrate the nature of this task, one might imagine all of the readers of this book envisaging everyone dying, save for them. If they had then to create a government and establish health care policy, it is unlikely that they would share a common understanding of the good life or proper moral authority. They will likely have divergent views regarding abortion, euthanasia, and the governmental support of health care. Still, they could frame a government that could with moral authority employ punitive and defensive force against those who use the innocent without consent (e.g., use people as subjects of experimentation without consent). It could as well enforce recorded contracts (e.g., agreements that physicians make with their patients). If they produce resources in common, they can also create whatever rules they wish in order to decide on how to distribute those resources. For example, they could rely on a two-thirds majority in a plebiscite. They could establish a directorate that could make choices by simple majority vote. They could establish a committee that, by a simple majority, would create a list of the ten most important endeavors to fund and then choose from that list by lot. One can even create welfare rights, in particular, governmentally funded rights to health care.

Although much in contemporary public policy, including health care policy, can be reunderstood and justified, much cannot. In particular, the modern secular myth of the special moral authority of a majority falls beyond justification. Even force by the consent of the majority is mere force without further justification. If such use of force is not to be understood as the *Realpolitik* of respecting overwhelming social forces, the legitimacy of secular moral authority in public policy-making must be derived from the consent of actual individuals. Instead of attempting vain arguments to justify the secular moral authority of government in terms of its organization, control of a particular territory, or its aspirations to a particular form of moral rectitude, one must determine the extent to which the moral authority of public policy (here policy bearing on health care) can be derived from the agreement of those involved.

The attempt to establish such authority at once discloses its limits. The secular moral limits on public authority can be expressed through a list of individual or "natural" rights, where "natural rights" are those that one can never presume individuals to have tacitly ceded, without threat of force, to a social organization.[89] These rights (which express or indicate the limits of public consent and the limited moral authority of governments) are indefinite and include such secular moral rights as the right to use contraception, to have a private tier of health care, and to commit suicide. These are not rights because these are necessarily good things to do (indeed, suicide is from the author's understanding a grave moral evil). It is just that their proscription falls beyond the secular moral authority of a secular state.[90] These rights are secure against majoritarian decisions. Even a vote of all save one for their abolition does not affect their secular moral standing. Such rights are reminders of the radical limits of a community's secular moral authority over individuals in their actions with themselves and consenting others. From a secular moral perspective such actions are private unless the individuals involved either violate the conditions for morally authoritative action among moral strangers or agree to submit their private lives to a particular community's regulation. For example, people have a secular basic moral right to sell their organs for transplantation.

Moral authority in secular health care policy is derived from permission and even in circumstances of complex collaborative undertakings is at its roots consensual or contractual. Moral controversies in biomedicine are public policy disputes to be resolved peaceably by agreeing to procedures for creating moral rules based on the principle that force cannot be used against the innocent without their consent. Since the web of explicit and implicit consent is usually very intricate, it will often be difficult to chart exactly when consent has occurred. It will frequently not be at all clear what one ought to do, or where and when secular moral obligations exist. However, one should do the best one can under prevailing circumstances. If conditions do not admit of greater perfection, anything worth doing well is worth doing poorly.

This view of the state and of public policy may appear exotic in that Western understandings of the state and political theory have been so influenced by the Aristotelian ideal of a state formed as a morally cohesive whole.[91] Aristotle had as his model the city-state, which as he argued should not be larger than can be taken in at a single view (*Politics* 7.4.1326b), that is, not more than one hundred thousand citizens (*Nicomachean Ethics* 9.10.1170b). It is ironic that Aristotle conceived of politics in looking back to the polis, although he tutored Alexander the Great for Philip of Macedon, who fashioned one of the first major large-scale states. The challenge is that of fashioning a large-scale state with secular moral authority and health care policy spanning numerous moral communities that have analogies with Aristotle's city-states, but which are not bound to particular geographical locations. A large-scale state must act as a neutral vehicle for spanning numerous communities with often diverse views of a proper content-full bioethics.[92] Against this now better developed account of general secular morality, we can return and revisit the contrasting content-full moralities of concrete moral communities.

## Morality and bioethics for friends;
## morality and bioethics for strangers

It is within communities, not large-scale societies, that one is embedded in a full matrix of moral content and structure. It is within particular moral communities that one lives and finds full meaning in life and concrete moral direction. It is within particular moral communities that one possesses a content-full bioethics. There one is a Southern Baptist, an Orthodox Catholic, a Roman Catholic, an Orthodox Jew, or a Maoist communist. It is only within such communities that life with its pleasures and sufferings can take on its full significance. Only in terms of the values that direct such communities does one learn which moral and nonmoral goods ought to be pursued and at what costs. On the general secular level one can discover that breaking promises to a patient is usually a form of using unconsented-to force against the innocent. It is in such communities that one learns what promises one should make. Within a particular community, one can also learn whether it is better to suffer the pains of a prolonged fatal illness or to avoid this through suicide, whether it is better to raise with love a defective child or to prevent its birth through prenatal diagnosis and abortion, whether it is better to accept sterility or to hire a surrogate mother. Such choices take substance from a concrete understanding of values, obligations, rights, and wrongs.

Young physicians and nurses learn particular values and virtues through "role models." By embodying the virtues of a particular moral viewpoint, "role models" show possibilities for understanding goodness, evil, and meaning in life. They teach by action and commitment regarding a particular understanding of good health care. From a general secular perspective, one might consider the various moral communities as experiments in the building of moral worlds, as creative endeavors to fashion views of the good life and alternative content-full bioethics. In their diversity they are instructive regarding the range of ways in which individuals can experience the good, understand the goods of health care, as well as practice medicine and the other health care professions. They also reflect the hunger of the human spirit for meaning in human sexuality, birth, growth, health, sickness, suffering, and death.

The differences in the composition of moral goods within competing moral views are best seen, appreciated, and experienced *in concreto*. One is usually best instructed regarding content-full moral character through stories of heroes and saints, through histories, novels, poems, and plays. But the possibilities are diverse, even within one moral community. One might think of a child seeking a model for a good life and of content-full moral obligations being sent to the lives of the saints, where he comes upon accounts of the holy monk St. Herman of Alaska and of the warrior-king St. Olaf of Norway. How ought he to choose between pursuing the virtues of St. Herman (1757–1837) in his love and kind attention to all animals,[93] human and nonhuman, or the virtues of St. Olaf Haraldsson (995–1030), who died at Stiklestad on Friday, July 29, 1030, trying his best to defeat the enemies of his nation?[94] General secular arguments will not provide conclusive guidance for the choice if one presumes Olaf did not employ unconsented-to force against the innocent. To appreciate a content-full understanding of virtue, one must see virtue incarnate in the life of a particular person within a particular community with its particular moral traditions and practices.[95]

Since there are no generally sustainable, secular arguments to establish as canonical a particular view of the good life and of content-full moral obligations, and as long as the ways of life under consideration respect the freedom of the innocent, then, from outside, the choice among any particular moral community will appear to be similar to an aesthetic choice. There will be a number of moral viewpoints unexcludable on the basis of secular moral arguments. That is, they will not involve using the unconsenting innocent. Within this constraint, choices among styles of morality or of moral orientation can be made on the basis of which appears to be the most beautiful or well composed. For example, is it better to be a devout Southern Baptist, a Texian deist, or a homosexual San Franciscan atheist? Each is likely to carry special risks and advantages with respect to future morbidity, mortality, and quality of life. Each also carries with it a particular understanding of the good. Secular morality can give no basis for choosing.

Is it better to practice medicine as an abortionist or an internist? Is it morally better to practice with profit as a central motive or, instead, as a part of a nonprofit church clinic? In these and many other circumstances, secular moral arguments will give no guidance. From the outside, for those unconverted to the canonical content-full moral community, such choices will not be moral choices in the strict sense of choices one could hope to universalize or justify in terms of content-full principles that should bind all. Instead, the choice is best understood as one among competing views of the good life and of content-full moral obligations, a choice that must be made according to particular sentiments, according to which alternative appears the richest, most encompassing, and most engaging. As was shown earlier, such choices cannot be decisively grounded in general secular terms as morally authoritative on the basis of sound arguments without already endorsing a particular moral sense or viewpoint.

A concrete moral community can seem quite different from within as opposed to how it is experienced from the outside. From within a particular religious group, it may be evident that it is wrong, with a wrongness sustained by the Deity's disapproval, to commit suicide, even when faced with the final weeks of debilitation due to incurable cancer. Those who live in such a moral community will recognize their position as that which all *ought* morally to embrace, but they will not have general secular moral arguments to demonstrate this wrongness to moral strangers. For those who agree with them regarding, for example, basic premises or rules of evidence and inference, such arguments will be successful. Otherwise, they can at best hope to convert through witness and persuasion. Since respect of freedom is core to the grammar of secular ethics, individuals will have a general, rationally defensible right to commit suicide in the narrow sense that it will not be possible in general secular terms to show that the state has secular moral authority to forbid suicide. From the outside, then, an individual derives moral instruction from considering a community that forbids suicide by attempting to assay how all of its commitments congeal into a coherent and full moral life. In the end, the outside observer may conclude that this particular way of life provides the best of lives and most fully endows death with meaning, so that it is clear that one ought not to commit suicide. However, that judgment will not be the assent of those who endorse a community's deeper truth (e.g., its transcendent foundation in the will of God). Nor will it be the conclusion of a decisive secular moral argument. It is instead the sort of quasi-aesthetic judgment of an individual at home in a secular, pluralist society, but who is seeking an understanding of life that will provide both meaning and community.

Such choices are often made by cosmopolitan individuals who "shop" for intellectual and moral insights from various religious and cultural "traditions."[96] One might think here of the ways in which Protestants, Roman Catholics, Jews, and Moslems in cities such as Atlanta, Buenos Aires, London, New York, Paris, and Sydney have come to depart from their "traditional" views regarding contraception, abortion, or artificial insemination by donor. They have incorporated moral intuitions with roots in classic pagan times and contemporary philosophical reflections, as well as various New Age and other popular understandings of religion and reality. One might think of how the religiously half-believing piece together from various quarters inchoate senses of the meaning of pain, suffering, and disease. To the true believer, such eclecticism is not simply shoddy and shallow, but lacking depth and substance. Such is the price of the peaceable tolerant community.[97]

On the other hand, some have the strong moral conviction that strong moral convictions should not be had. Belief, commitment, and firm moral convictions are regarded as divisive at best and evocative of violence at worst. The world, they firmly believe, would be better off if there were less belief and moral conviction. They believe instead that most issues are better regarded more on the model of aesthetic choices. Such individuals tend to be intolerant of those who would merely tolerate (condemn but use no violence against those they condemn) instead of accepting the diversity of moral convictions that mark our condition. Ironically, such partisans of the value of moral diversity can be as intolerant as many of the religious communities they will not tolerate because of their strong moral convictions.

For those who believe truly, know morality rightly, and correctly experience what they should do, the choice of moral content will not be arbitrary. Moral content will not simply be the result of an aesthetic choice. These believers will not endorse the discounting of the seriousness of moral differences. Morality will be a truth given. Consider, for example, this account of receiving moral content through participation in the Liturgy. It offers a discursive invitation to a mystical encounter.

You are not isolated and separated from other people and things. You are not enclosed in the prison of space. You are not stifled by the condemnation of living in time. Your life is not a glass of water which does not quench your thirst if you drink it, and goes bad before your eyes if you do not. You are not a mechanically operating section of a limitless whole, nor an individual in an anonymous multitude. The Author of life has shattered the bonds of purely mechanical existence. You are an organic part of a theanthropic mystery.[98]

With such a context, one will implicitly possess a bioethics. One will have a casuistry fashioned and directed for oneself by a spiritual father. Within such a context, one will learn to understand the differences and the underlying unity in the hagiographies of Herman of Alaska and Olaf of Norway. One will learn how one should use them in the development of one's own moral life. This content with all its richness will not gear in or touch the elements of a general secular ethics. It will live in the interstices, in the exclaves within the fabric of a secular morality.[99] It will not provide a morality or bioethics for moral strangers.

We are left with a dialectical understanding of the nature of ethics and bio-ethics. While on the one hand recognizing a universal though content-less secular fabric or grammar of ethics and bioethics, we must as well recognize a plurality of concrete moral viewpoints and of content-full bioethics. Although from the perspective of this general secular morality the content of particular ethics and bioethics is irremediably subjective and relative, there is a secularly objective, in the sense of intersubjective, morality. There is an intersubjective fabric to secular ethics in virtue of the very understanding of ethics as an authoritative alternative to the resolution of disputes through force. For example, because there will not be a generally defensible basis to forbid the rich from purchasing health care not available to the poor, the purchase of such care will be a right sustainable in general, secular ethics, even if within particular states, particular moral communities have succeeded in forbidding the exercise of this secular moral right. Although from the outside the plurality of moral understandings and communities will appear as a diversity of content-full moral alternatives, from the inside truth can be seen and this very moral diversity recognized as a pluralism of error.

## Communities, secularity, and bioethics: providing health care in a morally fragmented world

The moral life is lived within two dimensions: (1) that of a secular ethics, which strives to be content-less and which thus has the ability to span numerous divergent moral communities, and (2) the particular moral communities within which one can achieve a content-full understanding of the good life and of content-full moral obligations. The first is defensible in terms of general secular moral arguments regarding the nature of ethics. This dimension offers some secularly absolute and universal secular moral conclusions, even if they are content-less. Since it is an attempt to secure moral authority and purpose for common action across moral communities, it presupposes the existence of a number of competing moral viewpoints and the richness of the moral life they contain. Taken by itself, secular bioethics would be an empty framework. The second dimension is that of competing content-full visions of the good life and of content-full moral obligations, including concrete accounts of virtues and vices. It is the first dimension that can establish secular rights of patients to refuse even lifesaving treatment. It is the second dimension that will indicate when one ought to exercise this right. There can be a tension between general secular ethics, which offers a procedure, and the ethics and bioethics of particular moral communities, which offer content, between ethics which at its conceptual core turns on respect for the freedom of moral agents as the source of permission or secular moral authority, and ethics and bioethics which in their concreteness involve the pursuit of particular goods and the honoring of obligations that can only be understood within particular moral visions. As a consequence, it will often be appropriate to say, ''The patient has a right to do that, but it is wrong.''

The contrast will often not be as stark as one might anticipate if one imagines the ideologically or religiously committed comparing their moral commitments with that of a contentless secular morality. Ever more individuals live more of an aesthetic than a moral life. They are reluctant to recognize many elements of their morality as making absolute claims. They are more likely to say, "Well, this bioethical claim is true for me. It might apply to you." They are more than tolerant. They are ecumenical cosmopolitans who have framed a morality of shifting content and unburdensome obligations. But they still possess a content that the morality of moral strangers cannot provide, though the content that they do possess is not that which is traditionally associated with the moral zeal of those who are truly committed to a particular ideology or religion. As a result, when contrasting the contentless morality of moral strangers with the content-full morality of moral friends, one must recognize that the moralities of moral friends are not all of one piece. In addition, content-full moralities do not all engender claims of the same character and intensity.

This may explain why many ecumenical cosmopolitans find it difficult to recognize the moral gulfs that separate those who live within robust moral communities.[100] They are able with ease to communicate with individuals of various cultures, religions, and backgrounds. They never notice that those with whom they usually collaborate as friends are rarely committed Christians, Jews, or Moslems, dedicated libertarians or egalitarians. Rather, their discussion partners are people of subdued moral commitment, who eschew fervor of belief. They may even avoid those with religious or ideological zeal as fanatics to be dismissed as morally deformed. As a result, the moral strangers they encounter and acknowledge are for them never really that strange. Given their own particular moral visions and understandings, they treat the observant committed believer or ideologue not as a stranger but as someone deranged, thus discounting the differences that do indeed divide and that announce the diversity of moral commitments.

This has important implications for the ways in which one understands the various bioethics. One might naively anticipate that the bioethics of a nominal Roman Catholic will sharply contrast with that of a nominal Presbyterian, Jew, or Buddhist, or that the bioethics of a nominal socialist and a nominal capitalist will be starkly contrasting. However, in actually delivering health care, one finds that the lived morality of many is quite distant from the moral commitment announced, or once announced, by that particular religious or ideological group. For many individuals, contrasts have been muted and the vigor of claims has abated. It may then be useful to distinguish among content-full bioethics as to whether they rest on a morality (1) that requires ultimate commitment, or (2) that simply offers a content-full understanding of life, suffering, and health care, however undemanding, as well as the degree to which particular individuals are committed to their moralities.

*The strangeness of moral strangers*

Because the division separating moral strangers is often obscured by (1) the political usefulness of ignoring or discounting differences, (2) the management of consensus and the projection of its existence through political processes, including bioethics committees, and (3) the existence of many individuals with muted commitments, many persons may doubt that moral strangers in fact frequently present themselves. Again to emphasize, moral strangeness does not require that the other be incomprehensibly other, only that the other be seen as other because of differences in moral and/or metaphysical commitments. Moral strangers can be the best of affective friends. Indeed, they can even be spouses (for that matter, spouses can be moral enemies). Still, to be moral strangers is to inhabit different moral worlds. An atheist physician in the Netherlands may regard the refusal of physician-assisted suicide by a patient in terminal agony as alien to the moral commitments of the physician. The atheist lives in a moral world alien to the believer, who endures illness as a submission to the will of God with the prayer, "I know, Oh Lord, that I justly deserve any punishment Thou mayest inflict upon me. For I have so often offended Thee and sinned against Thee."[101] Indeed, to many it is not only wrongheaded but offensive to regard illness as a divine punishment. Moreover, such submissiveness may be seen to be in conflict with the morality of an enlightened democratic culture. So, too, the woman who on religious grounds refuses abortion after rape may be regarded not as a brave witness to exemplary moral convictions, but as a woman exploited by a false and patriarchal understanding of values.

    The strangeness of moral strangers does not show itself only when atheists and believers meet. Consider two groups of atheists: one holds that prostitution, commercial surrogacy, and the sale of organs are exploitative, whereas the other holds that the proscription of prostitution, commercial surrogacy, and the sale of organs is exploitative. The first may see an improper balance of power between the buyer and the seller of sexual services, reproductive services, or organs. The second may see an improper imbalance of power between the proscribing state and the buyers and sellers of sexual services, reproductive services, or of organs. The first may in secular terms regard sexuality, reproduction, or the body as having a special standing. The second may see the sale of sexual services and reproductive services as no different from selling services as a singer or a ballet dancer, as well as the sale of organs, as in principle no different from consenting to manual labor. Or, one might think of the contrasting understanding of those who hold a just society to be one that gives all an equal opportunity to succeed or fail on the basis of their talents, as well as their luck at the natural and social lotteries (*laissez faire, laissez passer*), versus those who hold that a just society is one that ensures, as far as possible, an equality of outcome. One group may not see anything unfair in the circumstance that the rich can buy lifesaving treatment, which the poor cannot afford. The other may regard this circumstance as blatantly unjust.

The recognition of moral strangers should be a recognition of the limits of secular moral authority. This recognition discloses a limit to the Enlightenment aspirations that led to the carnage of the French Revolution, and the rationalist excesses that culminated in the October Revolution. Reason cannot deliver a content-full morality or vision of justice. This recognition sets limits to plausible state power. These limits must be recognized in the face of strong temptations to embrace particular philosophies and ideologies as if they were delivered from reason itself.

Here one finds, perhaps, the greatest source of contemporary moral fanaticism: the notion that one must at all costs, even at the cost of using others without their permission and as means, achieve a particular vision of fairness, justice, or equality. Like religious fanatics who will employ the force of the state if it is available to them to coerce conversion, so, too, such ideologues will deploy state force thoroughgoingly to achieve their understandings of justice, fairness, and equality, even in areas where others freely associate around contrary moral understandings. Like fascists who in the service of achieving law and order create an all-intrusive state, so, too, fairness fascists in the service of their understanding of justice wish to leave no private area untouched by their intrusions. In the area of health care policy, they will find it morally opprobrious that individuals should be free to use their own resources to purchase better basic or luxury health care. They will not be able to tolerate the existence of those moral strangers who wish freely and peaceably to create alternative understandings of fairness, justice, or equality in health care.

There are real differences among moral visions. They ground substantially different understandings of bioethics. These differences flow from the availability of different premises and rules of evidence for participants in a moral controversy, so that such disputes cannot be resolved by sound rational argument or by an appeal to a commonly acknowledged moral authority (i.e., a person who is recognized as appropriately in authority by virtue of a common moral vision, not merely through a particular agreement, as one might agree to the services of an arbitrator). It is this inability to resolve moral controversies except by agreement that marks the distance between moral strangers even when the distance is not experienced emotionally as strangeness. Only contentless general secular morality can reach across such gulfs and allow collaboration in the absence of content-full moral concurrence.

## The health professional as bureaucrat and geographer of values

Physicians, nurses, and other health care workers play complicated moral roles because of the variegated character of morality. First, they must live their moral lives within at least two moral worlds, within at least two moral dimensions. The first is that of the moral community from which they draw personal content-full meaning and live out their content-full moral undertakings. It is in terms of this moral world that they know what commitments they ought to make, what things are worth living and dying for (e.g., how much risk of infection with the AIDS virus one ought to assume in order to treat patients). It is within such a moral context that they learn about concrete virtues and vices and are instructed in the formation of a good character. However, insofar as health professionals acknowledge that the moral presuppositions that structure their own concrete moral world cannot be justified in general secular terms with a general secular moral authority canonical for all, they must appeal to the possibility of a neutral lingua franca for a secular pluralist society.

Even if they practice medicine or nursing within a Seventh Day Adventist community and hospital, or in a devout Roman Catholic community and hospital, they must recognize that they have created, and are sustaining, a special moral exclave. This does not mean that such exclaves may not be quite substantial. Indeed, they might very well foresee special health care systems directed by their own concrete moralities and protected by special civil and criminal law governing only their own facilities and personnel (e.g., abortion would be a crime on their premises). The more they come in contact with others who do not share their moral presuppositions, the more they will recurringly be forced to recognize that they live not only within their own community, but also within a secular pluralist moral context and within a secular moral fabric that reaches across communities and binds individuals of disparate moral communities in common moral presuppositions. For instance, the Roman Catholic gynecologist opposed to contraception and abortion will need to come to terms with the fact that women will have a secular pluralist moral right to abortion, although abortion is deeply morally wrong. Such physicians will need to develop means of warning patients about the range of expected services they will not offer and information they will not provide. They will need as well to secure legal recognition of their right not to collaborate with what they recognize as immoral.

In giving such warnings, health care professionals take on the role of quasi bureaucrats who remind patients of their rights and regarding circumstances under which their claims may be limited. They are obliged to seek lines of authorization or permission (e.g., look for instructions in living wills, advance directives). This metaphor of the health care worker as bureaucrat can clarify the role that physicians and nurses must play when they meet patients as moral strangers. Where one in fact does not share the moral presumptions of those with whom one works, one must seek ways of protecting against misunderstandings. Bureaucratic rules and formulations are inevitable in such circumstances. They provide formal guidance where informal agreement cannot be presumed. Bureaucratic rules often function to protect rights when individuals meet as moral strangers, as they characteristically do in large-scale secular pluralist societies. Here one might think of various stylized rules for obtaining free and informed consent (e.g., Institutional Review Boards and consent forms). Such are needed when it is not clear that all involved share the same assumptions concerning the best interests to be secured by medical interventions and research.

Physicians and nurses will also play the role of geographers of values and rights. They come to know, through their experience, what it is to be sick with particular diseases, or to be dying in particular ways. They know the consequences of different choices of treatment, and the likely outcomes of adopting particular illness or dying styles. To play this role as geographers, they will also need to know the moral fine texture, not only of the secular pluralist moral framework, but also of the particular moral communities of particular patients.

As the next chapter shows, such geographies of bioethical quandaries reveal major points of tension within the moral life not simply between content-full morality and the secular morality of moral strangers, but also between the cardinal principles of morality: (1) one should use persons only with their consent (the principle of permission), and (2) one should act to achieve the good (the principle of beneficence). Physicians and nurses are recurringly confronted with conflicts between respecting the freedom of patients and doing what is in their patients' best interests. As geographers of values and rights, health care workers must become expert in introducing patients to the character of these tensions and to their moral implications. It is to this sort of conflict that we will turn in the next chapter.

## Bioethics in the face of moral diversity: a summary

We began this chapter by facing the seemingly unbridled nihilism and relativism that threatened, given the failure of the Enlightenment project. Western morality and the moral authority of public policy had been grounded in the assumption that reason could justify a canonical content-full morality and bioethics for moral strangers and thus convey the authority of reason to that public policy framed in conformity with the moral principles reason secured. This assumption has been shown to be untenable. Still, although reason fails to convey moral authority, a moral authority binding moral strangers can be derived from the permission of those who choose to collaborate. A sliver of the Enlightenment hope can be realized. A limit can be given to the nihilism that challenges us: general canons of secular morality can indeed be articulated. A limit can be given to what appeared to be an unrestricted relativism: the canons of secular morality, although they possess no content, allow for morally authoritative collaboration. But the limits set to nihilism and relativism ground limitations on the moral authority of secular public policy, including health care policy.

Because the Enlightenment project's collapse is due to the failure of the epistemological claim that one can by reason know what one ought to do, nothing follows about the existence of an ultimate truth or the ability to come to know that truth through grace. As a consequence, over against the contentless morality and bioethics that binds moral strangers, there remain numerous moral communities with their content-full bioethics. Again, because of the distance between secular morality and the morality of moral friends, and because of the limits of secular moral authority, it will often be appropriate to say, "*X* has a moral right to do *A,* but it is wrong." Most importantly, some communities still have vigor and make robust claims on their members. However, the large-scale societies created by moral strangers do not provide the community within which individuals can discover the full fabric of the moral life, understand true solidarity, or transcend the anomie of content-less individualism.

## Notes

1. Plato, *Republic* 5.459e, 5.461c.
2. Aristotle, *Politics* 7.16, 335b20–26.
3. *Republic* 3.405–10, and *Laws* 4.720b–e.
4. For a presentation of Hippocratic ethos, see, for example, *The Art, Decorum, Law, Physician,* and *Precepts.* An ethos should be understood as a lifeworld of taken-for-granted moral expectations. One ethos will differ from another as a different way of life, not as a different set of moral appeals within a common moral lifeworld. For an account of the constitution of the lifeworld, see Alfred Schutz and Thomas Luckman, *The Structures of the Lifeworld,* trans. R. M. Zaner and H. T. Engelhardt, Jr. (Evanston: Northwestern University Press, 1973).
5. See, for example, Samuel A. Cartwright, "Synopsis of Medical Etiquette," *New Orleans Medical and Surgical Journal* 1, no. 2 (1844): 101–4; and Medical Association of North Eastern Kentucky, *A System of Medical Etiquette* (Maysville, Ky.: Maysville Eagle, 1839). For a study of the development of American codes of medical ethics, see Donald E. Konold, *A History of American Medical Ethics, 1847–1912* (Madison: State Historical Society of Wisconsin, 1962).
6. *Code of Medical Ethics Adopted by the American Medical Association at Philadelphia in May, 1847, and by the New York Academy of Medicine in October, 1847* (New York: H. Ludwig, 1848). For a study of such rules of ethics and etiquette, see Jacqueline Jenkinson, *Scottish Medical Societies 1731–1939* (Edinburgh: Edinburgh University Press, 1993), especially pp. 53–67.
7. Although rules of etiquette are often dismissed as merely manners, they sustain an important element of ethics. See, for example, an article coauthored by Miss Manners: Judith Martin and Gunther S. Stent, "I Think; Therefore I Thank," *American Scholar* 59 (Spring 1990): 237–54.
8. As Tony Honoré indicates, the Greeks in close-knit city-states did not draw a sharp contrast between custom and law; *nomos* meant both. In contrast, Latin possesses *mos* (manner, custom, fashion) and *consuetudo* (custom, habit, usage) set apart from *jus* (right, law, justice) and *lex* (law). See Tony Honoré, *Tribonian* (Ithaca, N.Y.:

Cornell University Press, 1978). Distinctions among customs, codes of etiquette, and law become necessary as one acts across communities of belief. A Greek city-state attempted to encompass one community. In contrast, Rome attempted to embrace various communities in one impartial system of laws. Rome also, with its developed polytheism, endeavored to embrace different religions, thus requiring further distinctions between what was law and what was required by particular customs.

9. The recognition that large-scale states are not simply one moral community is in accord with Hegel's view of the state as a neutral matrix of freedom spanning numerous communities with different views of blameworthiness, the good life, and of content-full moral obligations. This account justifies Hegel's defense of toleration in which he argues against the anti-Semites of his day by holding that Jews should have civil rights. The state should not be Christian or Jewish, but a neutral framework that can peaceably embrace various communities of diverse belief. Hegel argued:

> The fierce outcry raised against the Jews from that point of view (that they should be considered a foreign race) and others, ignores that fact that they are, above all, *men;* and manhood, so far from being a mere superficial, abstract quality, is on the contract itself the basis of the fact that which civil rights rouse in their possessors is a feeling of oneself as counting in civil society as a person with rights, and this feeling of selfhood, infinite and free from all restrictions, is the root from which the desired similarity in disposition and way of thinking comes into being.

Hegel, *Hegel's Philosophy of Right,* trans. T. M. Knox (London: Oxford University Press, 1965), sec. 270, p. 169. This view of the state as a neutral matrix spanning communities is suggested also in the passage in which Hegel characterizes civil servants as the universal class. See *Philosophy of Right,* sec. 303.

10. The contemporary age is marked by a neopaganism and a rebirth of polytheist sympathies. See, for example, David L. Miller, *The New Polytheism: Rebirth of the Gods and Goddesses* (New York: Harper and Row, 1974). Indeed, much of New Age sentiments can be understood as an attempt to recapture the resonances of paganism and its bonds with the forces of nature and the earth. One finds as well psychological guides speaking of spirituality and the Greco-Roman gods and goddesses. See, for example, Thomas Moore, *Care of the Soul* (New York: HarperCollins, 1992). This polytheism is not celebrated by the author. Rather, with St. Gregory Palamas (1296–1359) he recognizes that the rational soul is not healthy but "sick in its cognitive faculty." Gregory Palamas, *The Triads,* ed. John Meyendorff, trans. Nicholas Gendle (Mahwah, N.J.: Paulist Press, 1983).

11. The "innocent" in the context of general secular morality are those who have not used moral agents without their permission.

12. J. Cook, *Captain Cook's Journal 1758–71,* ed. Capt. W. S. L. Wharton (London: Elliot Stock, 1893), pp. 91–95.

13. Colin M. Turnbull, *The Mountain People* (New York: Simon and Schuster, 1972), p. 135.

14. How the world appears to us is shaped by our expectations. N. R. Hanson, *Perception and Discovery* (San Francisco: Freeman, Cooper, 1969). In our approach to reality we are guided by both epistemic and nonepistemic values. See H. T. Engelhardt, Jr., and A. L. Caplan (eds.), *Scientific Controversies* (New York: Cambridge University Press, 1987). In addition, much of our systematic approaches to reality are guided by

both explicit and implicit agreements regarding *ceteris paribus* conditions. Scientific reality is in significant measure a social construction.

15. I. Lakatos and A. Musgrave (eds.), *Criticism and the Growth of Knowledge* (Cambridge: Cambridge University Press, 1970). The work of Fleck with regard to the history of syphilis is also pertinent: Ludwik Fleck, *Entstehung und Entwicklung einer wissenschaftlichen Tatsache, Einführung in die Lehre vom Denkstil und Denkkollektiv* (Basel: Benno Schwabe, 1935); *Genesis and Development of a Scientific Fact*, ed. T. J. Trenn and R. K. Merton, trans. F. Bradley and T. J. Trenn (Chicago: University of Chicago Press, 1979). On this work see Lothar Schäfer, "On the Scientific Status of Medical Research," pp. 23–38, and Nelly Tsouyopoulos, "The Scientific Status of Medical Research," pp. 39–46, in Corinna Delkeskamp-Hayes and Mary Ann Cutter (eds.), *Science, Technology, and the Art of Medicine* (Dordrecht: Kluwer, 1993); and Robert S. Cohen and Thomas Schnelle (eds.), *Cognition and Fact: Materials on Ludwik Fleck* (Dordrecht: Reidel, 1986). See also Thomas Kuhn, *The Structure of Scientific Revolutions* (Chicago: University of Chicago Press, 1962; 2d ed. 1970).

16. This is a well-discussed problem. Philosophers from A. J. Ayer in *Language, Truth, and Logic* (London: Peter Smith, 1935) to Charles Stevenson in *Facts and Values: Studies in Ethical Analysis* (Westport, Conn.: Greenwood Press, 1962; repr. 1975) have raised the issue in modern times of whether moral claims can in any sense be true or false or whether they simply express emotions or function as ways of persuading others to join in common action.

17. Henry Sidgwick, *The Methods of Ethics*, 7th ed. (London: Macmillan, 1907), pp. 338–42.

18. For an excellent example of the moral project of being sensitive to the various different competing moral appeals and then to the ways in which they can be meshed together, see Baruch Brody, *Life and Death Decision Making* (New York: Oxford University Press, 1988). Brody offers an example of very refined and nuanced intuitionism.

19. Appeals to casuistry are often made in the vain attempt to find a nonfoundationalist approach to resolving controversies in bioethics. As is shown, casuistical analyses presuppose a set of framing moral commitments. Secular appeals to casuistry are misguided. See, for example, Albert Jonsen and Stephen Toulmin, *The Abuse of Casuistry* (Berkeley: University of California Press, 1988). First, such appeals cannot operate without a commonly accepted framework of moral content that can interpret particular cases. In Roman Catholicism there was both a body of authoritative teaching as well as individuals in authority. Second, the secular appeal to cases occurs not within one moral understanding, but across moral visions in the hope to determine which should govern. To borrow a metaphor from Thomas Kuhn, secular moralists who appeal to casuistry engage in crisis casuistry, not normal casuistry. The latter was the domain of Roman Catholic casuistry. The challenge is to find a framework to resolve the moral controversies faced by secular casuistry. For a study of the difficulties, see Kevin Wm. Wildes, S. J., *A View from Somewhere* (in manuscript). As an example of Roman Catholic casuistry and its thickly contextual character, consider the following exploration of the problem faced by a Roman Catholic confessor.

On a certain Sunday morning the place is even darker than usual, owing to the rainy day. To the confessional there comes an aged woman, as the confessor learns by her voice and speech. She is just through confessing, when at the near altar the bell is rung for elevation. The confessor tells the woman to pause a little while, until after the elevation, and the woman answers, "Yes, Father." The confessor makes the sign of the cross and gathers his thoughts for admonition. After the elevation he turns again to the woman, admonishes and consoles her, etc., gives her her penance and pronounces absolution, ending with his customary "Blessed be the Lord" to the penitent, from whom, to his great surprise, comes the word Amen in a man's deep voice. The confessor, quickly looking up, perceives a young man leave the confessional and disappear. How did this young man get there in place of the aged woman? There is only one explanation. The aged woman must have misunderstood her confessor when he suggested to wait until after the elevation. When the confessor then made the sign of the cross, she probably understood this to be the absolution. Softly she left the place, and just as softly it was taken by the young man, who received the absolution of the priest probably in some astonishment. He may have been agreeably surprised by the imagined fact that this confessor did not even require the telling of his sins. This would raise now the following questions: 1. Has the confessor rendered himself guilty of *laesio sigilli,* by addressing his admonition, referring to sins of the aged woman, to the young man? 2. Has the woman been absolved? 3. Has the young man been absolved?

As to the first question, the confessor is held to have violated the seal of the confessional *ob errorem invincibilem* and therefore not to be guilty. That is, he could not have known that he was possibly informing someone else of the woman's sins. As to the woman, the answer is that the priest, when he said "Ego te absolvo," meant the old woman when he said "te." The priest may presume that the woman has not yet left the church and therefore would be in striking distance of the absolution. As to the third question, the young man is not absolved because, through not confessing his sins, he did not conform to the essentials of the sacrament. The commentary concludes "Suppose, however, the young man thought *bona fide* he had been absolved, and with this thought, although possibly in the state of mortal sin, went to receive Holy Communion? In this case it is to be held that through Holy Communion his mortal sins were forgiven *per accidens* if he approached the Holy Sacrament *bene attritus.*" Anonymous, *The Casuist* (New York: Joseph Wagner, 1906), vol. 1, pp. 73–74. This approach contrasts with that of the Orthodox Church that has as its exemplar confession to a geron or staretz who gives guidance through the Spirit. The entire analysis presupposes that the priest is in authority to forgive sins and that there is authoritative information about the scope of the priest's capacities. No such thick web of content or moral authority exists for the analysis of cases within a general secular context. One of the most engaging attempts to escape the problems that beset secular casuistry is provided in Baruch Brody, *Life and Death Decision Making* (New York: Oxford University Press, 1988).

20. Baruch A. Brody, "Intuitions and Objective Moral Knowledge," *The Monist* 62 (Oct. 1979): 455. There are numerous proposals about how to balance and judge competing moral appeals or versions of moral inquiry. Alasdair MacIntyre to the contrary notwithstanding, there is no moral appeal, tradition, or perspective that, if it has content, is not yet one more particular moral appeal, tradition, or perspective. To choose contentfully is to choose within a particular moral tradition or perspective, although particular versions of moral inquiry may merit being discussed as internally contradictory. Alasdair MacIntyre, *Three Rival Versions of Moral Enquiry* (Notre Dame, Ind.: University of Notre Dame Press, 1990).

21. Roderick Firth, "Ethical Absolutism and the Ideal Observer," *Philosophy and Phenomenological Research* 12 (1952): 331–41.

22. Richard B. Brandt, *A Theory of the Good and the Right* (Oxford: Clarendon Press, 1979).

23. Rawls's account is offered as a "theory of rational choice" which is to take account of agreement in the face of multiple conceptions of the good. John Rawls, *A Theory of Justice* (Cambridge, Mass.: Harvard University Press, 1971), p. 16. The choices of the contractor depend, *inter alia*, on their having a particular thin theory of the good (pp. 396–97).

24. Ibid., pp. 17–22, 126–42. An exposition of the original position in more ahistorical terms is found in the chapter entitled "The Kantian Interpretation of Justice 'as Fairness'" (pp. 251–57). See also pp. 195–201 for an exposition of the relationship between the original position and the framing of a constitution and laws.

25. As Rawls puts it, "persons in the original position have no desire to try for greater gains at the expense of the equal liberties" (*Theory of Justice*, p. 156).

26. For Rawls, an acceptable amount of the primary social goods is that amount distributed in accord with the two principles of justice. See, in particular, his formulation of the Second Principle, part (a), p. 302, in *Theory of Justice*. Rawls incorporates into his notion of contractors a particular understanding of what constitutes appropriate risk-aversiveness. See, for example, John C. Harsanyi, "Can the Maximin Principle Serve as a Basis for Morality?" *American Political Science Review* 6 (1975): 594–606.

27. *Theory of Justice*, p. 137.

28. Ibid., p. 302.

29. "An equal division of all primary goods is irrational in view of the possibility of bettering everyone's circumstances by accepting certain inequalities." Ibid., p. 546. For an account that is developed on the basis of quite different intuitions regarding inequality, see Larry S. Temkin, *Inequality* (New York: Oxford University Press, 1993).

30. Rawls gives the following account of envy. "To some extent men's sense of their own worth may hinge upon their institutional position and their income share. If, however, the account of social envy and jealousy is sound, then with the appropriate background arrangements, these inclinations should not be excessive, at least not when the priority of liberty is effectively upheld." *Theory of Justice*, p. 546.

31. Applications of Rawls to health care differ in terms of whether they place considerations of health care under the liberty principle (see, e.g., Ronald Green, "Health Care and Justice in Contract Theory Perspective," in R. Veatch and R. Branson [eds.], *Ethics and Health Policy* [Cambridge, Mass.: Ballinger, 1976], pp. 111–26, and "The Priority of Health Care," *Journal of Medicine and Philosophy* 8 [Nov. 1983]: 373–80) or the principle of fair equality of opportunity (see, e.g., Norman Daniels, *Just Health Care* [New York: Cambridge University Press, 1985]).

32. See Rawls, *Theory of Justice*, p. 396.

33. Ibid., pp. 152–58.

34. Ibid., pp. 143, 546.

35. Ibid., p. 128.

36. For an account of the BaMbuti, see Colin Turnbull, *Forest People* (New York: Simon and Schuster, 1961); and *Wayward Servants: The Two Worlds of the African Pygmies* (West, Conn.: Greenwood Press, 1965).

37. Rawls acknowledges the limited force of his conclusions. For example, he states at the end of *Theory of Justice:*

> It is perfectly proper, then, that the argument for the principles of justice should proceed from some consensus. . . . Certainly, the argument for the principles of justice would be strength- ened by showing that they are still the best choice from a more comprehensive list more systematically evaluated. I do not know how far this can be done. I doubt, however, that the principles of justice (as I have defined them) will be the preferred conception on anything resembling a complete list. (Here I assume that, given an upper bound on complexity and other constraints, the class of reasonable and practical alternatives is effectively finite.) Even if the argument I have offered is sound, it only shows that a finally adequate theory (if such exists) will look more like the contract view than any of the other doctrines we discussed. And even this conclusion is not proved in any strict sense. (p. 581)

In *Political Liberalism* (New York: Columbia University Press, 1993), he develops the point by tying his conception of justice to that of a modern constitutional democ- racy.

> While such a conception [i.e., a political conception of justice] is, of course, a moral concep- tion, it is a moral conception worked out for a specific kind of subject, namely, for political, social, and economic institutions. In particular, it applies to what I shall call the "basic struc- ture" of society, which for our present purposes I take to be a modern constitutional democracy. (I use "constitutional democracy" and "democratic regime," and similar phrases interchange- ably unless otherwise stated.) (p. 11)

Much content is packed into "modern," "constitutional," and "democracy." *Theory of Justice* reconstructs one among many views of justice or fairness.

38. For an exploration of various competing notions of liberalism, see John Gray, *Liber- alisms* (New York: Routledge, 1991).

39. For an exploration of how ethical theories differ in terms of the ways in which they appeal to notions of equality, see Amartya Sen, *Inequality Reexamined* (New York: Russell Sage Foundation, 1992). Indeed, much of contemporary ethics has come implicitly to recognize the ambiguities of notions of equality and freedom, even when those dealing with these topics have attempted to set these ambiguities aside. See, for example, Thomas Nagel, *Equality and Partiality* (New York: Oxford University Press, 1991), and Susan Wolf, *Freedom within Reason* (New York: Oxford Univer- sity Press, 1990).

40. Bruce A. Ackerman, *Social Justice in the Liberal State* (New Haven, Conn.: Yale University Press, 1980).

41. Robert Nozick, *Anarchy, State and Utopia* (New York: Basic Books, 1974).

42. Jürgen Habermas, *The Theory of Communicative Action* (Boston: Beacon Press, 1984), trans. Thomas McCarthy, vol. 1, p. 42.

43. Ibid.; also *Moral Consciousness and Communicative Action,* trans. Christian Lenhardt and S. Nicholsen (Cambridge, Mass.: MIT Press, 1990), p. 65.

44. *Theory of Communicative Action,* vol. 1, p. 115.

45. Ibid., vol. 2, p. 399.

46. For an engaging, game-theoretical account of morality, see David Gauthier, *Morals*

*by Agreement* (Oxford: Clarendon Press, 1986). Gauthier also provides in this vein an account of Hobbes not as providing a hypothetical-contract theory, but a social contract account, in which "each recognizes the need for sanctions, for penalizing non-compliance, and this makes the agreement to institute a sovereign part of a social *contract.*" "Taming Leviathan," *Philosophy and Public Affairs* 16 (Summer 1987): 296. A social contract thus becomes a solution to a cluster of social problems and in this sense a game-theoretical resolution of the problems of framing peaceable public policy. See, also, Jean Hampton, *Hobbes and the Social Contract Tradition* (Cambridge: Cambridge University Press, 1986), and Gregory S. Kavka, *Hobbesian Moral and Political Theory* (Princeton: Princeton University Press, 1986).

47. Tom L. Beauchamp and James F. Childress, *Principles of Biomedical Ethics* (New York: Oxford University Press, 1979).

48. Theoretical frameworks will demand some revisions in the original moral sentiments. Thus, if two individuals attempt to analyze the issue of deception of patients, one a follower of Bentham, the other a follower of Kant, the first will find circumstances in which deception may be allowed (and will indeed be obligatory), while the Kantian will find that all deception is always immoral. I am very much in debt to the Reverend Kevin Wm. Wildes, S.J., for discussions on this point, as well as with respect to the significance of appeals to middle-level principles.

49. At times two different moral visions reconstructed in two different theoretical fashions will still in particular instances endorse the "same" moral conclusion. The significance of the conclusions will not be the same. For example, a deontologist may hold that it is obligatory to refuse extraordinary treatment, because accepting such treatment would be contrary to the maxims for action of a rational individual. Such a choice would be regarded as heteronomous, as Kant would understand the matter. A consequentialist may see the refusal of treatment as equally obligatory, given the psychological and other costs involved. Both may endorse the refusal of treatment. But, the deontologist considers the action to be appropriate, independently of the consequences. The consequentialist will have no such sense of rightness independent of the consequences, but will endorse the same action. The context within which the moral decisions are made shapes the significance of the choice and the action. The actions or choices to an uninformed observer may appear to be the same, but they will have quite different significance.

50. Rawls, *Theory of Justice,* p. 8.

51. John Rawls, "Justice as Fairness: Political Not Metaphysical," *Philosophy and Public Affairs* 14 (Summer 1985): 223–51.

52. John Rawls, *Political Liberalism,* p. 369.

53. See the discussion Rawls gives of reasonableness, equality, and overlapping consensus in *Political Liberalism,* especially pp. xix-xx, 25, 39–40, 51, as well as 150–54. Also see his list of liberal values on p. 224. Much could be said about the ways in which Rawls smuggles in particular norms to buttress his account of political liberalism. For example, Rawls trades on a prior notion of reasonableness in order to identify the consensus that he wishes to anoint as normative. "Such a consensus consists of all the reasonable opposing religious, philosophical, and moral doctrines likely to persist over generations and to gain a sizable body of adherents in a more or

less just constitutional regime, a regime in which the criterion of justice is that political conception itself." Ibid., p. 15. Much turns on the meaning of "reasonable."

54. Here my analyses regarding deceptive senses of consensus are deeply in debt to discussions I have had with the Reverend Kevin Wm. Wildes, S.J.

55. Nozick, *Anarchy, State, and Utopia*, p. 160.

56. I am much in debt to the Reverend Kevin Wm. Wildes, S.J., for our discussions regarding the ways in which the appearance of consensus can be constructed.

57. Karl Marx and Frederick Engels, *The German Ideology* (New York: International Publishers, 1967), p. 39.

58. John Gray, *Post-Liberalism* (New York: Routledge, 1993), p. 82.

59. Ibid.

60. For a study of some of the ambiguities of consensus, see Kurt Bayertz (ed.), *The Concept of Moral Consensus* (Dordrecht: Kluwer, 1994).

61. The collapse of the Soviet bloc revealed how what appeared to be a large-scale consensus, or overlapping consensus, was in fact but a dominant ideology. After seventy years of Communist rule, many of the parties that were in existence prior to the October Revolution surfaced again to claim a place in political life. Whole countries that appeared to be somewhat stable have sundered around understandings that many thought forgotten. Force and circumstance had crafted what was surely not an enduring consensus.

62. See, for example, Michael Oakeshott, *Rationalism in Politics and Other Essays* (Indianapolis: Liberty Press, 1991).

63. As to Rorty's interpretation of Hegel, which suggests that he accepts the merely given of the morality within which he lives, see H. T. Engelhardt, Jr., "Sittlichkeit and Post-Modernity: An Hegelian Reconsideration of the State," in H. T. Engelhardt, Jr., and T. Pinkard (eds.), *Hegel Reconsidered: Beyond Metaphysics and the Authoritarian State* (Dordrecht: Kluwer, 1994), pp. 211–24. *Pace* Rorty, Hegel can be regarded as critically appreciating the contingency of particular morality without simply endorsing the contingent.

64. Richard Rorty, *Contingency, Irony, and Solidarity* (Cambridge: Cambridge University Press, 1989), p. 59.

65. Ibid., p. 61.

66. Rorty appears of the view that the centrality of democracy and the character in which he understands it can simply be accepted as a gift of history and need not be shown to have authority. "I have been urging that the democracies are now in a position to throw away some of the ladders used in their own construction." Ibid., p. 194. In my account of the morality of moral strangers, a ladder is provided, the authorization given by participating individuals, which ladder should not be thrown away.

67. Ibid., p. 196.

68. Singapore Ministry of Health, "Overview of Singapore Health Care System," Apr. 1993.

69. The actions of the International Military Tribunal during the Nuremberg trials presuppose some notion of natural law. The charter for the tribunal, in describing war crimes (i.e., crimes against peace) and crimes against humanity, does not explicitly

make mention of natural law or of the *ius gentium*. Still, it is a reasonable way to understand the full authority of the tribunal. In article 6, the tribunal clearly states that it will not be a defense against charges of crimes against humanity that the actions were "not in violation of the domestic law of the country where perpetrated." "Charter of the International Military Tribunal II, Art. 6c," *Trial of War Criminals* (Washington, D.C.: U.S. Government Printing Office, 1945), p. 16. In the "Report of Robert H. Jackson to the President," published as a preface to the *Trial of War Criminals,* an attempt is made to justify the tribunal's jurisdiction on the basis of past treaties; Jackson as well appeals to Hugo Grotius's distinction between just and unjust wars, a distinction drawn from natural law arguments.

70. As Gaius states, "Quod uero naturalis ratio inter omnes homines constituit, id apud, omnes populos peraeque custoditur uocaturque ius gentium, quasi quo jure omnes gentes utuntur." *Institutes of Gaius,* trans. Francis De Zulueta (London: Oxford University Press, 1976), p. 3, vp. 1.

71. In Justinian's words, "The law of nature is that law which nature teaches to all animals. Though this law does not belong exclusively to the human race, but belongs to all animals." Flavius Petrus Sabbatius Justinianus, *The Institutes of Justinian,* trans. Thomas C. Sandars (1922; repr. Westport, Conn.: Greenwood Press, 1970), 1.2, p. 7.

72. Blackstone speaks of the laws of nature as discoverable by reason. These laws of nature are "the eternal, immutable laws of good and evil, to which the creator himself in all his dispensations conforms; and which he has enabled human reason to discover, so far as they are necessary for the conduct of human actions. Such among others are these principles: that we should live honestly, should hurt nobody, and should render to every one his due; to which three general precepts Justinian has reduced the whole doctrine of law." See William Blackstone, *Commentaries on the Laws of England,* ed. St. George Tucker (New York: Augustus and Kelly, 1969), vol. 1, p. 40. One should note that the laws of nature so put are extremely abstract. The nature of honesty is not specified nor the nature of harm to others, much less what is due to another. Such specification would require a particular moral sense.

73. An assessment of the consequences of the collapse of the Christian and Enlightenment hopes is provided by Alasdair MacIntyre in *After Virtue* (Notre Dame, Ind.: University of Notre Dame Press, 1981). *Pace* MacIntyre, I argue that there is a vindication for a shred of the Enlightenment dream: the possibility for a general morality through resolving moral controversies by agreement. MacIntyre makes a major contribution in outlining the modern predicament, which is defined in part by the remnants of its predecessor cultures. Postmodernity provides bits and shards of once-integral moral visions. It is the rationalist presumptions of both the Western Christian synthesis and the Enlightenment, which has misled ethics into a search for definitive rational grounds for establishing as morally authoritative a particular content-full moral viewpoint.

74. I am very much in debt to Tom L. Beauchamp for his article, "Ethical Theory and the Problem of Closure," in Engelhardt and Caplan, *Scientific Controversies,* pp. 27–48. Indeed, the conversations with those who contributed to the *Controversies* volume helped guide me in the development of *The Foundations of Bioethics.*

75. During the Western Middle Ages there were disputes as to whether the pope of Rome or ecumenical councils possessed final authority (the Church of the East denied final authority to either). An endorsement of the preeminence of conciliar authority is found in the statement of March 30, 1415, by the Council of Constance, which affirmed the traditional view (i.e., prior to the eleventh century) that an ecumenical council was in fact superior in authority to that of the pope. It held that the council "had authority directly from Christ, and that everyone of whatever status or dignity, even if he were the pope, is bound to obey it in that which pertains to faith." *Conciliorum Oecumenicorum Decreta* (Basil: Herder, 1962), p. 384 (author's translation). This assertion of conciliar authority over the church as a whole departed in some points from traditional teaching. In any event, Roman pontiffs generally took the opposite view. In fact, the views of the conciliar movement were explicitly condemned. See, for example, the bull *Exsecrabilis* of January 18, 1460. Henricus Denzinger (ed.), *Enchiridion Symbolorum,* 33rd ed. (Rome: Herder, 1965), p. 345. A good overview of this dispute is provided by Heiko A. Oberman et al. (eds.), *Defensorium Obedientiae Apostolicae et Alia Documenta* (Cambridge, Mass.: Harvard University Press, 1968). The current Roman Catholic dogma of papal supremacy was articulated by the First Vatican Council on July 18, 1870, when the doctrine of papal infallibility was promulgated. For an account of the conciliar movement, see Antony Black, *Political Thought in Europe 1250–1450* (New York: Cambridge University Press, 1992).

76. Roman Catholic doctrine, as it developed, saw reason as able to disclose the fundamentals of natural law or the *ius gentium.* See, for example, the encyclical of Pope Pius XII, *Summi pontificatus* of October 20, 1939. This point is also made by the First Vatican Council.

   The Roman Catholic understanding of natural law turns on a rationalistic interpretation of elements of the original Christian teaching. St. Paul speaks of the Gentiles having "the requirements of the law . . . written on their hearts" (Romans 2:15). The Orthodox interpretation is that Paul was in fact talking about the human heart, a facility of the soul able, with proper disposition, to appreciate the guidance of God. See, for example, John S. Romanides, *Franks, Romans, Feudalism, and Doctrine* (Brookline, Mass.: Holy Cross Orthodox Press, 1981), pp. 45ff. The Roman Catholics, in contrast, came to hold that reason, not the heart, could discern the law of God.

77. As an example, see Thomas Paine's critique of Christianity in *The Age of Reason.*

78. To talk this way about reason and grace is to put matters in terms that developed within and came to characterize Western Christianity. It led to the view that moral and theological reasoning can function with at least partial success outside of the context of true faith and worship. This has supported the peculiarly Western view that even atheists can be theologians. In contrast, the traditional view underscored an "inseparable relationship between theology and spirituality." Archimandrite Vasileios, *Hymn of Entry,* trans. Elizabeth Briere (Crestwood, N.Y.: St. Vladimir's Seminary Press, 1984), p. 24. Theology is both the expression and result of prayer and fasting. Thus, Abbot Damian states "Our Faith is not intellectual, of the head; it is mystical, supernatural, and spiritual, of the heart. For it is in a *broken and contrite*

*heart* that the Holy Spirit dwells and from which He heals, directs, and teaches. It is the heart, in that place and in that place alone, broken and contrite, where our vocal prayers learn silence and where we can be still and know God." *Dawn* 15 (Oct. 1992).

79.  In the Middle Ages it was accepted that heretics, in particular heretics who would not repent or who had lapsed for a second time into heresy, were to be killed. This view is clearly enunciated in St. Thomas Aquinas's *Summa Theologica* 2 Q. xi arts. 3 and 4. As already noted, it is also reflected in the constitutions of the Fourth Lateran Council (1215), which held that "Catholics who truly take up the cross and give themselves over to the extermination of heretics, shall enjoy the same indulgence, which is given by sacred privilege to those who go to the Holy Land." *Conciliorum Oecumenicorum Decreta*, p. 210 (author's translation).

The issue of who counted as a heretic became more complex after the Reformation. Not only the Roman church but those who left it in heresy proceeded to exterminate heretics. The use of the writ "de haeretico comburendo" (the writ issued for the burning of a heretic) continued into the seventeenth century. No doubt such a writ would have been issued by the authorities of those times against both the author of this volume and many of its readers.

80.  Indeed, it has been argued that Western Christianity undermined its very own roots by attempting to establish Christianity by reason. By vainly attempting through reason to prove what faith should show, Western Christianity invited atheism. Michael Buckley, *At the Origins of Modern Atheism* (New Haven, Conn.: Yale University Press, 1987). The failure of Western Christendom's hope for a rational justification of a content-full morality discloses a fundamental crisis in the justification of content-full morality.

81.  One cannot coherently treat of oneself except as free. This is a Kantian point. Though one does not know that one is free, one must think of oneself as free. Thus, one cannot coherently state, "I know that I am free." All one can state is, "Given all my past causal conditioning, and given my character, and given my current exposure to stimuli, I am caused to say, 'I am determined.'" One cannot hold that it is true that one is determined. One can only engage in the behavior of stating that one is determined. Which is to say, it is impossible to think of oneself as making knowledge claims for moral choices, save insofar as one thinks one is free. Moreover, it does not appear possible for us as humans not to engage in making knowledge claims or moral choices. Even determinists paradoxically wish to suggest that we *should* acknowledge the truth of determinism.

82.  "Transcendental" is used to identify an argument that lays out the conditions for the possibility of a major domain of human experience of action. As defining conditions, transcendental conditions are a priori. Here I borrow from Kant, who underscores morality's presupposition of freedom (e.g., *Critique of Pure Reason*, Bxxviii–Bxxix; *Critique of Practical Reason*, 31, 43f, 46).

Kant restricts transcendental claims to areas of theoretical knowledge and does not extend them to claims about morality. "I entitle *transcendental* all knowledge which is occupied not so much with objects as with the mode of our knowledge of objects in so far as this mode of knowledge is to be possible *a priori*." *Critique of Pure Reason*,

A11 = B25, p. 59. However, one need not restrict the realm of transcendental arguments so narrowly. See especially Klaus Hartmann, "On Taking the Transcendental Turn," *Review of Metaphysics* 67 (Dec. 1966): 224–25. See *The Critique of Pure Reason,* A12 = B25. Here I extend the notion of transcendental claims to the sphere of moral experience. That one cannot but think of oneself as free is a transcendental condition, not an empirical fact or metaphysical claim.

83. Appeals to intersubjectivity as objectivity have a kinship with the transcendental arguments of Immanuel Kant. Kant despaired of being able to settle arguments concerning the nature of reality by appeals to reality as it is in itself (i.e., reality unframed by the conditions of human experience, reality as it is known by the Deity). Instead, he appealed to the conditions of human experience. Knowledge of a spatiotemporal, sensible world has conceptually expressible preconditions. For there to be experience, there must be points of permanence in that experience. Changes must occur according to some pattern or rule. The points of permanence with their changes must be in correlation with each other. These are necessary conditions for the possibility of coherent experience, for there being a commonly shared phenomenal world. "The principle of the analogies is: Experience is possible only through the representation of a necessary connection of perceptions." A176 = B218, p. 208. Also, "The conditions of the *possibility of experience* in general are likewise conditions of the *possibility of the objects of experience.*" Norman Kemp Smith (trans.), *Immanuel Kant's Critique of Pure Reason* (London: Macmillan, 1964), A158 = B197, p. 194. Though my account of the categorial conditions for knowledge and morality has a highly Kantian accent, it can in principle be recast with benefit in more Hegelian terms. A Hegelian categorial account places the argument within the terms of reason and avoids the Kantian difficulty of mediating between the sheer givenness of the object and the predicament of the finite knower. Here is not the occasion to show how the concerns of the finite knower can be placed within a general categorial understanding. The reader may wish to consult sections 445 through 450 of G. W. F. Hegel's *Encyclopaedia of the Philosophical Sciences* (1830). See also Klaus Hartmann, "The 'Analogies' and After," in L. W. Beck (ed.), *Proceedings of the Third International Kant Congress* (Dordrecht: Reidel, 1972), pp. 47–62; and "On Taking the Transcendental Turn," pp. 223–49.

Kant attempted to sketch the general conceptual framework within which particular empirical claims can be framed and tested. For Kant the structure of the empirically experienced known comes from the knower, not the thing-in-itself. "Hitherto it has been assumed that all our knowledge must conform to objects. But all attempts to extend our knowledge of objects by establishing something in regard to them a priori, by means of concepts, have, on this assumption, ended in failure. We must therefore make trial whether we may not have more success in the tasks of metaphysics, if we suppose that objects must conform to our knowledge." Kant's *Critique of Pure Reason,* Bxvi, p. 22. "We can know a priori of things only what we ourselves put into them." Ibid., Bxviii, p. 23.

This account involved a singular shift of philosophical attention. Kant's point of departure for justifying his account of the nature of reality is not the divine perspective, but that of the possible community of finite knowers who know spatiotemporally and sensibly. Kant provides an account of reality (i.e., reality as it is for us) in terms of the conditions of human experience.

> It [the transcendental unity of apperception] is indeed the first principle of the human understanding, and is so indispensable to it that we cannot form the least conception of any other possible understanding, either of such as it is itself intuition or of any that may possess an underlying mode of a sensible intuition which is different in kind from that in space and time. (B139, p. 157)

> We can therefore have no knowledge of any object as thing in itself, but only in so far as it is an object of sensible intuition, that is, an appearance. (Bxxvi, p. 27)

I will not be quite as confident as Kant that there is only one such finite perspective for humans. Kant never considered that there might be, as in cosmology and in quantum physics, modes of non-Euclidean and non-Newtonian understandings. Kant, however, realized that our mode of intuition need not be unique.

> This mode of intuiting in space and time need not be limited to human sensibility. It may be that all finite, thinking beings necessarily agree with man in this respect, although we are not in the position to judge whether this is actually so. But however universal this mode of sensibility may be, it does not therefore cease to be sensibility. (B72, p. 90)

With certain qualifications, there is no conflict between my position here and that of Kant. I will proceed with the recognition that (1) there may be many special human realities (e.g., the realities of macro- versus microphysics), (2) that the portrayal of the conditions of reality in any detail is itself conditioned by the perspective of a particular historical period, and (3) that secular science and morality constitute two major areas of human reality, each with its own conditions for its possibility.

84.   Here I may appear to be in agreement with Amartya Sen, who contends that

> It is convenient to begin with the observation that the major ethical theories of social arrangement all share an endorsement of equality in terms of *some* focal variable, even though the variables that are selected are frequently very different between one theory and another. It can be shown that even those theories that are widely taken to be "against equality" (and are often described as such by the authors themselves) turn out to be egalitarian in terms of some other focus. The *rejection* of equality in such a theory in terms of some focal variable goes hand in hand with the *endorsement* of equality in terms of another focus.

> *Inequality Reexamined* (Cambridge, Mass.: Harvard University Press, 1992), p. 3. His contention is false if it is meant to include all ethical systems, including those of a theological nature. God and humans are not equal. See, for example, St. John Chrysostom's homilies "On the Incomprehensible Nature of God."

85.   For the notion of grammar at stake, think here of Ludwig Wittgenstein's remarks relating grammar and ontology: "Essence is expressed by grammar." *Philosophical Investigations,* trans. G. E. M. Anscombe (Oxford: Basil Blackwell, 1963), sec. 371. Or, "Grammar tells us what kind of an object anything is" (sec. 373). In this sense, grammar shows the possibility for the coherence of a dimension of human meaning. For a consideration of transcendental arguments in Wittgenstein, see Stanley Cavell, "Availability of Wittgenstein's Later Philosophy," in George Pitcher (ed.), *Wittgenstein: The Philosophical Investigations* (New York: Doubleday, 1966), pp. 151–85. Cavell states, for example, that "we could say that what such answers are meant to provide us with is not more knowledge of matters of fact, but the

knowledge of what would count as various 'matters of fact'. Is this empirical knowledge? Is it a priori? It is a knowledge of what Wittgenstein means by grammar—the knowledge Kant calls 'transcendental' '' (p. 175).

86. Nozick's presentation of freedom as a side constraint is inadequate. It is offered in his account somewhat as a surd given. See Nozick, *Anarchy, State, and Utopia*, pp. 30–34. I have come to a somewhat similar notion but through exploring the possibility of grounding a secular morality in a special variety of transcendental argument.

Because of the theoretical needs ingredient to his particular approach to showing the compatibility of physical necessity and moral freedom (as well as because of other presuppositions), Kant fails to distinguish between freedom as a value and freedom as a side constraint. Following Kant, I underscore the presupposition of respect of freedom as the necessary condition for the possibility of justified blame and praise. Justified blame and praise (e.g., blame and praise that is due another, not just useful to assign), as well as acting with moral authority, presuppose grounds for showing some actions to be right or wrong. The minimum foundation required for this moral nexus is provided by using persons only with their permission. This principle provides the minimum basis for the coherence of a general secular morality. More would need to be said to address the similarities and dissimilarities with Kant whose argument is quite different in the *Metaphysik der Sitten* over the *Kritik der praktischen Vernunft*.

87. My account of ethics portrays it as one among a number of major domains of possible experience and action. Again, unlike Kant, I underscore the conditions for thinking oneself part of the kingdom of ends, not just those of experience. Even in Kant's writings there are some suggestions as to how to proceed with regard to giving a transcendental account of moral reality. In addition to the ways in which one might regard Kant's writings concerning ethics, one should note that in the preface to the second edition of the *Critique of Pure Reason* Kant notes that we can have a priori knowledge either through determining the object of our knowledge or through making the object actual (Bix–x). What is provided in this chapter is an account of the necessary conditions for the possibility of fashioning a secular moral world. Whatever strengths or weaknesses transcendental accounts may possess in other areas, at least here they offer a means for understanding how the conditions of moral reality are grounded in our character as persons. For an account of some of my views regarding the development of transcendental arguments, see *Mind–Body: A Categorial Relation* (The Hague: Martinus Nijhoff, 1973). See, for example, *Critique of Pure Reason,* A783 = B811 through A790 = B818; and A808 = B836.

88. One might think here of Hegel's argument that philosophy justifies itself within a circle of thought. The more encompassing the circle, the more powerful the explanation. See, for example, *The Encyclopaedia of the Philosophical Sciences* (1830), sec. 17.

89. The early government of Texas provides an interesting example of how such ideas of basic or natural rights developed within one variant of the American tradition. When the founders of the Texian republic came to conceive of the authority of the state, they were even more powerfully influenced by deist and anticlerical sentiments than were the founders of the American republic. The Declaration of Independence (Mar. 2,

1836) characterizes "the army and the priesthood" as both "the eternal enemies of civil liberty, the ever-ready minions of power, and the usual instruments of tyrants." The Texas Declaration of Independence, Mar. 2, 1836, in Ernest Wallace (ed.), *Documents of Texas History* (Austin: Steck, 1963), p. 98. The Texians are best interpreted not as denouncing simply a particular priesthood, but any moral orthodoxy imposed by force. Further, the Texian Bill of Rights, articulated in the Constitution of the Republic and repeated in the first Texas State Constitution (1845), portrays the government as the creation of free individuals, and fundamental rights as those prerogatives free individuals can never be presumed to have ceded to a government. Thus, the Declaration of Rights outlines a right to revolution: "All political power is inherent in the people, and all free governments are founded on their authority, and instituted for their benefit; and they have at all times the inalienable right to alter, reform, or abolish their form of government in such manner as they may think expedient." The same exists as the first Right in the Bill of Rights of the 1845 Constitution. The Constitution of the Republic of Texas, Mar. 17, 1836; see also the Texas Constitution of Aug. 28, 1845, and the Bill of Rights; *Documents of Texas History*, pp. 106, 149.

This passage occurs as well, with only slight alterations, in the current Constitution of the State of Texas.

All political power is inherent in the people, and all free governments are founded on their authority, and instituted for this benefit. The faith of the people of Texas stands pledged to the preservation of a republican form of government, and, subject to this limitation only, they have at all times the inalienable right to alter, reform, or abolish their government in such manner as they may think expedient. (Constitution of the State of Texas, art. 1, sec. 2)

If a Bill of Rights lists natural rights in the sense of authorities over oneself that have not been ceded to a government, a government has no authority to amend or change them. Section 21 of the Constitution of 1845 states: "To guard against transgressions of the high powers herein delegated, we declare that every thing in this 'bill of rights' is excepted out of the general powers of government, and shall forever remain inviolate." Texas Constitution of Aug. 28, 1845, art. 1, sec. 21, *Documents of Texas History*, p. 150. This passage exists as well in the current Constitution of the State of Texas. See art. 1, sec. 29.

The authority of the government in this account is derived neither from God nor from a particular vision of the good life and of content-full moral obligations, but from the uncoerced consent of moral agents who fashion a common thing, a *res publica*. The most general characteristics that mark legitimate public policy are not its goals but the procedures for its fashioning. The state and other societal endeavors can first and most generally be identified as having moral authority in terms of its springing from the consent of those involved.

The example of Texas is heuristic. Unlike Athens, which can be taken as the metaphor for the political assumption that the concrete character of the good life and of content-full moral obligations can be rationally disclosed, and Jerusalem, which can be taken as the metaphor for the political understanding that the concrete character of the good is disclosed in a communal and personal relationship with God, Washington-on-the-Brazos (the first capital of Texas) presents the image of all-too-human persons (i.e., all-too-fallen persons) acting within the moral constraints of mutual respect (in the limited sense that general secular morality can justify, i.e., using persons only with their permission) to create a political fabric with which individuals can, with willing others, fashion the concrete substance of various peaceable understandings of the good life and of content-full moral obligations. The Texian Republic stood as an inheritor of the political traditions that guided the pagans who gathered in the Althing in A.D. 930 at Thingvellir, a site chosen by Grim Goat-Shoe, thirty miles east of Reykjavik. It is from elements of that pagan tradition, of which the Icelanders were a part, that the Anglo-American jury system is drawn along with many of the Anglo-American understandings of individual rights (i.e., "the rights of Englishmen"). However, one does not need to choose among Athens, Jerusalem, and Reykjavik. Reykjavik (or Washington-on-the-Brazos) affords a peaceable place for the pursuit of either Athens or Jerusalem—a place where people can decide on their own whether and how they will attempt to go to heaven or hell.

90. Within particular moral communities, the secular government may be understood as having an authority that is not secular. Consider, for example, St. Paul in his letter to the Romans (13.1): "Let every soul be subject to the governing authorities. For there is no authority except from God, and the authorities that exist are appointed by God." Here one finds a theme salient in traditional Christianity: one should submit in humility to authority. Still, it is clear from the tradition that St. Paul's injunction did not mean that one should obey the Roman emperor when asked to renounce Christianity. Submission has its limits, which must at times be expressed in martyrdom.

The question then arises, what ought the religious attitude to be when the state is not secular or pagan, but Christian. Again, the tradition forbids force in the service of converting others to the truth. "You cannot compel people to become what you are. . . . One has to not be ashamed of being what one is. But that does not mean that we should use unlawful ways of bringing people to join us, or to impose our faith on people. No, it is in the spirit of liberty and full lucidity and serenity that we should proclaim what we are." Patriarch Ignatius IV of Antioch, *Again* 15 (June 1992): 17–18. However, when there is an anointed emperor, though he is bound by such limitations, he also has secularly unjustifiable authority. As the Liturgy of St. Basil prays,

Have in remembrance, O Lord, our most God-fearing and Christ-loving Ruler, N., to whom thou hast given the right to reign in the earth. Crown him with the armour of truth, with the panoply of contentment. Overshadow his head in the day of battle. Strengthen his arm, exalt his right hand; make mighty his kingdom; subdue under him all barbarous nations which seek wars; grant unto him peace profound and inviolate; inspire his heart with good deeds toward thy Church, and toward all thy people; that through his serenity we may lead a quiet and tranquil life, in all godliness and soberness.

*Service Book of the Holy Orthodox-Catholic Apostolic Church,* trans. Isabel Hapgood, 6th ed. (Englewood, N.J.: Antiochian Orthodox Christian Archdiocese, 1983), p. 109.

The difference between the morality (and bioethics) given through belief and the morality (and bioethics) that can be justified to moral strangers to bind moral strangers is troubling for those whose ideology or belief would ground the legitimacy of an Inquisition and the forcible conversion of the politically and religiously incorrect.

91. The Aristotelian view of the state is admittedly much more complex than this quick encapsulation suggests. Still, it trades on a content-full moral vision, which cannot with secular moral justification span contemporary large-scale societies with their plurality of moral visions. For a perceptive account of Aristotle's treatment of community, see Bernard Yack, *The Problems of a Political Animal* (Berkeley: University of California Press, 1993).

92. The difference between state and community and between society and community is explored in Engelhardt, "Sittlichkeit and Post-Modernity: An Hegelian Reconsideration of the State," pp. 211–24.

93. The following is one of the many vignettes concerning St. Herman of Alaska.

> Father Herman, when the river fish appeared in the spring, would start digging in the sand so that the fish could only just get past and as soon as the fish made for the shore they would come into this trap. Then the Elder would adopt the following procedure, as related by Ignatii: The Apa (elder) would order the fish to be caught and stunned and then gutted and cut into two strips—of these he would take a very small portion for himself and order the remainder to be placed on a board and cut into strips to feed the birds which were constantly around his cell, and, what was even more remarkable, the mink which lived and had their litters under his cell! It is strange that it is normally impossible to approach this little animal when it has pups, yet Father Herman would feed them by hand. Was what we saw not miraculous, Ignatii would ask. After Herman's death the birds and animals left.

Michael Oleksa (ed.), *Alaskan Missionary Spirituality* (New York: Paulist Press, 1987), p. 79.

94. Sigvat is quoted by Snorre Sturlason in the *Heimskringla* as giving the following characterization of Olaf Haraldsson:

> Some leaders trust in God—some not;
> Even so their men; but well I wot
> God-fearing Olaf fought and won
> Twenty pitched battles, one by one,
> And always placed upon his right
> His Christian men in a hard fight.
> May God be merciful, I pray,
> To him—for he ne'er shunned the fray.

Olaf Haraldsson is regarded by the Orthodox Catholic, Roman Catholic, and Protestant religions as the patron saint of Norway. See Snorre Sturlason, *The Heimskringla*, trans. Samuel Laing (London: Norroena, 1906), vol. 2, p. 645.

95. Stanley Hauerwas, *A Community of Character: Toward a Constructive Christian Ethics* (Notre Dame, Ind.: University of Notre Dame Press, 1981).

96. This attitude toward religion renders faith into a variety of cultural habit or tradition. Thus, one can present religious commitments as varieties of traditions. See, for example, David M. Feldman, *Health and Medicine in the Jewish Tradition* (New York: Crossroad, 1986); Martin E. Marty, *Health and Medicine in the Lutheran Tradition* (New York: Crossroad, 1983); Robert Peel, *Health and Medicine in the Christian Science Tradition* (New York: Crossroad, 1988); Fazlur Rahman, *Health and Medicine in the Islamic Tradition* (New York: Crossroad, 1989).

97. For some ideological and religious zealots, the situation may be frustrating, if not intolerable: they will be restrained from intruding into the freedoms of others. Some former believers may experience their lives as lacking a meaning that only selfless and unrestrained commitment can provide. They may falsely interpret that their own needs for commitment include a need to constrain others to be committed as they are. Perhaps many of the middle-class children who join revolutionary groups do so as part of a quest for an all-consuming dedication. The balance—the tolerance, the sophrosyne required by secular pluralist societies—is empty, insipid, and effete in comparison to the consuming commitment that can be felt as a member of the Baader-Meinhof gang, of Communist movements such as the Shining Path, of the National Socialist Party, of the Inquisition, or of any ideological or religious group that requires aggressive consecration of self and all to the truth, even to the coercive conversion of the unbelieving. Such individuals seeking this form of total commitment may find themselves in a society with muted tones of dedication. They do not feel able to pursue their goals within moral exclaves as do the Hassidim or Amish, aspiring at most to convert through witness, never force. Finding no opportunity given to them to die as martyrs, they invoke force to martyr others.

98. Archimandrite Vasileios, *Hymn of Entry,* trans. Elizabeth Briere (Crestwood, N.Y.: St. Vladimir's, 1984), pp. 75–76.

99. There will not be a collision with general secular morality in this case because of the traditional Christian's commitment to peaceable submission. Indeed, the call of Christ is, in the end, to absolute submission and love.

> But I tell you not to resist an evil person. But whoever slaps you on your right cheek, turn the other to him also. If anyone wants to sue you and take away your tunic, let him have your cloak also. And whoever compels you to go one mile, go with him two. Give to him who asks you, and from him who wants to borrow from you, do not turn away. You have heard that it was said, *You shall love your neighbor* and hate your enemy. But I say to you, love your enemies, bless those who curse you, do good to those who hate you, and pray for those who spitefully use you and persecute you. (Matthew 5:39–44)

It is for this reason that one is excommunicated for killing a person, even if one kills in self-defense or in a just war. See the sixty-sixth Apostolic Canon, as well as Canon 5 of St. Gregory of Nyssa (Sts. Nicodemus and Agapius, *The Rudder of the Orthodox Catholic Church,* trans. D. Cummings [1957; repr. New York: Luna Printing, 1983], pp. 113–16, 874–76). Other religions, as well as secular ideologies, with other understandings of the proper relationship to power and to the licitness of imposing their moral vision without consent will find themselves in collision with the constraints of general secular morality.

100. For an exploration of the lifeworld of the ecumenical cosmopolitans and its expression in one genre of the taken-for-granted experience of yuppies, see H. T. Engelhardt, Jr., *Bioethics and Secular Humanism: The Search for a Common Morality* (Philadelphia: Trinity International Press, 1991), especially pp. 33–40.

101. "Prayer of a Sick Person," in *A Pocket Prayerbook for Orthodox Christians* (Englewood, N.J.: Antiochian Orthodox Christian Archdiocese, 1990), pp. 22–23.

# 3

## The Principles of Bioethics

At the very roots of ethics and bioethics there are profound tensions. Ethics is not one practice. The different practices, related by family resemblance, often collide. As the last chapter shows, there are deep and important differences between the morality and bioethics that can bind moral strangers and the moralities and bioethics that can bind moral friends. The morality that can bind moral strangers hinges on the authority that individuals convey through permission. This morality has a negative structure. It discloses rights and duties of forbearance. The requirement to use individuals only with their consent sets limits. On the other hand, this morality justifies morally content-full joint endeavors through agreements to collaborate. The morality of moral strangers is the focus of this volume.

Just as important, indeed more important than the morality of moral strangers, is that which can bind moral friends. This morality gives content. However, there are diverse moral communities framed by different moral visions. These moral visions give rise to content-full bioethics and offer substantive guidance about how one should properly act as a patient, physician, nurse, or citizen framing health care policy. This volume does not address these moralities and the bioethics they support. It does not explore the particular content-full morality that ought to shape the bioethics and guide the health care policy through which moral friends can collaborate.

The morality of moral strangers shows the extent to which individuals from different moral communities can collaborate. It shows as well the limitations to their authority when they act together. The morality of moral strangers shows that which is important but must rely on conversion, not force. It may not coerce its acceptance. Therefore, one often understands the wrongness of another's action or situation but does not have the secular authority to force things aright. Because the morality of moral strangers has no content but sets limits to the authority of others to act on the unconsenting, there is often a tension expressed in the observation, X has a right to do A, but A is grievously wrong.

A second fundamental tension springs from the difference between respecting the freedom and securing the best interests of persons. This tension is recurringly expressed in health care. Patients frequently choose to engage in behaviors that physicians and nurses know to be dangerous, possibly disabling, and in the end perhaps lethal. Out of respect for those persons, physicians and nurses must often, if not usually, tolerate noxious lifestyles or failures to comply with treatment. Yet physicians and nurses, in joining the health care profession, have committed themselves to achieving the best interests of patients. This tension can be appreciated as the conflict between two ethical principles: that of permission and that of beneficence. It is in terms of the contrast between these two principles that the moral tension felt in many choices regarding abortion, treatment compliance, or refusal of health care is to be understood.

Permission and beneficence are principles in two senses. They function as chapter headings or indexes directing one to clusters of issues. In this case, the principles function as rules, perhaps as rules of thumb, which direct the inquirer to a particular approach to the solution of a problem. As such, the principles are, even if not fundamental, at least useful. These principles also function to indicate the sources of particular areas of moral rights and obligations. In this sense they are *principia:* they indicate the source, beginnings, commencements, or origins of particular areas of the moral life. They are principles in the sense of indicating two different roots for the justification of moral concerns in health care.

## Permission and beneficence: the conflict at the roots of bioethics

### *The will to morality and the problem of intersubjectivity*

As the last chapter shows, there are major problems in reaching a rationally justified resolution of bioethical quandaries in secular pluralist societies. When the premises held in common are insufficient to frame a concrete understanding of the moral life, and if rational arguments alone cannot definitively establish such premises, then reasonable men and women can establish a common fabric of morality only through mutual agreement. The concrete fabric of morality must then be based on a will to a moral viewpoint, not on the deliverances of a rational argument. The secular moral point of view in its most generally definable sense will be that intellectual standpoint from which one understands that conflicts regarding the propriety or impropriety of a particular action can be resolved intersubjectively by mutual agreement, and which viewpoint one then embraces in order to enable an intersubjectively grounded practice of blaming and praising, of mutual respect, and of moral authority. The moral fabric sustaining the various forms of the moral life is then a general practice that is as unavoidable as is the interest in resolving moral disputes. In terms of that morality, mutual respect becomes understood as using others only with their permission.

One can find a similarity with the practice of intersubjectively establishing empirical knowledge claims. Though one cannot guarantee that the principles of induction will succeed in the future, if one is interested in the intersubjective establishment of knowledge claims, one can then in general terms provide the canons for justifying particular empirical knowledge claims, should such ever be possible.[1] Insofar as such knowledge claims can be established intersubjectively, they will presuppose approaches that can be described as inductive. One can without any metaphysical presuppositions or assurances indicate the necessary conditions for a very general and human practice: the development of empirical generalizations.[2] So, too, one need not be sure that an actual moral community will ever be formed. However, one can sketch its necessary conditions while recognizing that actual interests in intersubjectively fashioning a moral world are required if moral communities are to be formed.

For a will to a moral viewpoint to be more than an inclination toward a particular moral viewpoint, it will need to be a will to a moral fabric as general as the very concept of morality itself. Yet an actual ethical life will require a particular concrete moral sense. In being tied to the notion of morality itself, the process of establishing a concrete morality by mutual agreement gains general rational justification in the sense of being coextensive with a generally available rationale that is ingredient in the very commitment to resolving moral disputes without recourse to force. If the practice of secular ethics is to be at least the endeavor of establishing the propriety of actions in ways other than through force, and if the moral senses of individuals are divergent, then the cardinal moral principle will be that of mutual respect in the common negotiation and creation of a concrete moral world.

Since moral fabrics gain particularity by commitment to a particular ordering of the goods of human life, the characterization of *the* moral fabric cannot provide the specification for such a particular ordering. If it did, it would lose its generality. On the other hand, the more the characterization of *the* moral fabric is tied to the very enterprise of being a person, the more firmly it can be generally justified. This is the case, for in asking a question about morals as a philosophical question, one is seeking a rational reply that is, as far as possible, inescapable. One is seeking a clincher to a dispute concerning which of the possible ways one can live life or practice medicine one *ought* to choose, where the sanction for violating the "ought" is not a threat of force or a feeling of guilt, but irrationality, worthiness of blame, or the failure to realize the goods one wishes to achieve. In seeking a characterization of the fabric of morality and bioethics tied to the fabric of rationality, one is unlikely to secure content to characterize the concrete nature of the moral life.

With the arguments to this point, one can understand why physicians should not treat, experiment on, or handle a competent patient without that individual's permission. One has established the basis for strong duties of mutual respect in health care. However, no duties of beneficence have been established. One does not know what goods one ought to pursue, only where one's authority ends. For example, ought one to provide health care for those who cannot pay for it? What are the noncontractual obligations of individuals and societies to do good, not just to refrain from unauthorized actions involving others? What is the good that ought to be done? Obligations to act with beneficence are more difficult to justify across particular moral communities than the principle to refrain from un-authorized force, in that one can have the possibility of coherent resolution of moral disputes by agreement without granting the principle of beneficence. The principle of beneficence is not required for the very coherence of the moral world, or of bioethics. It is in this sense that this principle is not as basic as what I will term the principle of permission. The principle of beneficence is not as inescap-able. One can act in nonbeneficent ways without being in conflict with the minimal notion of morality.

## How Kant smuggled content into his moral conclusions

The difficulty of finding a general justification for beneficence is appreciated if one examines Kant's attempt to justify morality. He endeavors to show that to act morally is to act rationally in the sense of acting in ways that are not self-contradictory.[3] In this fashion, Kant can show that one cannot speak consistently of self-respect and of oneself as worthy of blame or praise (i.e., worthy of happiness or unworthy of happiness) without regarding similar entities with simi-lar respect. Kant elaborates an ethics of respect for persons. However, an appeal merely to self-contradiction does not provide a justification for a principle of beneficence. In fact, as Hegel[4] and Alasdair MacIntyre[5] following Hegel show, Kant does not have an argument that can provide content for ethics. Kant attempts to gain content for his ethics through arguments that depend for their success on (1) a failure to distinguish between freedom as a value and freedom as a side constraint (by securing respect of persons, Kant thinks he has secured the obliga-tion to value autonomy), and (2) an appeal to a form of contradiction, which can be termed a contradiction in will. Under the latter he includes actions, the affir-mation of which does not involve a conceptual contradiction (affirming the notion of the peaceable community, in the sense of a community whose authority is not based on force, while at the same time deciding to use force against the unconsenting innocent, would involve a conceptual contradiction), but which Kant believes one could not in fact will for others without later willing the contrary for oneself (e.g., a refusal to be beneficent to others, although in the future one might wish such beneficence to be shown to oneself).

As to the first point, Kant's principle of respect for his moral law is not simply a constraint on acting against persons without their consent. It affirms freedom as a cardinal value. It thus steps beyond the support of Kant's actual arguments; the argument would require an appeal to a particular moral sense. Since Kant's arguments employ such an appeal, Kant does not allow suicide, although in the case of a competent person there is surely consent.[6] As the preceding chapter showed, to make any value, including the value of freedom, the cardinal value is to endorse a *particular* ethic. Valuing freedom does more than elaborate and justify the fabric of morality itself. One can consistently treat all persons as ends in themselves while affirming as a moral maxim that individuals may freely decide when to cease to be free by choosing suicide or a term in the French Foreign Legion. Respect of freedom as the necessary condition for the very possibility of mutual respect and of a language of blame and praise is not dependent on any particular value, or ranking of goods, but requires only an interest in resolving issues without recourse to force. When one has distinguished between freedom as a condition for morality, and freedom as a value, one loses the basis for duties to oneself as well. Or to put it another way, one can freely release oneself from one's duties to oneself, if such secular duties were to exist.[7] In not highly valuing freedom for oneself, one acts within the constraint of not using unconsented-to force against the innocent. In contrast, a bioethics based on Kant's assertions would lead one not to respect the choices of patients unless they affirmed a content-full principle of autonomy. Patients would not be free to choose in ways that did not affirm freedom as a value (e.g., by committing suicide).

As to the second point, by claiming one cannot without contradiction will to abandon what I term the principle of beneficence, not because of any formal contradiction, but because of a contradiction in one's will, Kant also seeks further content for ethics.[8] Indeed, Kant acknowledges that arguments for duties of beneficence are based not on the impossibility of thinking their opposite. He claims, instead, that one cannot consistently will not to respect the principle of beneficence. To underscore, Kant sees here a contradiction in will, not in logic. This difference marks duties of beneficence, as he acknowledges, not as strict duties, but as meritorious duties. Kant portrays the sentiments of someone who would take this position in the following way: "What concern of mine is it? Let each one be as happy as heaven wills, or as he can make himself; I will not take anything from him or even envy him; but to his welfare or to his assistance in time of need I have no desire to contribute."[9] In response, Kant argues that though one can consistently conceive such as a universal law of nature, it would still be impossible to *will* that such a principle should hold everywhere as a law of nature. "For a will which resolved this would conflict with itself, since instances can often arise in which he would need the love and sympathy of others, and in which he would have robbed himself, by such a law of nature springing from his own will, of all hope of the aid he desires."[10] It is in this sense that Kant relies on a contradiction of will rather than a conceptual contradiction in order to ground a principle of beneficence.

This suggestion by Kant is heuristic. The moral world can be divided into one dimension admitting of strict justification in that it is tied to the notion of the rational life, and a second tied to a notion of sympathy. If one recasts Kant, matters can be put this way: one can regard the misfortune of others and consistently hold that the principle of beneficence as grounded in the notion of ethics spanning various moral communities does not provide strict moral obligations, but only a reasonable moral ideal. Moreover, one will not be provided with one canonical ideal. This is the case in that nonbeneficent actions do not conflict with the notion of the peaceable community, but rather only with that of the beneficent community, and there are numerous content-full understandings of beneficence. As a consequence, the use of force against peaceable, nonbeneficent individuals is without authority, for it is against the notion of the peaceable community, which is the core of secular ethics. In fact, it would render those using such force blameworthy in terms of the core of secular morality. The principle of beneficence is exhortatory and undetermined, whereas the principle of permission is constitutive. As a result, it is easier to determine international standards for free and informed consent in terms of respect of persons, but harder to establish a criterion for a decent or basic level of health care.

The principle of beneficence can at least suggest that it would be good to benefit persons in need, even if the principle cannot justify the use of force to compel beneficence or specify the content of beneficence. Thus, it is good for physicians to provide health care free to indigent patients. Its violation can at least justify the withdrawal of beneficence not owed out of contract or agreement. The principle reminds one of what the moral life can be about—fashioning webs of sympathy through a commitment to providing goods to fellow persons in need. Yet what should count as needs generating moral claims can be determined only in a particular context and often only by multilateral agreement. The obligations of physicians become more substantial, once all members of a medical society have agreed that physicians should attempt, where practical, to provide a certain range of free services to those in need.

One could be tempted to read Kant as unwittingly making a point of prudence in defending his principle of beneficence.[11] However, the issue is more forcefully and more consistently to be understood as a reminder of the necessary condition for the possibility of understanding morality as a reciprocal web of sympathy. The moral life is not exhausted by an account of it as the fabric of a peaceable community. It is also the fabric of mutual sympathy. The question is, how inescapable is this second understanding and what is its content?

## The sanctions for immorality

One should note here the moral sanctions for misconduct. Secular morality lacks the sanctions of the law and of religion. It cannot of itself execute, imprison, fine, or damn to hell. Secular morality can demonstrate that certain ways of acting justify blameworthiness or impede the realization of the goals of the actors. Secular morality can also show when defensive or punitive force is justifiable.[12] But in itself it has no physical force. The sanctions of morality are tied to its justification. To use unconsented-to force against the innocent is incompatible with holding that others are wrong in using such force against oneself, or meaning anything more by terming another wrong or blameworthy than that one dislikes the other's conduct and wishes that he and others would refrain from it.[13] In short, the notion of the peaceable community as fashioned by the principle of permission is a cardinal element in the lives of persons. One embraces it as soon as one attempts to talk about morality across moral communities. Not to adopt it is to lose the basis for coherent moral discourse in a secular, pluralist society. The principle of permission grounds the morality of mutual respect in the sense that it requires that others be used only with their consent. The sanctions are intellectual. To raise an ethical question is to raise an intellectual question regarding justifications for action.

The case for beneficence depends not on the coherence of morality, but on the need for content. Unlike the principle of permission, which justifies the process for generating content, the principle of beneficence identifies the content of the practice of morality. The principle of permission shows that patients may not be used as means merely; the principle of beneficence supports the concrete moral goals to which medicine ought to be directed. However, particular moral senses establish competing rankings of the goods of life. The principle of beneficence in its most general form simply signals that moral arguments center on questions of what is good or proper to do. The difficulty with the principle of beneficence lies in the circumstance that any specific ranking of goods depends on a particular moral sense and is, therefore, not able to reach across moral communities. Its content is bound to a particular agreement, moral vision, or community. This indeed is the core of the difficulty. For example, under what circumstances, and to what extent, do obligations to aid others outweigh the good of having free time at one's disposal to pursue one's own goals? To put things more concretely, how much of one's office practice ought one to devote to free care for the indigent? Ethical disagreement regarding beneficence separates communities of moral commitment because there are no conclusive secular rational arguments to establish a particular moral sense. The problem of justifying any particular view of beneficence is under such circumstances insuperable.

Insofar as a portrayal of a general secular ethics is possible, which in its generality marks it as integral to the endeavors of persons, then that account of ethics is justified in being an inescapable element of life. It is in this fashion that the principle of permission has been justified: it is the necessary condition for the possibility of resolving moral disputes between moral strangers with moral authority and for sustaining a minimum secular ethical language of praise and blame. It is in this sense formal. It provides the empty process for generating moral authority in a secular pluralist society through mutual agreement. It can show that abortion, contraception, and suicide may not be forbidden with moral authority, but it cannot show that it is good to pay for abortion and contraception for the indigent or to assist rational individuals seeking to commit suicide who need aid. One may contend that the rational life is in addition concerned with the common pursuit of the good. But unlike the appeal to mutual respect through the principle of permission, the principle of beneficence needs to be specified within a *particular* moral community in order to be of any practical use.

The principle of beneficence is, as a result, more qualified than the principle of permission for yet another reason. If someone asks, "Why ought I to do to others their good?" one will not be able to respond, "Because if you don't, you will deny the very possibility of moral authority, for you will have denied the principle of respect to persons generally, including yourself." Instead, one can at best retort, "If we do not do to others their good, we will not have affirmed the possibility of what could be termed the kingdom of beneficence, or the beneficent community." The principle of beneficence reflects an interest in the common pursuit of the good life and of mutual human sympathies. It is the ground of what might be termed the morality of welfare and social sympathies.

Humans are social animals, and consequently they tend to conceive of goods socially. However, if some do not, what can one say of them beyond the obvious fact that they are not sympathetic persons? [14] What, in terms of morality, is the sanction for lack of sympathy or beneficence? In the case of violation of the principle of permission, the sanction is blameworthiness to the point of losing grounds for objecting to retaliatory force. The individual who violates the principle of permission is placed outside the peaceable community. Anyone who uses defensive force against such a guilty person does not violate secular moral authority, for guilty persons cannot consistently appeal to a principle they have rejected in order to condemn the users of force. The sanction is thus a major one. But if one fails to be beneficent, one has at most cut oneself off from the beneficent community. It is true that one cannot be unsympathetic and consistently claim the sympathy and support of beneficent persons—unless they have contracted to supply such support. In that case, their support would be grounded, not in the principle of beneficence, but in the principle of permission. Rejecting beneficence as a principle leads to an essential impoverishment of the moral life, not to its full rejection. Moreover, most will not reject the principle of beneficence outright, but rather only wish to substitute *their* principle for someone else's.

However, when an individual does not simply refuse to will or do the good, but wills to do evil to another person, then the malevolent individual renounces the moral community, even when acting with permission. There are two important variations. In the first, the malevolent individual wills to do what another holds to be good and to which that individual consents, but which the malevolent individual understands to be evil. Consider, for example, a physician who knows that abortion is evil and who performs an abortion on a consenting woman who considers the act good. Imagine that the physician does it out of a vindictive desire to involve the woman in evil. The physician acts malevolently, though from the point of view of the woman benevolently and, in this case, with permission. In the second instance, the malevolent individual wills to do a good to another, which the other holds to be evil but still consents to receive. One might this time imagine the previous physician's sibling giving a blood transfusion to a Jehovah's Witness whom the physician hates. The physician, not being a Jehovah's Witness, holds the blood transfusion to be an unalloyed physical good for the Jehovah's Witness. The Jehovah's Witness, on the other hand, accepts the blood transfusion out of a weakness of faith because of the physician's cajoling. The physician's hope is that the Jehovah's Witness will live from that point on with a bad conscience.

What can one say of such malevolence? First, the obligation to be non-malevolent is stronger than the obligation to be beneficent. In the case of the failure to be beneficent, one does not live up to the core goal of morality, achieving the good. But in the case of malevolence, one acts against this goal. This much seems plausible even without an appeal to any content-full understanding of good or evil. One can recognize the principle of nonmalevolence as the most binding element of the moral concern with beneficence, with achieving the good, because malevolence is the rejection of the good. Does this mean that one is then licensed to use force against the malevolent? When the person who is the object of malevolence consents to the malevolent act, then evil is done with permission, trumping any general secular basis for using defensive or punitive force, because the core of secular moral legitimacy is authorization. Still, actions done malevolently against future persons who cannot consent, and even against moral subjects that are not moral agents, plausibly legitimate defensive force. Defending against malevolence does not require presupposing a particular moral vision. Moreover, anyone who acts malevolently and without permission has no grounds to protest when visited with defensive force.

With these reflections in hand, one can now reappraise the sanctions for immorality. First, as has been noted, philosophical arguments will not deliver the sanctions available through certain religious arguments. Philosophers will not be able to demonstrate that particular forms of immorality will lead to eternal pain. Nor does philosophy have the sanctions of the law. It cannot provide fines, imprisonment, or the lash. The arguments examined earlier show that acting against the very notion of the peaceable community makes one blameworthy in the eyes of rational beings anywhere in the cosmos. As a result, one loses any ground for protesting against their defensive, punitive, or retaliative force. As soon as one is interested in ethics as an alternative to the resolution of moral disputes through force, one has committed oneself to mutual respect. And, if one rejects the principle of mutual respect, one cannot rationally protest when others respond with force. Since the questions regarding the sanctions for immorality are intellectual, the sanctions are intellectual. They pronounce outlawry upon the offending individual, a charge against which that person cannot consistently protest as long as he continues in affirming the immoral action. Reflections on autonomy lead to the justification of a morality of mutual respect, whose sanctions are the loss of the grounds for respect and for protest against defensive and punitive actions by others. Reflections on the morality of beneficence, however, focus on the morality of common welfare. To affirm the morality of beneficence is to affirm the enterprise of the common good, of the fabric of mutual sympathies, which fashions the morality of welfare. To reject beneficence outright is to lose all claim to the sympathies of others. However, to reject a particular principle of beneficence is only to lose claims to the sympathies of others within a particular context or community. In summary, violations of the principle of permission justify circumscription of the autonomy of the offender. Violations of the principle of beneficence eliminate claims by the offender to the kind of beneficence rejected for others.

## Giving authority and content to the principle of beneficence

What, then, can be said of the principle of beneficence? Was it proper for the owner of this book to have expended money in its purchase, rather than to have helped the starving poor? What if the choice was between this book, contributing to saving endangered species, feeding the starving in the third world, or contributing to a fund to help a child in Australia to receive a high-cost treatment with a possibility of less than 50 percent of saving the patient's life? On the basis of what principle can one determine how much beneficence is required and what form it should take? The difficulty lies in determining when it becomes obligatory to be beneficent, not just act in a praiseworthy fashion. There appears to be no clear answer in the abstract. The range of goods to be achieved and harms to be avoided for humans, as well as other animals, is wide and complex. The correct ordering is in dispute, as well as the point at which needs and desires impose particular obligations. It is important to note that this leads to two major difficulties with duties and rights of beneficence. One must establish (1) their content (which will depend on a particular view of the good life), and (2) their authority (i.e., the authority to require one, rather than another, view of beneficence, including the significance of the circumstances under which inconveniences or contrary inclinations properly excuse one from discharging a duty of beneficence).

The bonds of beneficence, if they are to be established, must be framed through mutual understandings, both implicit and explicit, which establish both content and authority. Only in particular social contexts, within the embrace of particular moral communities, can one discover what are in fact the bonds of beneficence. The bonds of beneficence that tie individuals in special roles of friend, colleague, spouse, parent, child, patient, and physician are *in part* contractual. By this I do not mean to suggest an explicit contract, but a web of usually implicit understandings. Some attempt to impart a special distinction to such understandings by employing the term *covenant*. They undoubtedly wish to suggest a quasi-religious meaning, though the biblical sense of covenant itself is derived from the notion of a treaty, usually made with a conquering force.[15] In any event, one fashions a web or nexus of commitments and understandings, both explicit and implicit, which sustain a fabric of moral understandings. These understandings are usually open to revision.

One can, in many circumstances, choose other friends, colleagues, patients, physicians, or health care delivery systems. One can even disown one's parents or children, or adopt children. One can emigrate or enter a social group with which one has more substantial agreement. One can change party affiliation and convert to a new religion. Though history, culture, and circumstance constrain such choices, life in a world containing a plurality of moral communities in intimate contact demonstrates daily the possibility of such fashioning and re-fashioning of social bonds. However, the principle of beneficence at stake here is not one sustained only by a particular moral community. Within a community of BaMbuti, Ik, patrician Romans of the Republic, or contemporary Orthodox Jews or Mennonite Christians, there is a web of moral understandings that sustains concrete, though often complex, principles of beneficence. In terms of such principles, one is able to sketch in detail the obligations of beneficence of physicians to patients. However, a principle of beneficence that would span the diversity of communities could not support a particular ordering of goods, but only the provision of goods in general to persons in general. The principle can at best indicate that special roles of beneficence should characterize such relations. The principle of beneficence is in general simply the principle of doing good.

Because of the divergent understandings of what should count as actually doing the good, one cannot understand in secular morality the principle of beneficence as the Golden Rule. If one does unto others as one would have them do unto oneself, one may in fact be imposing on others against their will a particular view of the good life. The Golden Rule can thus be (and in fact has been) the basis for the tyrannical imposition of particular concrete understandings of the good life. To avoid such tyranny, one will need to phrase the principle of beneficence in this positive form: "Do to others their good." However, insofar as one attempts to do to others what they would hold to be their good, not what one or one's own moral community would hold to be their good, the sense of obligation to be beneficent weakens. First, one's own understanding of beneficence within one's own moral community will set standards for when one is obliged to shoulder what burdens to do good to others. Second, one will need to transfer that view of the proper exchange of burdens for the benefits of others to doing good to an individual in another moral community with a different view of the hierarchies of goods and harms and of the boundary between obligatory and supererogatory actions. Third, within one's own moral community one may understand that what others take to be their good is an evil that may not be abetted or a harm that should not be inflicted.

Consider a physician in community A, which holds that it is important to save life, even if the probabilities of success are very low and the costs very high. In this community, over 3 percent of the gross domestic product (GDP) is expended for critical care alone, and some 18 percent of the entire GDP goes to health care. When visiting community B, which invests only 4 percent of its gross domestic product in health care, and some $3/10$ percent of its GDP in critical care, while investing 5 percent in philosophy and the fine arts, the physician is shocked. Are the people in community B wrong? Do they have a misguided sense of medical beneficence? Or do they instead have a correct sense of how to be beneficent towards others through providing easy access to good art as well as better scholarship in the humanities (presuming that such excellence is achieved by greater expenditure).

Expressing the principle of beneficence in the maxim "Do to others their good" recognizes that any talk of the best interests of others presupposes a particular judgment about what constitutes those best interests. When one speaks across moral communities, different judges of best interests with different moral senses are presupposed. Moreover, the morality of mutual respect gives to individuals the right to veto the provision of a good they do not want. On the other hand, the moral insights of one's own moral community may forbid doing to others what they hold to be good but which one knows to be evil or harmful. The maxim "Do to others their good" must then be understood as "Do to others their good, unless one recognizes (1) the purported good to be a harm or (2) the provision of the good to be in some sense wrong." Because of conflicts among the diverse visions of the good, the good one recognizes that one ought to do to others will frequently be seen by those others as a harm. One may then be forbidden by the principle of permission to do to others what one sees to be their good, but which they regard as harmful. The ambiguity of "their good" lies at the roots of concerns regarding paternalism, a topic to which attention will be given in chapter 7. In general, the more individuals share a moral community and a single moral sense, the more clearly defined the moral obligations of beneficence become, and the more there will be an agreement between the giver and the receiver regarding the nature of the good.

An individual may properly claim not to be obliged to provide a benefit to another because it would more seriously harm others or because it would in fact harm the individual seeking aid. The second case involves an instance of the principle of nonmaleficence, a special application of the principle of beneficence. It underscores the fact that one will not be obliged to provide to others a service one finds to be a violation of the principle of beneficence. Here I use the principle of nonmaleficence as not doing to another a harm to which the individual does not object (and to which the individual presumably consents). Consider a college sophomore who at the end of a passionate love affair reads Goethe's *Die Leiden des jungen Werther* and comes to the house of a friend to borrow a sixteen-gauge shotgun with which to commit suicide. Although the principle of permission would not forbid the provision of the shotgun on request, the principle of nonmaleficence would. Medical examples may include requests for unjustified surgical procedures, drugs, or other treatments. It will be obligatory or supererogatory to do to others their good, as long as the provision of that good in terms of one's own moral sense is not seen on balance to be a harm.

Consider, for example, the surgeon who is convinced that the only proper treatment for carcinoma of the breast is radical mastectomy. If that surgeon is confronted with a patient wanting a surgical excision of the carcinoma, followed by radiation and chemotherapy, may the surgeon comply, even if the surgeon does not believe this maximizes the patient's good with respect to survival? The answer here can be yes, in that the surgeon may also recognize the patient's concerns with function and cosmetic appearance, and may hold that the patient simply has a different hierarchy of values within which she balances maximal life expectancy, maximal cosmetic appearance, maximal use of her arm, and maximal realization of liberty values. The physician may regard the act of providing to the patient the treatment she requests, given its full context, as beneficent. The same may be the case when a fifteen-year-old girl seeks contraceptive information from a physician who does not believe that sexual activity among teenagers is good for them. The physician may even hold that the provision of the information might increase the likelihood of adolescent sexual activity. Still, the physician might properly judge that the consequences of an unwanted pregnancy make the provision of contraceptive information and materials on balance a beneficent act.

Here again one must remember the context for the discussion of these moral principles: the attempt to reach across particular moral communities. Just as one must seek a foundation for moral authority across moral communities, one must also seek a characterization of moral content across such communities. The principle of permission signals, for example, the need for consent. So, too, the principle of beneficence, one would hope, would signal across moral communities what is proper to do for patients, such as providing a minimal basic package of health care for the indigent. This does not appear to be possible, at least in any concrete fashion. One is left, rather, with the principles of permission and beneficence, which contrast as a general principle of authority and a general principle of the good. As principles spanning particular moral communities, they possess only a minimal content. This circumstance makes the principle of beneficence a general concern for providing others with the goods of life. Even if it is somewhat vacuous, the principle of beneficence is central. Moral quandaries are not just quandaries about who has the authority to resolve moral disputes; they concern as well the character of the goods to be pursued. Indeed, a concrete understanding of the good life presupposes an ordering, vision, or understanding of goods and harms, as much as any peaceable society presupposes authority from its members. As a consequence, morality in a secular pluralist society is the practice of doing the good within the bounds of moral authority across communities with disparate moral visions.

The necessary conditions for the possibility of a *particular* moral community are, then, (1) an interest in pursuing the good and avoiding harm within (2) the constraints of moral authority, that is, permission. Goods and harms take on a concrete moral significance within the context of a community with a particular moral vision. The principle of permission marks the very boundary of all moral communities. To violate it is to be an enemy of moral communities generally. However, to honor it is not quite yet to be a member of a moral community. This is the case, in part, because the principle of permission is a principle of forbearance only. It is a negative principle. In general secular morality, the principle of permission is not beyond, but it is before, any concrete good or evil. It is only through the positive principle of beneficence that content is acquired for the moral life. Thus, not being beneficent is not to be an enemy of the moral community, but neither is it to be a member of a moral community. An individual who pursues his own solitary good, but without violating the rights of others, falls into a sort of moral limbo. It is only in affirming the principle of beneficence that one commits oneself to the enterprise of fashioning a moral community and to giving content to beneficence.

For bioethics this means that understanding the restraints due to the requirement of authority through permission is central, but insufficient for an account of proper health care. One must ensure consent, one must forbear from preventing access to abortion and contraception, and one must respect the rights of individuals to sustain a private tier of health care services. However, this necessary web of duties of forbearance in general secular morality will be insufficient for a picture of the moral life. One will need in addition to determine the obligations of physicians and society to provide care and support to patients.

In order to appreciate the ambiguities with respect to beneficent action and the difficulties in acquiring substantial moral authority for health care policy, one must note the differences between moral communities and societies or polities. Full-fleshed moral communities enjoy intact moral traditions, practices, and understandings of the good life, replete with individuals who are in moral authority as well as those who are moral authorities. Their members meet as moral friends, sharing in common sufficient moral premises and rules of evidence and inference to resolve moral controversies by sound rational argument or by appeal to commonly recognized moral authority. Sometimes the community and the polity will be nearly identical. Perhaps at times this was the case in Greek city-states. Perhaps it is still the case in many Japanese villages. But city-states can be rent into importantly different communities as is illustrated by the history of the Ghibellines and Guelphs and their dual administration of northern Italian cities. In any event, large-scale polities are not moral communities, but the alliance of individuals and at times diverse communities in certain common undertakings. Large-scale polities compass diverse communities with divergent views of justice, fairness, community, moral probity, and the good life. Large-scale polities compass individuals and communities with divergent moral, political, ideological, and religious commitments. It is possible for large-scale societies to establish programs of beneficence (e.g., the provision of health care), but there will not be *one* communal understanding of the beneficence undertaken. Some will see, for example, the health care provided as speaking to a basic human right or need. Others will see the care provided as an arbitrary commitment to a particular set of services. Yet others will understand the health care provided as a commitment made politically in exchange for a commitment to improving highways.

The contrast of the terms *society* and *community* is, to an extent, stipulative. Many communities have disengaged from the practices and traditions that frame their moral understandings so that their moral commitments appear as intuitions and prejudices unsustained by a coherent framing context of meaning. As Alasdair MacIntyre has observed, their moral convictions have become like the taboos of late eighteenth- and early nineteenth-century Hawaiians.[16] Their communities have become more like associations. On the other hand, those who hunger after the purpose and moral authority available within a community endeavor to regard their polities as if they were or could become moral communities and share in a common content-full vision of beneficence.

*Justifying the principles of morality*

The justifications that have been offered for this principle of morality are not simply psychological claims regarding dispositions to be respectful or sympathetic. They are conceptual points regarding what it means coherently to think of ourselves within particular inescapable conceptual frameworks. For example, to ask how to determine the causes of cancer or whether a berry is poisonous is to ask a question presupposing points of relative permanence, changes according to patterns or rules, and a reciprocity among the points of permanence and change. Here one should recall Kant's arguments regarding the necessary conditions for the possibility of experience.[17] Asking about (or thinking about) the nature of empirical reality (or even having a coherent experience) commits one to such a set of presuppositions regarding empirical coherence. Such principles are so inescapable that to reject them is tantamount to endorsing a psychosis with full-blown autism.[18] Experience has a set of presumptions that are conceptually statable because it is the experience of a rational being.[19]

So, too, thinking about blaming or praising with justification presupposes a framework in terms of which there can be a criterion or authority for evaluation. The minimal condition for this possibility is mutual respect, which grounds both a sense of moral authority and a justification for blame and praise in the principle of permission. To establish a more concrete moral sense requires premises that are impossible to secure in general secular terms. Such premises would require committing oneself to a particular community with its already accepted metaphysical, ideological, or religious presuppositions. Mutual respect in the sense of the requirement of permission is barely sufficient, but still quite sufficient for the minimum grammar necessary for a secular fabric of moral authority. The principle of permission as a summary of the core of the morality of mutual respect must be embraced insofar as one coherently thinks of oneself as making claims to respect, or regarding persons in terms of their worthiness of blame and praise, or as able to recognize moral authority in a secular pluralist context—that is, in a context where special religious, metaphysical, or ideological premises are not granted. If one does not participate in this world of mutual respect, then one is left with using force without even a purported general secular justification, or with an alleged justification (i.e., in terms of special religious, metaphysical, or ideological assumptions), which cannot be secured in general secular terms. Hence, persons anywhere in the cosmos interested in giving general justifications for respect, worthiness of blame or praise, and moral authority would have grounds for recognizing as immoral persons who employ such unjustified force. The morality of mutual respect, through the principle of permission, sets the boundaries to morality generally. It discloses those who are outlaws from that morality and therefore cannot protest against defensive or punitive force. As such, it is a restraining principle.

The morality of welfare and social sympathies, which is summarized under the rubric of the principle of beneficence, discloses the nisus of morality, the interest in securing the good of persons and of sentient beings generally. To understand morality is to understand that it is concerned with achieving the good for persons. (1) The general limits on the capacity of reason to disclose a justified concrete view of the good and (2) the restraints due to the morality of mutual respect (expressed in a negative principle of autonomy) set limits to secularly morally justified actions on behalf of beneficence. However, if one were to understand bioethics only in terms of these restraints, one would have forgotten why one had decided to engage in health care to begin with, namely, to achieve a set of important goods for patients and potential patients.

The principle of beneficence is as unavoidable as the question, What is good or bad to do. To be interested in an intersubjective answer to such a question is to presuppose a concern for the good of persons and sentient beings generally. To raise the question of the good and the bad in this fashion is to attempt to take a general perspective, an anonymous perspective, one that belongs as much to all as it does to any particular person. It involves stepping away from particular personal interests and advantages so as to judge which lines of conduct should generally be affirmed as good and which should generally be condemned as evil. To answer such a rational question is, after all, not to determine what is true idiosyncratically for me, but what is true for inquirers generally. Within the general perspective of secular morality, one steps away from bias, prejudice, and personal distortion towards anonymous appreciation, which is intersubjective.[20] This commitment to generality is a goal, the expression of a regulative principle, and never fully realized.

Because of the unlikelihood of a general agreement about what is the proper concrete understanding of the good life, the question of what is good or bad to do cannot receive a concrete or content-full answer. The question is heuristic: it aims individuals toward as rationally justifiable an account as possible of good and bad consequences. However, such accounts will vary, as different individuals accept different hierarchies of benefits and harms. It will vary as well, depending on whether the good is regarded as agent-neutral or agent-relative. It will also vary depending on how highly one ranks the goal of people being able to act on their own vision of the good and the like. The best one can do is to articulate the principle of beneficence, Do to others their good, in the concreteness of particular moral communities. Particular understandings of good and harm must be pursued, while not forgetting the absoluteness of the general concern for doing good and avoiding evil. The principle of beneficence is thus dialectical. It speaks of a goal that cannot be directly articulated in general secular terms: a true and final understanding of what is good or evil to accomplish. This understanding can only be fully realized within a particular moral community, indeed, only within the right one.

The principles of permission and beneficence ground and summarize two central moral points of view: (1) that in terms of which one considers what it means to act with authority, within one's rights, and (2) that in terms of which one considers what it means to do good and avoid evil. Each is justified through being tied to an inescapable element of meaning. The principle of permission is inescapable, insofar as one asks whether one (or another) has acted (or will act) rightly in the sense of with moral authority. The principle of beneficence is inescapable insofar as one asks regarding the good one ought to achieve or evil one ought to avoid for others. The principles express the circumstance that the moral point of view is one of beneficence within the constraint of respect for persons.

## The tension between the principles

Neither the principle of permission nor that of beneficence is justified in terms of its consequences. They rather disclose unavoidable areas of personal conduct. They are in this sense deontological principles: their rightness is not defined in terms of, or justified in terms of, their consequences. However, concrete rules of beneficence are likely to be teleological in being justified in terms of their consequences. Concrete applications of the principle of permission, in contrast, bind, even if they have negative consequences for liberty. The principle of permission, which is justified in terms of the morality of mutual respect, does not focus on freedom as a value, but on persons as the source of general secular moral authority. It is not goal- or consequence-oriented (i.e., teleological). Physician–patient agreements (e.g., a physician's agreement to keep a patient's disclosures confidential) bind in general secular morality in terms of the principle of permission, independently of their consequences. In contrast, a rule for distributing health care resources on grounds of beneficence would be defeated if it failed to provide more benefits than alternative rules.

The two principles thus lead to contrasting spheres of moral discourse: one deontologically oriented, the other teleologically oriented.[21] This contrast can produce moral tensions and irresolvable conflicts. An act can be justified within one dimension of morality but not within the other. Thus, one has conflicts of the general sort, "X has a right (obligation) to do A, but it is wrong." For example, "Physicians have a right to do what they want with their spare time, even when they could easily contribute a small portion of that spare time to aiding indigent patients, even when others hold that it is wrong not to use some of that time to aid those patients." One has a conflict between the morality of mutual respect and the morality of welfare. It is not just that one cannot specify the morality of welfare without appealing to mutual agreement and therefore to the morality of mutual respect (e.g., the physicians may accord a high value to the free use of spare time and disagree regarding [1] proper comparison of benefits and harms, including [2] the burdens to self that make particular exertions unreasonable). It is also the case that failure to be beneficent does not warrant defensive or punitive force.

First, goods and harms become intersubjectively moral goods and harms either in the embrace of a community with a common moral vision or through the agreements made in fashioning and sustaining an association or society. Such communities and societies have secular moral authority for themselves and for the ways in which they treat goods and harms only through respecting the principle of permission. Further, the principle of permission requires acquiescing in the choice by others of harms they hold to be goods, which may be at odds with the views of a moral community. One might think of a young man deciding to commit suicide after sustaining nonfatal but disfiguring burns or of individuals choosing within the rules of a medical insurance system in ways that will in the end subvert that very system through escalating costs. Respect for freedom and interest in the good conflict.

Since views of the good are divergent, and no particular view can in general secular terms be established as morally canonical, there will be no moral authority to stop persons from peaceably pursuing their own views of the good life alone or with consenting others. One might think of a society attempting to bring its members to realize a higher level of health and to lower certain health care costs by stopping smoking and engaging in exercise programs. What of the sedentary smokers who do not judge that such is worth the effort, because the health achieved is not worth the increased costs from more people living longer? What of those who hold that nonsmokers will in the end destroy the financial stability of the community by extending life, increasing the need for welfare payments in old age (e.g., social security payments), not to mention long-term nursing care as more individuals live long enough to develop Alzheimer's? The achievement of the societal view of the good will often fall prey to the free choice of individuals not to aid its prospering. Such dissenters from an orthodox vision of the good can be characterized as having valued personal freedoms higher than other goods or as having embraced a different view of the good life with a different schedule of the relative significance of costs and benefits. Such dissenters also underscore the tension between respecting freedom and acting benevolently, especially on a social level.

Dissenting communities within the embrace of large-scale associations, societies, and polities remind us of the limits of the secular moral authority of such polities. Limited democracies are morally neutral by default. They cannot acquire the authorization to establish a particular moral vision, religion, or ideology. After all, given the failure of reason to discover the rational, canonical, content-full moral vision, establishing a morality or ideology as a government's concrete morality or moral vision has no more secular moral plausibility or authority than would the establishment of a particular religion. Limited democracies are therefore morally committed to not being committed to a particular vision of the good; they are committed rather to being the social structure through which, and with whose protection, individuals and communities can pursue their own and divergent visions of the good. As far as possible, limited democracies should enable individuals and communities to pursue their own visions of the good, while not compromising the moral commitments of other individuals and communities. As we will see in chapter 8, this supports the right to establish parallel and morally different health care systems.

## The principle of justice

Most appeals to the principle of justice can be understood as being at root a concern with beneficence. Principles of justice that support the distribution of goods under a particular moral vision are special instances of attempting to do the good. Justinian in his *Institutes* characterized justice as "the constant and perpetual wish to render every one his due."[22] The problem, of course, lies in what is due to whom and why. On the one hand, principle-of-permission-based understandings of justice, such as Robert Nozick's, construe just distributions as those that occur without violence to the free choices of owners.[23] In contrast, there are views of justice based on appeals to ideal distributions of goods. These presuppose particular views of the good life. As we shall see, these disparate foundations for claims about justice undergird major moral conflicts concerning the distribution of both privately and commonly owned goods.

These disparate foundations are at the root of complex claims such as those presented in the following statement: "It is your right to use your own private funds for the health care of those you choose and no others, but it is wrong in the sense that it shows no acknowledgment of the needs of others." The first clause, in its appeal to rights, signals the limits of public authority. It appeals to the principle of permission. The second clause, in its notion of wrongness, appeals to a particular moral vision of the good life and of just distributions. It appeals to a particular principle of doing good, of being beneficent. This same conflict can recur in the allocation of commonly owned goods: "I know that we voted according to commonly agreed-to procedures regarding the ways in which we would invest our common resources. However, investing them as agreed, primarily in the development of good vineyards rather than in health care research and health care, is wrong." The first clause appeals to a view of the good as fashioned through the common agreement of an association. The second clause appeals to a particular view, not so sanctioned, regarding the proper use of resources. And of course, there are numerous competing particular views of distributive justice and obligatory beneficent action. Such views are rooted in the various content-full moral philosophical understandings of the proper use of resources or in a religion or traditional moral vision.[24]

## The principles of bioethics

In approaching the problems of moral judgment in bioethics, we have then two major moral principles. Their character reflects the circumstance that they are principles for resolving moral disputes among individuals who do not share a common moral vision. They guide us through the moral division of secular pluralism. They sustain the possibility of moral discourse in secular pluralist societies where no one moral sense can be established. They function also as guides for tracing the lineage of supposed secular moral authority for public policy. Public policy that lacks a morally justified authority is without secular moral force. One might think here of laws forbidding commercial suicide services for competent individuals.[25] Such laws are without secular moral authority (here again one experiences the agonizing gulf between content-full morality and what can be established in general secular terms), at least as long as the individuals have not explicitly ceded their right to suicide (e.g., one might imagine that officers in the armed forces might be required to relinquish that right under specified conditions as a condition for their commission). On the other hand, laws protecting human research subjects against being used in experimentation without their consent carry moral authority in that they are grounded in the very notion of protecting the peaceable community. They spring from the notion of the morality of mutual respect.

Other areas of public policy have less certain moral authority. It will be clear how to use commonly owned resources in ways that support the common good. The provision of a mix of preventive and primary health care out of common funds would appear reasonable. However, arguments can reasonably be advanced for various mixtures, including a major preponderance of either preventive or primary health care. The actual character of public health policy will thus have to be created by common agreement and will not be discoverable by an inspection of the principle of beneficence in isolation. One will need to appeal to the principle of permission as the basis for the common fashioning of particular programs of beneficence. In most cases, one finds both principles intertwined. These two principles are principles in the sense of being *principia*. They indicate foundations for major elements of the moral life. (Further derivative principles will be introduced in chapter 4.)

---

PRINCIPLE I. THE PRINCIPLE OF PERMISSION

Authority for actions involving others in a secular pluralist society is derived from their permission. As a consequence,

    i.  Without such permission or consent there is no authority.

    ii.  Actions against such authority are blameworthy in the sense of placing a violator outside the moral community in general, and making licit (but not obligatory) retaliatory, defensive, or punitive force.

  A. Implicit consent: individuals, groups, and states have authority to protect the innocent from unconsented-to force.

  B. Explicit consent: individuals, groups, and states can decide to enforce contracts or create welfare rights.

C. Justification of the principle: the principle of permission expresses the circumstance that authority for resolving moral disputes in a secular, pluralist society can be derived only from the agreement of the participants, since it cannot be derived from rational argument or common belief. Therefore, permission or consent is the origin of authority, and respect of the right of participants to consent is the necessary condition for the possibility of a moral community. The principle of permission provides the minimum grammar for secular moral discourse. It is as inescapable as the interest of persons in blaming and praising with justification and resolving issues with moral authority.

D. Motivation for obeying the principle is tied to interests in acting in a way i) that is justifiable to peaceable persons generally, and ii) that will not justify the use of defensive or punitive force against oneself.

E. Public policy implications: the principle of permission provides moral grounding for public policies aimed at defending the innocent.

F. Maxim: Do not do to others that which they would not have done unto them, and do for them that which one has contracted to do.

G. The principle of permission grounds what can be termed the morality of autonomy as mutual respect.

## PRINCIPLE II. THE PRINCIPLE OF BENEFICENCE

The goal of moral action is the achievement of goods and the avoidance of harms. In a secular pluralist society, however, no particular account or ordering of goods and harms can be established as canonical. As a result, within the bounds of respecting autonomy, no particular content-full moral vision can be established over competing senses (at least within a peaceable secular pluralist society). Still, a commitment to beneficence characterizes the undertaking of morality, because without a commitment to beneficence the moral life has no content. As a consequence,

    i.   On the one hand, there is no general content-full principle of beneficence to which one can appeal.

    ii.   On the other hand, actions without regard to concerns of beneficence are blameworthy in the sense of placing violators outside the context of any particular content-full moral community. Such actions place individuals beyond claims to beneficence. In particular, malevolence is a rejection of the bonds of beneficence. Insofar as one rejects only particular rules of beneficence, grounded in a particular view of the good life, one loses only one's own claims to beneficence within that particular moral community; in either case, petitions for mercy (charity) can still have standing. Actions against beneficence constitute moral impropriety. They are against the content proper to the moral life.

A. Implicit contract: content for a principle of beneficence is acquired by fashioning a community with a common view of the proper account or ordering of goods and harms.

B. Explicit contract: content for duties of beneficence can be derived as well from explicit agreements. In this case, as in the previous case, the content of a duty of beneficence is grounded in the principle of permission.

C. Justification of the principle: the principle of beneficence reflects the circumstance that moral concerns encompass the pursuit of goods and the avoidance of harms. Since such disputes can be resolved in secular pluralist societies only by an appeal to the principle of permission, the principle of permission is conceptually prior to the principle of beneficence. One can know when one is violating the morality of mutual respect, even when one cannot know, because of its lack of content, whether one is violating the principle of beneficence. However, recognition of the principle of beneficence provides the minimal characterization of the content required for moral concerns.

D. Motivation for obeying the principle is tied to interests in acting in a way: i) that is justifiable to beneficent persons generally, and ii) that will not justify one in being characterized as an unsympathetic individual who may be excluded from a particular or any community's beneficence.

E. Public policy implications: the principle of beneficence provides the moral grounding for refusable welfare rights drawn from common holdings.

F. Maxim: Do to others their good.

G. The principle of beneficence grounds what can be termed the morality of welfare and social sympathies.

---

## Moral tension and the centrality of forbearance rights

In light of these two principles, one can appreciate better the character of conflicts in health care. The conflicts are often deep, if not intractable, because they reflect profound tensions within the project of morality itself. Concerns with mutual respect and concerns with common welfare are sufficiently distinct so as not to allow a means for a mediation of their tensions.[26]

Diverse claims with regard to rights and obligations, and with regard to the rightness or wrongness of actions, can be generated on the basis of different elements of secular morality (i.e., permission-regarding morality versus beneficence-regarding morality), as well as in terms of conflicts between secular philosophical ethics and moralities based on particular religious or moral viewpoints. In addition, considerations regarding beneficence are themselves complex. There appears to be a number of competing reasonable accounts of what it means to be beneficent, to act to support a web of mutual sympathy, to support the common welfare.

Different ways of articulating concerns to achieve the good or avoid evil will lead to different claims regarding what is good to do. This includes the circumstance that different lexical orderings of goods will produce different views of what it means to act beneficently. Which is more important, to control pain fully but at the risk of addiction, or to avoid any substantial risk of addiction, but at the price of substantial pain? One might think of the conflicts that occur between financial interests and concerns to achieve optimal health, or optimal chances of curing disease and restoring function. Such conflicts exist both on a societal level as well as for individuals. As we have noted, there are conflicts between interests in maximizing the chances of cure and prolonging life expectancy, versus risks of pain and suffering that confront a patient in choosing among various means for treating cancer. How does one compare a lower chance of a five-year cure for cancer of the larynx with a greater chance of maintaining acceptable vocal function? And from whose point of view? When one examines the principle of beneficence, one finds it fragmenting into a number of senses of beneficence. There is no single secular canonical sense of what it is to do the good, for the goods open to persons are multiple and often incompatible. As a consequence, different rules for acting beneficently will conflict.

Consider the comparability of concerns to maximize health and longevity versus interests in living a relatively unrestricted, unfettered existence. One might term this the mountain climber's quandary. At what point does it become irrational to risk one's life in order to be the first to scale a particular face of a mountain in a particular season of the year? Similar questions arise for the individual with chronic obstructive pulmonary disease who wishes to continue to smoke a little, or for the individual with hypertension or diabetes who wishes not to be fully compliant with a physician's suggestions regarding optimal treatment. These cases present a conflict between various liberty and other values and the values of health and longevity.

One finds as well conflicts between interests in health and short-range concerns to avoid anxiety that occur when patients choose to deny that they have a disease and pretend instead that they are well. Such choices lead to the noncompliance of patients with hypertension and similar diseases. One can surely list other conflicts as well. Medicine is an arena of conflicting values and conflicting understandings of values, which in many circumstances appear even to a great number of rational and prudent individuals to be incommensurable. A canonical lexical ordering is not discoverable, at least in general secular terms. It is not possible to disclose a general rational hierarchy of such goods and harms so as to indicate in general what choices should be made by rational and prudent individuals.

This is not to say that a careful analytical examination of choices and their consequences will not be helpful. The more one is able to display for individuals the consequences of their choices, as well as the reasons for and against competing possible choices, the more they will be enabled to choose rationally. One should, as far as possible, play the role of a geographer of values, mapping the various consequences of placing oneself at a particular place in the terrain of possible outcomes. Such a geography will obviously be complicated. One will need to chart a multidimensional world of various possible outcomes tied together by various probabilities. Most choices in medicine do not lead to a particular outcome with a probability of 1. This will itself raise issues in value theory. How does one compare a very high probability of a very disastrous outcome with a low probability of a very disastrous outcome? As the stakes come close to being those of life or severe impairment, the usual assessment of what counts as prudent bets appears to change. Thus, an individual might be willing to accept a one in a thousand chance of being killed in order to earn fifty thousand dollars, but not a nearly 100 percent chance of dying for fifty million dollars outright. However, in terms of straightforward objective calculations, the two "bets" are comparable.

To find one's way around a moral world defined in terms of obligations to respect free choice, and interests in achieving the goods of persons, one will need to attend carefully to these complexities. One will need to recognize in addition that the conflict between concerns for respecting the free choices of individuals and concerns with achieving the best interests of individuals is complicated not only by numerous senses of best interests, but also by the fact that moral concerns are framed within a secular dimension, as well as within numerous particular religious and other moral communities. The moral world fragments into numerous tiers and dimensions. To find one's way around in a multitiered, multi-dimensional moral universe, one will need to fashion as best one can accounts or geographies of the terrain of moral rights and obligations, of right-making and wrong-making conditions. For example, how patients and physicians see the proper trade-off between control of pain and risk of addiction will be influenced by their particular views of the character of the good life and of rational choice. Though it will be impossible to fashion general uncontested geographies of moral relations in many cases, some guidance still will be better than none.

For this reason it is often useful to indicate the basis for claims regarding rights and obligations, or regarding the rightness or wrongness of actions, by making reference to the morality of mutual respect and the moralities of welfare. This distinction itself is a complicated one, since various senses of well-being constitute our notions of welfare or best interests. Further, one should note that customary distinctions may not be justifiable, at least in some areas. For example, the principle of beneficence places concerns with liberty as a good under the rubric of beneficence. The principle of permission concerns the rights of individuals to choose freely even when that freedom is directed not to valuing freedom but to trading liberties for other goods. Finally, the morality by which we can collaborate peaceably with moral strangers contrasts with those contexts where we live our concrete moral lives informed by particular religious and/or other metaphysical and ideological understandings that provide us with a concrete portrait of the good life (e.g., as a politically liberal Methodist).

The morality that binds moral strangers is contentless in being committed to no particular ranking of values, thin theory of the good, or vision of proper action. Because the morality of moral strangers derives the only common secular moral authority from the agreement of those who collaborate, it does have content-full moral implications (e.g., one may not use competent individuals as living organ donors without their permission). But these implications follow from the centrality of this practice that can with general moral authority bind moral strangers in common endeavors: persons are to be used only with and through their permission. It is not that this practice is good, worthwhile, or to be valued. Even peaceable action is not to be valued. At least, no such judgments can be justified in general secular moral terms. It is rather that those who step into this practice can still share a discourse that can bind moral strangers. As members of different moral communities, each will have a community-determined understanding of why it is important, good, useful, or at least tolerable to step within this morality of moral strangers. But the morality itself makes no judgments regarding values. It instead sustains a fabric of moral authority, which derives from bare consent.

In the context of general secular morality, the principle of permission always trumps the principle of beneficence. The obligation to do to others their good is a fundamental one. However, the obligation as such is unspecified. Only in concrete contexts can one determine the extent of the obligation, and how to rank or order the various goods that can be at stake. The general obligation not to use force without authority has a greater governance in that it can be clearly disclosed in particular situations without an appeal to anything more than the understanding of the individual who would be subject to such force. The principle of permission can be applied without an appeal to the principle of beneficence. Thus, the right not to be treated without one's consent gains applicability at once from the wishes of the possible patient. It is enough for that individual to refuse in order to indicate that the authority of the physician does not extend to that patient. In contrast, the claim that one should out of beneficence support someone's health care costs rather than give the funds to friends for a trip to Nevada to gamble, eat well, and drink, requires an agreement about the relative importance of these goods. In a general secular context, the principle of beneficence requires an appeal to the principle of permission in order to be applied.

Rights to do with oneself or with consenting others as one chooses are not only fundamental, but function without an appeal to a particular social understanding. This is because such rights are justified in terms of the perspective of moral agents in general, that is, persons who do not share a common moral vision but who resolve disputes authoritatively without recourse to force. It is this perspective that justifies the morality of mutual respect. No particular view of the good life is presupposed. It is for this reason that obligations of forbearance do not require a community's concurrence, but only the dissent of the individuals about to be subjected to force. The individual's refusal is sufficient to give applicability.

Of course, things are never simple: particular notions of particular boundaries support special rights to forbearance and often will require the particular understandings of particular communities. Still, there will remain a general range of actions where the reasonable presumption will be that the persons about to be subjected to force must first be asked for permission, because they cannot be presumed already to have consented (e.g., before performing a colonoscopy to screen for polyps). Yet there are exceptions (e.g., giving emergency medical help that must be supplied at once to avoid loss of life, mutilation, or compromise of bodily or psychological function). Standing community assumptions can defeat these general presuppositions. And there are limits. To walk up in a line of persons receiving vaccination and proffer one's arm can be enough to constitute consent, but not enough to create a right to the vaccination. In short, a difference between duties of forbearance and beneficence derives from the fact that another's refusal is sufficient to create an obligation of forbearance, whereas mutual agreement is required for a concrete duty of beneficence. Rights and obligations to forbearance as a result possess a greater absoluteness, a greater capacity to hold in a transcultural fashion, than do rights and obligations to beneficence. It is easier to establish the claim that women have a right to refuse an abortion than that they have a right to have others pay for that abortion, should they not be able to afford one.

It is in this sense that negative rights and duties are stronger than positive rights and duties. Thus, the duty not to kill and the right not to be killed without one's permission are stronger than the duty to provide resources to save a life or the right to have access to resources in order to save one's life. For example, the duty of physicians not to kill patients in human experimentation has greater secular generality than the duty to provide sufficient care and resources in order to save lives, at least when persons meet as moral strangers. One need not know anything about another in order to know that one may not kill that person without permission. However, when one meets a stranger in need of expensive health care to whom one has not made prior commitments, the issue is not as clear. (How much trouble are we obliged to go to?) General negative duties based on mutual respect hold without any special agreements or understandings. Thus, one has prima facie obligations to obtain consent for the use of human subjects in medical research, wherever one might be engaged in such endeavors. Contractual obligations to provide a good or service (e.g., expensive medical treatment) can be just as strong, but they require a special prior understanding (an insurance policy, a health maintenance organization's commitment to certain levels of care, and so on). Consider the difference between a physician vacationing at a posh hotel in Calcutta and the same physician on duty in an HMO. While in the hotel the physician has a less defined set of obligations (if any) to patients in need in Calcutta than to patients *of* the HMO. Obligations of beneficence appear to depend on special contractual agreements and/or special interpretations of the principle *of* beneficence. The principle of beneficence, it should be noted, also generates negative duties, as well as a duty not to harm others, even with their permission. Thus, the principle of nonmalevolence requires that physicians ought not to provide treatment they judge to be harmful, unless liberty or other interests of the patient outbalance the harm. These negative duties will have the same imprecision as positive duties of beneficence.

## Conflicting rights and obligations

It will not be possible to decide in many circumstances which obligation or right ought to be honored. If one is attempting to distribute goods in a beneficent fashion in health care, how does one rank the needs of individuals in end-stage renal failure versus the needs of those who have a high likelihood of being exposed to measles or polio and have not been vaccinated? How does one compare the claims of preventive medicine and specialty care medicine, or claims of those wishing to treat cancer and those wishing to treat arthritis or the everyday aches and pains of living? Ranking obligations of beneficence is, as has already been acknowledged, extremely difficult.

Further, what does one do in cases where there appear to be conflicts of promises and contracts? One must, as carefully as possible, draw out the geography and genealogy of rights and obligations to see which likely have precedence. Consider the case of a couple seeking counsel regarding the possibility of having a second child with an inherited recessive birth defect. If tests indicate that in fact the husband cannot have been the father of the first child, what obligation does the physician have, and to whom, and why, regarding a disclosure concerning the risks of future children with the disease for that couple? May the physician simply reassure the couple that they have no risk of having another child with the disease and privately inform the woman of the risks of further reproduction with the lover who sired the child in question? Must the physician inform the husband that he is not the father of the first child, especially if raising the child will entail special financial, psychological, and social costs?

One of the ways to approach an answer would be to determine with whom the physician has the primary patient–physician relationship, the husband or the wife. Such priority could perhaps be determined by who contacted the physician first, or by who is paying the physician. Is the matter changed in any way if the physician is reimbursed through a third party? What if the third party is the government? Must one instead turn to the ways in which the physician agreed initially to aid the couple? At times, perhaps, the physician will be lucky enough to have the relationship so structured that the lines of obligation are clear. Perhaps the physician is the woman's obstetrician, with primary obligations to her. In other cases, the issue may be irresolvable. Important moral questions may have at times no clear secular resolution.

## TEYKU: the opacity of some problems to moral reasoning

Classic examples of moral quandaries can be found in Western religious texts. Consider Judas Maccabaeus's solution to the disposition of the stones of the altar of the Second Temple, which had been desecrated by the Hellenic Syrians during their occupation. Since he could not determine how to dispose of these holy but desecrated stones, he ordered them to be placed on the Temple hill until a prophet should come and indicate what should be done with them (1 Maccabees 4:44–46). The unresolved problem in moral reasoning has been underscored in the Talmudic notion of TEYKU. TEYKU problems involve disputes regarding the law that do not admit of resolution, in that the arguments on either side balance each other. TEYKU problems stand indefinitely in a state of insolubility. Or as some of the mystical literature suggests, Elijah, the herald of the Messiah, will come to solve the TEYKU problems.[27] Which is to say, in concrete moral communities there may be a person in authority who can decide how to resolve the unclarity. Otherwise, one is left with an appreciation of the fact that some important moral problems may in fact be insoluble, either due to the unclarity of the facts of the situation, or due to unclarities regarding moral principles themselves.

To return to the case of the child with the genetic disease, it may be unclear in principle whether one's obligations of beneficence to the husband or to the wife are stronger. In questions of moral conflict where issues are truly TEYKU, one is surely free to flip a coin, follow one's inclinations, or choose on the basis of prudential self-interest. However, there are often differences in consequences. In such circumstances one should act so as to lose as few goods as possible and to violate as few rights as possible (the satisfaction of rights grounded in mutual respect will have first claim). Since medicine is a discipline practiced in tragic circumstances where all patients die and most suffer illness before death, physicians are often faced with choices where not all rights can be satisfied and surely not all goods realized, and where a definitive and all-encompassing hierarchy of rights and goods cannot be established.

The concept of TEYKU indicates the limits of reason in resolving moral quandaries. At times, it may not be clear what one ought to do. Such unclarity will at times spring from the tensions within morality itself: between the concern to act with authority and to do the good. In most cases, it will be clear that individuals will not have authority to use force to achieve their view of the good against the protests of innocent persons. However, one might ask, what if the existence of a nation or of a corporation such as IBM or Texaco were at stake? Or for that matter the world, or perhaps the cosmos? May one enslave one individual in order to achieve such an important beneficent goal? May one torture *one* unwilling individual to save the cosmos? When does the good at stake become so important as to override the secular notion of a peaceable moral community? Would it be reasonable in secular moral terms to shoot an innocent stranger to save one's family of three? What if one has a family of twelve? What if the lives of a hundred are at stake? Of ten million? Of ten billion? Of a hundred trillion? Such cases, perhaps, are not so much TEYKU as deeply tragic. An individual who violated the morality of permission even for such an important and beneficent good would be blameworthy. If the good at stake is so overwhelming, most would show special mercy and understanding. But one would still need to recognize that a violation of the moral order had occurred. Such limiting cases reveal the limits of secular morality and the guidance it can provide in a world that is always at some tension with moral aspirations and at times deeply opaque to our moral hopes.

The tragic nature of medicine is thus accentuated by conflicting values and moralities. Medicine treats individuals, all of whom will die, some of whom will suffer greatly, in circumstances where medicine can often not postpone death or greatly alleviate suffering. The character of medicine is such that one must often make choices among alternative possibilities of different forms of suffering and death without knowing with certainty what will happen. One may choose to operate in order to save a life only to have the patient die of the anesthesia. One may give antibiotics to a patient only to have the patient develop a life-threatening allergic reaction. The character of the choices physicians must make carries the possibility of leading inexorably to unwanted painful outcomes. In addition, the character of secular morality through which one must make choices regarding approaches to treatment is itself flawed in the sense that the moral obligation to respect persons will often constrain physicians to acquiesce in patients' choices— choices that most likely will lead to the loss of important goods. In medicine, one is recurringly confronted with the loss of goods.

## Notes

1. Hans Reichenbach, *Theory of Probability* (Berkeley: University of California Press, 1949), pp. 470–82.
2. This view of inductive knowledge does make ontological presuppositions in the sense that its deliverances presume a general conceptual structure.
3. Consider the first formulation of the categorical imperative: "Act as though the maxim of your action were by your will to become a universal law of nature." Immanuel Kant, *Foundations of the Metaphysics of Morals*, trans. L. W. Beck (Indianapolis: Bobbs-Merrill, 1976), p. 39; *Grundlegung zur Metaphysik der Sitten*, AK IV 421.
4. G. W. F. Hegel, *Hegel's Philosophy of Right*, trans. T. M. Knox (London: Oxford University Press, 1965), sec. 135.
5. Alasdair MacIntyre, *A Short History of Ethics* (New York: Macmillan, 1973), pp. 190–98.
6. Karen Lebacqz and H. Tristram Engelhardt, Jr., "Suicide," in D. J. Horan and D. Mall (eds.), *Death, Dying, and Euthanasia* (Washington, D.C.: University Publications, 1977), pp. 669–705; Kant, *Grundlegung*, pp. 421–22.

    On a number of intertwining grounds Kant rejects the notion that one may consent to one's own suicide. Six merit special mention. They all cluster around Kant's very content-full understanding of morality, which has much more content than a general secular ethics can justify. First, personhood for Kant is not the source of moral authority but the object of a concrete duty: "a man is still obligated to preserve his life simply because he is a person and must therefore recognize a duty to himself (and a strict one at that)." *The Metaphysical Principles of Virtue: Part II of the Metaphysics of Morals,* trans. James Ellington (Indianapolis: Bobbs-Merrill, 1964), p. 83, AK VI 422. Second, according to Kant, in disposing of oneself one disvalues oneself. "If he disposes over himself, he treats his value as that of a beast. He who so behaves, who has no respect for human nature and makes a thing of himself, becomes for everyone an object of freewill. . . . Suicide is not abominable and inadmissible because life should be highly prized. . . . But the rule of morality does not admit of it under any condition because it degrades human nature below the level of animal nature and so destroys it." *Lectures on Ethics,* trans. L. Infield (Indianapolis: Hackett, 1963), p. 152. Third, suicide is forbidden because in self-destruction one undermines existence, the condition for doing one's duties. "In taking his life he does not preserve his person; he disposes of his person and not of its attendant circumstances; he robs himself of his person. This is contrary to the highest duty we have towards ourselves, for it annuls the condition of all other duties." *Lectures on Ethics,* p. 149. Fourth, Kant regards the decision to commit suicide as willing the nonexistence of the moral community. "To destroy the subject of morality in his own person is tantamount to obliterating from the world . . . the very existence of morality itself." *Metaphysical Principles of Virtue,* p. 83, AK VI 422. Kant conflates having a moral community and the existence of a moral community with deciding to will or act against its very notion or existence. He conflates a material condition with a formal contradiction. Kant likely also sees a contradiction in rationally deciding no longer to be rational. Fifth, Kant also holds the choice to commit suicide to be a contradiction of impulses. "One immediately sees a contradiction in a system of nature whose law would be to destroy life by the feeling whose special office is to impel the improvement of life. In this case it would not exist as nature; hence that maxim cannot obtain as a law of nature, and thus it wholly contradicts the supreme principle of all duty." *Foundations of the Metaphysics of Morals,* trans. L. W. Beck (Indianapolis: Bobbs-Merrill, 1976), p. 40, AK IV 423. Sixth, because of duties to self, suicide occurs without permission, so that it counts as self-murder. "That man ought to have the authorization to withdraw himself from all obligation, i.e., to be free to act as if no authorization at all were required for this withdrawal, involves a contradiction." *Metaphysical Principles of Virtue,* p. 83, AK VI 422. All of these considerations by Kant cluster around his account of determinism and moral choice. Kant excludes from autonomous choice all decisions made on the basis of an inclination. For a choice to be free, it must follow from the character of what it is to be a rational agent. Autonomous choices are not those we wish to make (i.e., to which we are inclined), but those that follow from the moral law. Kant is committed to this position because of his solution to the problem of freedom and determinism.

In summary, Kant's position on suicide makes it very clear that his account of autonomy is in opposition to the principle of permission. His account of autonomy is embedded in a particular solution to the problem of free will versus determinism. Unnoticed by Kant, this account incorporates into his notion of rational action numerous positive understandings of acting rationally. As a result, for Kant choices regarding one's self are not different from choices regarding others. Kant therefore concludes that anyone who would commit suicide would have no principle basis for not murdering others. "If man were on every occasion master of his own life, he would be master of the lives of others." *Lectures on Ethics*, p. 151.

7. Marcus Singer, "On Duties to Oneself," *Ethics* 69 (1959): 202–11.
8. Kant, *Grundlegung*, p. 424.
9. Kant, *Foundations of the Metaphysics of Morals*, p. 41; *Grundlegung*, p. 423.
10. Kant, *Foundations*, p. 423.
11. Kant generally does not see concerns of prudence to be truly ethical concerns. Indeed, he would not have acknowledged concerns with beneficence to be merely concerns of prudence.
12. What is offered here is an account of the basis of retributive justice. However, the account is in a negative form. It shows simply when certain actions of punishment would not be forbidden. This understanding reveals similarities between ancient Germanic and Kantian theories of retributive justice. The criminal who acts against the very fabric of the moral community repudiates mutual respect, rejects the law of the peaceable community, and becomes an outlaw who can neither appeal to the peaceable community for protection nor consistently protest the use of defensive or punitive force.
13. In such a circumstance one would be left with only an emotive account of ethics. Charles L. Stevenson, *Facts and Values* (New Haven: Yale University Press, 1967), especially pp. 1–70.
14. For Hume, sympathy is the powerful principle in human nature that produces our moral sentiments. As he argues:

> Now justice is a moral virtue, merely because it has that tendency to the good of mankind; and, indeed, is nothing but an artificial invention to that purpose. The same may be said of allegiance, of the laws of nature, of modesty, and of good manners. All these are mere human contrivances for the interest of society. And since there is a very strong sentiment of morals, which in all nations, and all ages, has attended them, we must allow, that the reflecting on the tendency of characters and mental qualities, is sufficient to give us the sentiments of approbation and blame. Now as the means to an end can only be agreeable, where the end is agreeable; and as the good of society, where our own interest is not concerned or that of our friends, please only by sympathy: It follows, that sympathy is the source of the esteem, which we pay to all the artificial virtues.

David Hume, *A Treatise of Human Nature* (Oxford: Clarendon Press, 1964), p. 577.
15. For an analysis of the biblical notion of covenant, see George E. Mendenhall, *The Tenth Generation* (Baltimore: Johns Hopkins University Press, 1973), and Diebert R. Hillers, *Covenant: The History of a Biblical Idea* (Baltimore: Johns Hopkins University Press, 1969).
16. Alasdair MacIntyre, *Three Rival Versions of Moral Enquiry* (Notre Dame, Ind.: University of Notre Dame Press, 1990), pp. 182–83.
17. Kant lays out the conditions of possible experience in general as that which is presupposed for the possibility of encountering objects. See *Critique of Pure Reason*, A158 = B197.
18. Eugen Bleuler defined autism as "this detachment from reality, together with the relative as absolute predominance of the inner life." *Dementia Praecox or the Group of Schizophrenias*, trans. Joseph Zinkin (New York: International Universities Press,

1950), p. 63. The reality of which Bleuler speaks is the one we must acknowledge for common endeavors. This reality has similarities with Kant's phenomenal reality. Bleuler holds that there is no way to demonstrate the existence of external reality in itself. One must take it for granted as the necessary condition for the possibility of intersubjective activities.

> But for the existence of the external world there are no proofs. That the table which we see has existence is only an assumption, even if of practical necessity. But if I once take for granted the existence of the table, and that of other people, and the external world, then this table can be shown to these other people. Like myself they can perceive it with their senses. *The reality of the physical world is therefore uncertain and relative, that is, it is not possible to prove it, but on the other hand, it is objectively demonstrable.*

Eugen Bleuler, *Textbook of Psychiatry* (New York: Macmillan, 1936), p. 8.

19. For the list of Kant's categories, see *Critique of Pure Reason*, A80 = B106.

20. Traditionally, for Christians the matter is quite different. In order to determine what ought concretely to be done, one turns not to an anonymous perspective, but to One Who is surpassingly personal. The relationship to morality is then not one of reasons and principles, but of grace, love, and living substance.

21. I distinguish here between deontological principles as those that cannot be reduced to interests in the achievement of particular goods or values, and teleological principles that can be so reduced. As John Rawls indicates, "A deontological theory [is] one that either does not specify the good independently from the right, or does not interpret the right as maximizing the good." *A Theory of Justice* (Cambridge, Mass.: Harvard University Press, 1971), p. 30. In contrast, within teleological theories, "the good is defined independently from the right, and then the right is defined as that which maximizes the good." Ibid., p. 24.

22. "Justitia est constans et perpetua voluntas jus suum cuique tribuens." Flavius Petrus Sabbatius Justinianus, *The Institutes of Justinian,* trans. Thomas C. Sandars (1922; repr. Westport, Conn.: Greenwood Press, 1970), 1.1, p. 5.

23. Robert Nozick, *Anarchy, State, and Utopia* (New York: Basic Books, 1974).

24. From the point of view of those inside of intact moral communities, their appreciation of morality is rarely seen simply as created or as the product of an agreement, though when seen from the outside the authority of such peaceable moral communities will be seen as springing from various genre of implicit or tacit consent.

25. H. T. Engelhardt, Jr., and Michele Malloy, "Suicide and Assisting Suicide: A Critique of Legal Sanctions." *Southwestern Law Review* 36 (Nov. 1982): 1003–37.

26. As Hegel would point out, this abstract conflict is mediated in the concrete ethical life, within *Sittlichkeit;* see *The Philosophy of Right*. For a contemporary exploration of these issues, see H. T. Engelhardt, Jr., and Terry Pinkard, *Hegel Reconsidered: Beyond Metaphysics and the Authoritarian State* (Dordrecht: Kluwer, 1994). Still, regarded abstractly, there is an antinomy in practical reason between the duties of autonomy and the duties of beneficence.

27. Louis Jacobs, *TEYKU* (New York: Cornwall Books, 1981).

# 4

## The Context of Health Care:
## Persons, Possessions, and States

Not all humans are equal. Health care confronts individuals of apparently widely divergent capacities: competent adults, mentally retarded adults, children, infants, and fetuses. These differences are the bases of morally relevant inequalities. Competent adults have a moral position not held by fetuses or infants. In addition, there are social inequalities among competent adults as a consequence of disparities in social power and wealth. The wealthy may buy goods and services not available to the less fortunate. These inequalities reach into the central fabric of health care decisions. Finally, special questions of equality and inequality among persons are raised by the existence of states. States frequently claim special moral prerogatives to regulate health care and to distribute health care resources. To come to terms with bioethical issues as they arise for patients and health care professionals within the embrace of states, one will need to know how seriously one ought to take the various moral and financial inequalities among humans and the supposed moral prerogatives of states.

### The special place of persons

Persons, not humans, are special—at least if all one has is general secular morality. Morally competent humans have a central moral standing not possessed by human fetuses or even young children. It is important to understand the nature of these inequalities in some detail, for physicians and medical scientists intervene

135

in numerous ways in the lives of adult humans, children, infants, fetuses, and laboratory mice. There is a need to understand in some detail why secular obligations of respect or of beneficence vary according to the moral status of the entities involved. It is also essential to recognize the agonizing gulf between general secular morality and the content-full canonical morality.

Only persons write or read books on philosophy. It is persons who are the constituents of the secular moral community. Only persons are concerned about moral arguments and can be convinced by them. Only persons can make agreements and convey authority to common projects through their concurrence. To choose, to make an agreement, is to be conscious of what one is doing. It requires the self-reflexivity of self-consciousness. Otherwise, there is a happening, not a doing. The choice to agree or disagree, to convey authority or to withhold authority, requires an appreciation of this basic difference involved in choosing. In this sparse sense, the self-consciousness of a moral agent must be rational. It must include seeing the *ratio*, the relationship between choices and their consequences or significance. Further, for an agent to be an authority giver or withholder, rather than merely an effect of forces, it must be regarded as imputable, not simply as caused. It must be free. Finally, the agent must be a *moral* agent, possessing moral rationality in the sense of being able to appreciate that actions can be tied to a sense of blameworthiness or praiseworthiness. An agent may reject all senses of blameworthiness or praiseworthiness. But, to be an entity with which one could in principle resolve or fail to resolve a moral controversy, such an entity must be able to understand choices as able to be morally regarded. This concept of person (as well as of moral competence) is thus defined wholly within the practice of moral strangers resolving moral controversies by agreement, by giving and withholding morally authoritative permission.[1]

The very notion of a general secular moral community presumes a community of entities who are self-conscious, rational, free to choose, and in possession of a sense of moral concern. It is only when such entities are interested in understanding when they or others are acting in a blameworthy or praiseworthy fashion that moral discourse is possible. Insofar as they wish to collaborate with common authority, they create the peaceable moral community. The peaceable secular moral community exists both actually and potentially. It exists potentially as a moral standpoint in terms of which self-conscious rational entities can speak of blame and praise, and through permission and agreement understand themselves bound by their mutual authority. It is an intellectual standpoint in the sense that once one understands what it means justly to blame or praise, one realizes that such activities presuppose entities worthy of blame and praise, beings that could have abided by the conditions for the possibility of a peaceable community. In terms of this possible moral standpoint, persons can at any time in any place conceive of themselves as belonging to, and being bound by the rules of the peaceable community. An examination of moral language reveals a very important intellectual standpoint: the *mundus intelligibilis* of Kant.[2]

Competent physicians and patients of any rational species anywhere in the cosmos can participate in this moral standpoint, which embraces not only the staff and patients of terrestrial hospitals, but also ships' doctors and their patients on flying saucers, should such exist. It is in terms of this intellectual possibility or standpoint[3] that persons can think of themselves as free; as Kant put it, "we think of ourselves as free, we transport ourselves into the intelligible world as members of it and know the autonomy of the will together with its consequence, morality."[4] When persons deport themselves in accord with the notion of the peaceable community, they can come to live in a general secular moral community with real boundaries, so that those persons that act against the peaceable community are by their own choices moral outlaws of all and any particular moral community. In summary, all persons can envisage *the notion of the peaceable (moral) community*. Insofar as they act in accord with this notion, despite inequalities in intelligence, power, and wealth, they participate with others in *the peaceable (moral) community* (i.e., defined by general secular pluralist morality). They also have the opportunity of fashioning with consenting others a *particular* moral community (defined in addition by its particular view of the good life).

By examining the foundations of morals, Kant offered what could be termed the grammar of a major dimension of human thought. It is impossible for rational, self-reflective entities coherently to construe themselves except as moral, responsible entities. To protest that they ought to have been treated differently, to blame themselves or others for their actions, is to enter the domain of moral discourse, and at once to place all entities that engage in that discourse in a special light. The self-reflective character of our thought commits us to certain ways of regarding ourselves and similar entities.

We cannot coherently regard ourselves solely as caused to do the things we do. An entity that asserted that all of its assertions were simply caused, not rationally affirmed, would at that point abandon any truth claim to that assertion regarding determinism. It would be holding, instead, that it had been caused to make that statement (i.e., "I am determined to say 'I am determined,' not because it is true, but because I am caused to say 'I am determined' ")[5] independently of considered reflections or rational bases for assent. The domain of morality in which we think of ourselves as free and responsible is inescapable. On the other hand, there is, as Kant correctly recognizes, the domain of scientific and empirical reflections where we do indeed treat the world as determined. This second standpoint is as equally unavoidable as the moral point of view.[6] Persons are put in the peculiar predicament of having to conceive of themselves as determined, caused to do the things they do, while on the other hand conceiving of themselves and other persons as moral entities, worthy of blame and praise and therefore free.[7] Kant's insight is the recognition that this understanding does not require a metaphysical claim (i.e., a claim about transcendent realities). There are rather two major and inescapable domains of human reasoning and experience. Our very notion of ourselves as self-conscious, rational entities requires us to treat ourselves as moral agents, as persons, and as knowers, not just as caused entities.

As a consequence, persons stand out as possessing a special importance for moral discussions. It is such entities who have secular moral rights to forbearance, because they can deny permission. Competent moral agents are those who participate in moral controversies and can resolve them by agreement. But they may also disagree. Because the fabric of authoritative cooperation among moral strangers depends on agreement, moral agents may not be used without their permission. This moral concern, it must be stressed, focuses *not on humans but on persons*. That an entity belongs to a particular species is not important in general secular moral terms unless that membership results in that entity's being in fact a competent moral agent.

This should be fairly clear if one reflects on what it means to be a human, a member of a particular species. First, one must note that there have in fact been a number of human species within the genus *Homo*. To identify an entity as a member of *Homo sapiens* is to place it in a particular taxonomic locus. The genus *Homo* shares with the genera *Ramapithecus* and *Australopithecus* membership in the family Hominidae of the suborder Anthropoidea of the order primates of the class Mammalia. In identifying an entity as human, one indicates that it possesses primate characteristics, such as long limbs and pentadactyl hands and feet, along with an increased specialization of the nervous system. With the family Hominidae one would want to note the development of tool-making capacities, language, and other symbol-related or -dependent behavior. If one were in the future to possess a galactic study of rational species in the cosmos, one might find that numerous, somewhat different biological bases lead to the ability to use tools, language, and abstract symbols. Humans would be distinguished primarily through their biological peculiarities as primates. But insofar as one characterizes the peculiar anatomical structures and physiological capacities of humans as primates, one advances a set of biological characteristics that take on moral significance only insofar as they support the special characteristics of persons, namely, their capacity to play a role in the moral community. It is because members of *Homo sapiens* are usually self-conscious, rational, and possess a moral sense that being a human is so significant—or at least in general secular moral terms.

As angels, not to mention science-fictional speculation regarding rational, self-conscious entities on other planets, indicate, not all persons need be humans. What distinguishes persons is their capacity to be self-conscious, rational, and concerned with worthiness of blame and praise. The possibility of such entities grounds the possibility of the moral community. It offers us a way of reflecting on the rightness and wrongness of actions and the worthiness or unworthiness of actors. On the other hand, not all humans are persons. Not all humans are self-conscious, rational, and able to conceive of the possibility of blaming and praising. Fetuses, infants, the profoundly mentally retarded, and the hopelessly co-matose provide examples of human nonpersons. They are members of the human species but do not in and of themselves have standing in the secular moral community. Such entities cannot blame or praise or be worthy of blame or praise; they cannot make promises, contracts, or agree to an understanding of benefi-cence. They are not prime participants in the secular moral endeavor. Only persons have that status.

Because of interest in a general secular morality, persons as moral agents claim moral centrality. One speaks of persons in order to identify entities one can with warrant blame and praise, which can themselves blame and praise, and which can as a result play a role in the core of the moral life.

In summary, in order to engage in moral discourse, in order to participate in moral controversies and be able to refuse or agree to resolve them, such entities need to reflect on themselves; they must be *self-conscious*. They need in addition to be able to conceive of rules of action for themselves and others in order to envisage the possibility of the moral community. They need to be *rational* be-ings. That rationality must include an understanding of the notion of worthiness of blame and praise: *a minimal moral sense*. Sociopaths would cease to be moral agents (persons in the moral sense) only if they lost the capacity to understand blameworthiness to the point that they could not blame those who might injure them. Finally, they must be able to think of themselves as free. These four characteristics of self-consciousness, rationality, moral sense, and freedom iden-tify those entities capable of moral discourse, capable of creating and sustaining a moral community, capable of giving permission. The principle of permission and its elaboration in the secular morality of mutual respect applies only to such beings. It concerns only persons, which notion (i.e., being a person) is defined in terms of the ability to enter into this practice of resolving moral controversies through agreement. The morality of autonomy is the morality of persons.

For this reason it is nonsensical in general secular terms to speak of respecting the autonomy of fetuses, infants, or profoundly retarded adults, who have never been rational. There is no autonomy to affront.[8] Treating such entities without regard for that which they do not possess, and never have possessed, despoils them of nothing that can have general secular moral standing. They fall outside of the inner sanctum of secular morality. Just as this concern with respecting moral agents excludes some humans, it may in fact include nonhuman persons. Although failing to treat a fetus or an infant as a person in the strict sense shows no disrespect in general secular terms to that fetus or infant, to fail to treat a peaceable extraterrestrial moral agent without such respect would be to act im-morally in a fundamental fashion. It would mean that one had acted against the very possibility of *the* peaceable community.

What is important, in general secular terms, is not our membership in the species *Homo sapiens* as such. It is the fact that we are persons. This distinction between persons and humans will have important consequences for the ways in which one secular bioethics will treat human personal life versus merely human biological life. Once these distinctions are clearly drawn, one can disclose some of the conceptual confusions that have plagued the secular moral debates regarding abortion.[9] These debates have in part failed to recognize the character and limitation of general secular bioethics. In general secular bioethics, one will not be interested in when human life begins, unless one is attempting to determine when the human species evolved. Life, it would appear, is an unbroken continuum some four billion years old, and human life a phenomenon some two million years or more old. In general secular morality, one is, or should be, concerned with determining when in human ontogeny humans become persons.

The world of general secular morality is quite different from what many think or hope it might be. It presses a fundamental reappraisal of what moral strangers can share as moral judgments regarding the status of fetuses, infants, the profoundly mentally retarded, and the severely brain-damaged. The full implications of secular morality in this area are yet to be realized in health care policy, and if they are, they will lead to an even further disengagement from traditional Judeo-Christian morality and the bioethics it supports. Still, it is worth underscoring that general secular moral reflections about the status of persons do not deny traditional religious or metaphysical views regarding the existence of the soul or its entrance into the human body at some particular point in human ontogeny. Nor do they deny the special value of life that can be appreciated in the religious perspective. After all, general secular morality discloses only what can be shared by moral strangers. In disclosing this, it reveals the painful gulf between general secular and content-full morality that should bind moral friends.

### A bias in favor of persons?

Although this approach simplifies matters by freeing discussions of metaphysical quandaries, it begets some special problems and puzzles of its own. First, one might object that this way of construing morality creates an unduly person-centered or person-oriented construal of the moral universe. What of animals, trees, and the environment? Doesn't the universe count more than persons? However, it is only persons who reflect on the world and fashion accounts of its meaning. Moreover, when they meet as moral strangers, they meet without grace or special moral insight. They meet with the possibility of acting authoritatively in the associations they create. Such moral collaboration places persons as the foundation of the secular moral fabric. Only persons can give permission and convey authority. This orientation marks the morality of welfare and social sympathies as well. It is persons who can define for themselves their own best interests. They can take account of themselves and their own concern, even if it is to value themselves less than other persons or even nonpersonal things. Still, it is they who judge themselves and others when they make any calculations made under the principle of beneficence. But for nonpersonal organisms, others must choose on their behalf. Others must determine for those entities what their best interests are. Competent adult patients can define their own best interests in their own terms. It is surely the case that rational individuals can make mistakes in such calculations. But their judgments about themselves have a cardinal significance in that persons can decide for themselves the ordering of costs and benefits that they wish to take seriously for their lives, including the risk they are willing to run.

Persons are in this very important sense self-legislating. This is not the case in the instance of infants, the profoundly mentally retarded, and other individuals who cannot determine for themselves their own hierarchy of costs and benefits. Persons must choose for them. Since such choices will depend on the moral sense of the chooser, and since there is not one univocal moral sense to deliver in general secular terms a single authoritative hierarchy of costs and benefits, nonpersons will have imposed on their destiny the particular choices of particular persons or communities of persons. Both the morality of mutual respect and the morality of welfare and mutual sympathies are inextricably person-centered.

When persons must calculate in general secular moral terms the weight that should be given to the interests of persons versus nonpersons, the position of persons is central. Persons can appreciate harm and good, pleasure and pain, in intricate, reflective fashions. It would appear likely that rational beings after careful reflection will hold that it is better first to test pain-killing substances on animals, even when such experiments will mean suffering for the animals, rather than to move directly to trials on persons. The greater good of persons will likely be seen as having a higher position in the hierarchy of goods than the good of experimental animals who will need to be sacrificed in the course of medical experimentation and research. The hunter will decide that the delectation of the hunt, and the refined recall of the kill in sharing stories with other hunters, is a good that outweighs the value of the life of the animal to be hunted and killed. The same will be the case for those individuals who plan to raise animals for food. There will be none but persons to adjudicate which goods are to be given greater weight. Animals who are not persons, and will never be persons, are thus placed inescapably within the bounds of a person-centered morality, dominated by person-centered interests.

One should note that prejudice in favor of persons is not like prejudice in favor of humans versus other possible rational species. If, for instance, we ever needed to compare the competing claims of human and extraterrestrial persons, we could never morally use them merely as means, as one may use animals.

## Potentiality and probability

What is one in general secular terms to make of those entities such as embryos, fetuses, and infants who will with great likelihood develop into moral agents?[10] It might appear that one could in such circumstances appeal to a notion of potentiality in order to argue that since fetuses and children are potential persons, they must *eo ipso* be accorded the rights and standing of persons. This argument cannot succeed. Nor was it the argument that took center stage for the theologians of the Western Middle Ages who approached the issue of abortion within the compass of an Aristotelian world view and its commitment to a doctrine of potentiality. St. Thomas Aquinas argued that taking the life of an early fetus did not involve the evil of murder, even though the early fetus or embryo was potentially a person.[11] This view was reflected in Roman Catholic theology and in canon law from the time of St. Thomas until 1869, except for a brief period between 1588 and 1591.[12] During that time, taking the life of an early fetus or embryo was held usually to be a mortal sin, somewhat analogous to the mortal sin of contraception.[13] However, for the Roman Catholics it did not involve the sin of murder.[14] The Roman Catholic church saw a sort of human life preceding the human life of persons.

Undoubtedly, the language of potentiality is itself misleading. It is often taken to suggest that an $X$ that is a potential $Y$ already in some mysterious fashion possesses the being and significance of $Y$. But, if $X$ is a potential $Y$, it follows that $X$ is not a $Y$. If fetuses are potential persons, it follows clearly that fetuses are not persons. As a consequence, $X$ does not have the actual rights of $Y$, but only potentially has the rights of $Y$. If fetuses are only potential persons, they do not have the rights of persons. To take an example from S. I. Benn, if $X$ is a potential president, it follows from that fact alone that $X$ does not yet have the rights and prerogatives of an actual president.[15] It is therefore perhaps better to speak not of $X$'s being a potential $Y$ but rather of its having a certain probability of developing into a $Y$. One can then assign a probability value to that outcome.

It follows from these considerations that, though one is bound in general secular morality to respect persons in the sense of forbearing from unconsented-to harms against them and acting to aid them in achieving their good, it does not follow that one is bound to increase the number of such entities to which one has obligations. One might very well come to the reasonable conclusion that there are sufficient persons already to whom one has obligations. Reflections on the consequences of overpopulation may lead to the rational conclusion that it would be best if there were not more persons to feed, care, and respect. In addition, one might conclude that persons of a particular sort, such as those with severe physical or mental impairments, would create particularly severe moral obligations, which would be best avoided. In such circumstances, one might decide to prevent such obligations from coming into existence by using abortion. That zygotes, embryos, or fetuses are human rather than simian or canine would be, in general secular morality, of significance primarily in terms of one's interest in having more humans rather than more individuals of a different species. One might indeed imagine circumstances in which persons would be very pleased regarding the high likelihood that a whooping crane embryo would go to term, but disvalue the likelihood that a human embryo (e.g., one likely to lead to the birth of a severely deformed infant) would go to term. General secular morality focuses on the centrality of persons. But general secular morality is not able to disclose the canonical value of human biological life.

The value of animal life, which is not the life of a person, must be determined by persons. Since in the case of such animals there is no person to respect, the issue is the value that must be imputed to the entity and the regard one must give to the pains and pleasures of that animal. The more an organism's life is characterized not just by sensations but by consciousness of objects and goals, the more one can plausibly hold that the organism's life has value for it. The more an organism can direct itself with appreciation and subtlety to certain objects and away from others, the more plausible it is that it has an inner life with some prereflective anticipations of values, as values are understood by self-conscious free agents. Adult higher mammals enjoy their lives, pursue their pleasures, and avoid sufferings in elaborate and complex ways. Their lives in this very straightforward sense can have both value and disvalue for them. But since they are not persons, they cannot require that they be respected. They cannot as persons set moral limits to the extent to which they can be used by others. They cannot refuse with moral authority to participate in the results of comparisons of the value of being beneficent to them versus being beneficent to other entities. They are not members of the moral community but are rather objects of its beneficence. The value of an animal's quality of life is thus set by persons in two senses. First, if that animal has no developed conscious life, persons may find little intrinsic value in such life and the predominant value may be the value that the life has as an object for persons. Second, even if the animal has an inward life that in a prereflective sense has a value for that organism, persons must still compare that value with other competing values.

It is for these reasons in general secular morality that the value of zygotes, embryos, and fetuses is to be primarily understood in terms of the values they have for actual persons. Zygotes, fetuses, and embryos do not have the rich inward life of adult mammals. Thus, if the zygote promises to be the long-awaited child of a couple that has been struggling for years to have another child, it is very likely to be highly valued by the couple and by all who are sympathetic with the would-be parents' hopes. On the other hand, if the zygote is in an unwed graduate student for whom the pregnancy would mean a major disruption of study plans, the zygote will likely be highly disvalued by her and by all who are sympathetic with her plans. Or if the zygote has a trisomy of chromosome 21, not only will the parents and those close to the parents likely disvalue the zygote, but so will many in society, who will need to participate in the costs of raising a defective child, should the pregnancy be uninterrupted. Some value is likely to be assigned to the zygote simply because it is human. However, one must remember that the sentience of a zygote, embryo, or fetus is much less than that of an adult mammal. One might still be concerned that the processes of abortion might cause pain to the fetus. But one must remember that the level of obligations one has to a fetus, *ceteris paribus* in general secular morality, is the same as one would have to an animal with a similar level of sensory motor integration and perception. For suffering to occur, there must be some fairly well developed frontal lobe connections to allow the entity not only to experience the pain, but to recognize the pain over time as a noxious quale that must be avoided.[16] The capacities of fetuses give no indication that they approach the capacities for suffering of adult mammals. As a result, one's general secular moral obligations will simply be to make sure that the good pursued, such as avoiding the birth of a Down's syndrome child, outweighs the evil of the pain to the animal organism to be killed. The evil of abortion cannot be further appreciated in general secular terms.

### An excursus regarding animals

Some have found this assessment of the comparative standing of persons and animals to be improper. Robert Nozick speaks critically of the maxim "Utilitarianism for animals, Kantianism for people."[17] He speaks against the notion that "human beings may not be used or sacrificed for the benefit of others; animals may be used or sacrificed for the benefit of other people or animals, *only* if those benefits are greater than the loss inflicted."[18] This position derives from the Kantian moral contrast between persons and things. This moral position, in fact, is presupposed by the industry of medical research and investigation that first studies drugs through animal models. Persons are then used only after animal research has indicated that such a course is relatively safe. Such an approach is Kantian. Persons for Kant are subjects whose actions can be imputed.[19] Some may find grounds for suspecting that certain nonhuman mammals are indeed not only animals but also persons as we are. If they are persons, then we owe them respect. However, the behavior of all but perhaps the higher apes shows no evidence of a rational appreciation of the moral life. Persons are moral agents, entities that can with justification be blamed and praised. They are entities that can be a part of the community of ends. In contrast, nonpersons are not worthy of blame or praise. As a consequence, "Every object of free choice that itself lacks freedom is therefore called a thing (*res corporalis*)."[20] For Kant one has duties to persons, and duties to persons regarding things, including animals.[21] This duty to other persons regarding animals is constituted in part out of an obligation to act in ways that will enhance and protect moral sensibilities. Thus, Kant argues that "tender feelings toward dumb animals develop humane feelings toward mankind."[22] Certain rules or practices of kindness and consideration toward animals may generally work to the advantage of moral practices established to secure respect for persons.

One must go beyond the Kantian perspective. One ought, in addition to recognizing duties to other persons regarding animals, recognize as well a duty directly to regard the pain and suffering of animals. One has duties of beneficence to animals, even if the strongest of such duties are usually simply negative ones of beneficence, that is, duties of nonmaleficence. Although one does not have duties of respect to animals because they fall outside the bounds of the morality of mutual respect, one has duties to them in terms of the morality of welfare and mutual sympathies. Here it might be useful to distinguish between persons, who ought to be objects of respect, and animals, which ought to be objects of beneficent regard. We owe to persons both respect and beneficent regard. To animals we owe only beneficent regard.

One can in part take account of Nozick's concerns and bring them within a reformed Kantian viewpoint in which one recognizes that it is only persons who are the judges of the relative significance of harms and benefits and the objects of our respect and beneficent regard, while animals are the objects of our beneficent regard. When persons are dealing with entities that are not persons, it is persons who will make the judgment regarding the significance of any exchanges of harms and benefits. It is persons who fashion actual moral communities with their particular moral senses, histories, and practices. Nonpersonal animals do not constitute moral communities, nor do they have a history. Moreover, there is no border of respect protecting organisms that are not persons. Animals are protected rather through a web of moral concerns regarding welfare and sympathies, which also protects persons. Respect of persons springs from the concern to act in ways in which persons can be justified as praiseworthy or blameworthy. In contrast, in general secular morality, caring for animals springs from the concern to have a world that maximizes welfare and sustains a web of sympathies.

This web of sympathies binds us most tightly to those animals with which we can actually share sympathies—usually mammals and perhaps some birds. These bonds of sympathy are most fully drawn between humans and mature primates. This web of sympathies justifies a wide range of beneficent action. They strongly support practices of kindness and sympathy toward animals. However, they do not foreclose the raising of animals for meat or hunting, much less for use in research, whether it be medical research in the strict sense or even the testing of the safety of new cosmetics. Indeed, as all accounts of goods, values, and sympathies, the concerns and sympathies associated with the use of animals must be placed within particular moral visions, accounts, and traditions that will all be equally acceptable from the perspective of secular morality as long as they are not malevolent.

In summary, animals are protected by the morality of beneficence. Since the range of the capacity for animals to suffer or achieve pleasure and fulfillment spans from that of the higher primates to that of one-cell animals, the strength of claims to beneficence will vary dramatically. The more animals can feel, suffer, and have affection for others, the more concerns of beneficence toward them plausibly have weight. On the other hand, concerns of beneficence with respect to roaches and amoebas are much less substantial than that to primates. Still, capriciously to torment a paramecium for sport, if one were of the opinion that paramecia can be the subjects of torment, would be an act against the morality of beneficence (unless one held that a proportionate good was to be realized in or through that sport) as a violation of the subprinciple of nonmalevolence. Malevolently to torture a paramecium is in general secular morality more clearly wrong than hunting great apes for sport, if one holds that the balance of goods is positive. One would need also to classify animals in terms of whether they are (1) owned by individuals or groups, or (2) unowned, in order to be clear with respect to one's duties regarding them.

### Infants, the profoundly retarded, and social senses of "person"

These conclusions raise a third and very vexatious difficulty. What is one in general secular terms to make of the status of infants, the profoundly mentally retarded, and those who are suffering from very advanced stages of Alzheimer's disease? Such entities are not persons in any strict sense. Yet many are concerned to accord such entities many of the rights normally possessed by adult persons. In the case of rules against maiming and injuring but not killing fetuses and infants, one can advance a justification of our moral concerns in terms of respect for the future person that such a fetus or infant will likely become. Even if one does not accord special moral rights to merely possible persons (e.g., the persons who could be conceived were the readers of this volume engaged in fruitful sexual congress rather than philosophical study) or probable persons (e.g., zygotes that would develop into competent persons, were the women carrying them not to seek an abortion in order to complete their graduate studies in modernist theology), one can still understand the status of fetuses in the light of the standing of future actual persons. Future persons can have the standing of actual persons who we know will in the future exist. If one plants a bomb in the foundations of a grammar school with a timing device so that it will explode in fifteen years, one is intending to murder actual persons who will in the future exist. So, too, if one injures a fetus or infant, but does not kill it, one then sets in train a series of events that will in fact injure a future actual person.[23] In these terms one can secure certain moral protections (and moral grounds for the legal protection) of infants.

Considerations of beneficence protect animals, which are not persons, against being tortured uselessly, whether or not they are human. Considerations of the contingent rights of future persons protect entities that will become persons from being maimed. They do not protect infants, the profoundly mentally retarded, or those suffering from advanced Alzheimer's disease from being killed painlessly at nonmalevolent whim. Once more one is brought to face the painful contrast between general secular morality and content-full canonical morality. When one seeks general secular grounds to justify practices through which infants, the profoundly mentally retarded, and the very senile might in general secular terms be assigned a portion of the rights possessed by entities who are persons strictly, including rights not to be killed nonmalevolently at whim, one is given little satisfaction.

Perhaps, one develops a suggestion from Kant regarding the need to support practices that will, in general, lead to the protection of persons. To find grounds for protecting such individuals, one will need to look at the justification for certain social practices in terms of their importance for persons so as to justify for a particular community a social role one might term "being a person for social considerations." Since this sense of person cannot be justified in terms of the basic grammar of morality (i.e., because such entities do not have intrinsic moral standing through being moral agents), one will need rather to justify a social sense of person in terms of the usefulness of the practice of treating certain entities as if they were persons. If such a practice can be justified, one will have, in addition to a strict sense of persons as moral agents, a social sense of persons justified in terms of various utilitarian and other consequentialist considerations.

Most societies in fact have such a social sense of person, which is usually assigned to human beings at birth, or at some time soon after birth. In ancient Greek law an infant could be exposed with impunity up to the time it would be admitted into the family through a special ceremony, the *amphidromia*. After that the infant had standing and received some of the major rights of persons.[24] In other societies the line has been less clearly drawn. To take one example, a strain of Jewish interpretation holds that the death of an infant during the first thirty days of life should be considered a miscarriage. Such an infant had not yet been given the full standing of children that have survived beyond this point.[25] Even in contemporary American society one can note a greater acceptance of the cessation of treatment for severely defective newborns than would be the case with young children fully socialized within the role of child. It is as if the full conveying of social personhood does not occur immediately for many neonates.[26] As we shall see in chapter 6, this informal distinction between the treatment accorded to neonates versus other children has come under critical attack.[27] An understanding of embryos and infants as having a moral status equivalent to adult competent persons depends on a moral insight that cannot be grasped in general secular moral terms.

Still, in general secular terms a protected social role might be justified, or at least established within particular formal or informal agreements, for embryos, infants, and others in terms of (1) the role's supporting important virtues such as sympathy and care for human life, especially when human life is fragile and defenseless. In addition, with respect to infants and other humans ex utero there is the advantage of (2) the role's offering a protection against the uncertainties as to when exactly humans become persons strictly, as well as protecting persons during various vicissitudes of competence and incompetence, while (3) in addition securing the important practice of child-rearing through which humans develop as persons in the strict sense.

Since the assigning of some of the status of person as a social role on the basis of such concerns must be justified in terms of utilitarian and consequentialist considerations, the justifications will be somewhat different, depending on whether the practice concerns (1) humans who in the past were persons in the strict sense (e.g., individuals now suffering from severe Alzheimer's disease); (2) humans who are likely to become persons and have been brought within a social role giving them special social standing (e.g., infants); and (3) those humans who have not, and never will, become persons in the strict sense (e.g., the profoundly mentally retarded). There are likely to be somewhat different justifications for the particular protections afforded in each instance. In each case, one will find in different secular societies different special social roles justified in terms of different considerations around which agreements are framed. Finally, particular communities will always have the secular moral right to act peaceably on their own moral visions of rights and duties, benefits and harms.

### Severely defective newborns: weakening the protections of the social role of person

These practices of assigning rights to humans who are not persons will not be absolute, at least in general secular terms. When a set of considerations shows that suspending the practice will achieve a greater balance of benefits over harms, such an exception will be justified. One may want to require that such exceptions be generated only in terms of well-drawn rules for weighing the goods at stake. One may even require what is tantamount to a conflict between practices. In any event, there are secular moral grounds for not imposing undue financial and psychological burdens on those who are persons in the strict sense. First and foremost, persons have a general secular moral right, unless they have agreed otherwise, to act at liberty as long as they are not employing unconsented-to force against innocent persons, or imposing unjustifiable suffering on innocent organisms. Parents who judge that a defective newborn should either be allowed painlessly to die (or even be aided in dying painlessly!) do not offend against either of these two constraints. Practices of protecting the interests of parents and guardians who are persons in the strict sense will at times conflict with practices of imposing duties on parents and guardians through fashioning a social role of persons for children. The obligations imposed by others in terms of the social roles of persons will thus at best in general secular morality be prima facie obligations, which can in particular circumstances be set aside.

The concrete nature of the web of beneficence that characterizes the obligations to provide welfare, including care for severely defective newborns, is determined within a particular community through the judgments of those who are persons in a strict sense. There is likely to be a range of sentiments in this matter. In addition, there is the issue of the extent to which families have committed themselves to the social constraints of the surrounding society so as to oblige them to treat infants against the choices of the family members. The more one takes seriously the failure of general secular morality to establish a canonical content-full content, the more one will need to take seriously the moral standing of the family as a free association of persons who have rights to judge regarding those of its members who are not persons in the strict sense. To force parents to treat a severely defective newborn may indeed count as imposing by force and without justification a particular view of beneficence.

The geography of obligations may shift as a family accepts an infant and assigns it the role of child within an established set of practices, perhaps by accepting social support in various fashions for the child's care and development. The infant may then acquire a moral standing within both the family and the larger society. It is before that point that matters are not clear. For example, under what circumstances might parents insist not only that they will not provide for the care of a severely defective infant, but moreover that that infant should (1) be allowed to die, or (2) be killed. We will return to these matters in the discussion of severely defective newborns in chapter 6.

Here it is enough to note that defective newborns confront us with one of the many implications of a content-less secular morality. They offer us an example of entities that may have a special attenuated standing as social persons, in contrast with those infants who have been brought fully within the social role of person. Infants, the profoundly mentally retarded, and the severely senile may accrue a moral standing through which they possess rights but no duties. There will be justifications in certain circumstances for withdrawing elements of that moral standing. For a rather clear example, discussed further in chapter 6, hopelessly severely senile individuals are often accorded the standing of social persons in an attenuated sense very similar to that of severely defective newborns, for whom also nothing but basic nursing care need morally be provided. Finally, the hopelessly comatose, and anencephalic infants, appear to have a moral standing, which imposes even fewer general secular moral obligations.

## Being a person: in the strict sense and in various social senses

In anticipation one can make the following distinctions for general secular morality and for its bioethics. There is a sense of person as moral agent, which I have termed being a person in the strict sense (one might call this person$_1$), which contrasts with a social sense of person to whom nearly the full rights of persons strictly are accorded, as in the case of young children (person$_2$). A social sense of person is also accorded to individuals who are no longer, but who once were, persons, and who are still capable of some minimal interactions (person₃), and a social sense of person is also assigned as in the case of the very severely and profoundly retarded and demented who never were and will never be persons in the strict sense (person₄). Some may also assign a social sense of person to certain severely damaged humans (i.e., severely and permanently comatose humans), who cannot interact in even minimal social roles (persons₅). The seeming unitary notion of humans as persons or moral agents fragments.

There is unavoidably a major distinction to be drawn between persons who are moral agents and persons to whom the rights of moral agents are imputed. One can blame and praise adult competent patients, for they hold both rights and duties. They are moral agents. One cannot blame and praise infants. They are bearers of rights, but not of duties. One can at best act in their best interests. Persons who are moral agents have rights that are integral to the very character of general secular morality. The rights of persons in a social sense are created by particular communities. In addition, there are real distinctions between the moral standing of humans that can at least play a social role and those who cannot play such roles (e.g., the permanently comatose, or anencephalic children). These distinctions reflect a geography of moral presuppositions already well in place. Moreover, this geography of moral presuppositions accords with what can be justified in these areas in general secular terms. Still, none of these considerations speaks against particular moral communities establishing, within their own associations (which may include facilities for the provision of health care), the recognition that embryos, infants, and the senile have a moral dignity they share with competent adult persons.

These conclusions are not forwarded in order to weaken the status of children or infants. The very opposite is the intention. The goal has been to provide the strongest grounds, justifiable in terms of general secular arguments, for the moral standing of humans. It is because a careful examination of the practice of secular morality reveals a central importance for persons in the strict sense, but not for humans as such, that one is forced to elaborate secondary social senses of person in the attempt to account for and perhaps to justify the moral standing of infants, the profoundly mentally retarded, and the senile, as one finds this even in the predominant secular moral traditions of the West. Still, it is disquieting that the strongest rights claims that can be advanced in favor of humans who are not persons in the strict sense can in general secular terms be at best appreciated in consequentialist, if not indeed on utilitarian, considerations established by particular formal or informal agreements.

These conclusions do not represent an assault on those who are not persons in the strict sense. The circumstances reflect the limits of secular philosophical reasoning. Only some of our moral convictions can be justified within general secular morality. One should be pleased (perhaps, indeed, *relieved*) that the arguments available at least support strong deontological rights for persons in the strict sense.

### Sleeping persons and the problem of embodiment

There is yet another major puzzle to face. What are we to make of the status of sleeping individuals? If being a person depends on being a moral agent, and if one does not have a metaphysical doctrine of the soul to explain where persons go when they are asleep, what is the secular moral standing of a sleeping person?[28] Do personhood and its rights go away while one sleeps? This puzzle can be answered without metaphysical assumptions concerning souls or similar substances by appealing to an analysis of what it means to be a human person possessing moral claims within a community of moral strangers. This analysis depends on two cardinal considerations. Either one should dispel the puzzle sufficiently to give sleeping human persons a standing tantamount to those who are persons strictly: (1) the manner in which human moral agents present themselves as spatiotemporal beings, and (2) the conditions necessary to derive morally authoritative collaboration from spatiotemporally extended moral agents.

The first point concerns what it means to be an embodied person. Persons do not appear to themselves as discontinuous.

Minds that are finite, spatiotemporal, and sensibly perceiving span spatial and temporal extensions as a part of their very being.[29] Their embodiment is their spatially and temporally extended place in this world. What one can mean by a person in such circumstances cannot be an unbroken godlike continuity of self-consciousness. Rather it is a self-consciousness, as a recurring integration of experiences spanning discontinuities, all of which is in a spatially extended body. Such beings must sew together their various episodes of wakefulness and presence within a single identity.

Alfred Schutz explores this in his phenomenological account of going to sleep and awakening.[30] The very sense of a human person includes its unifying various temporally discontinuous episodes into one life. Of course these attempts can fail in whole or in part. John Hughlings Jackson was one of the first clearly to recognize that our integration as one continuous person is a precarious and difficult undertaking.[31] It is indeed an accomplishment. To be a finite, spatiotemporal, sensibly intuiting person is to have the task of constantly constituting temporally diverse experiences as one's own. This point is appreciated by Kant in his characterizations of persons or subjects in terms of the transcendental unity of apperception, the capacity to unite experiences under an "I think," to make a diverse manifold of experiences one's own. Those experiences that one can unite within one's unity of apperception under one's "I think," one's "I experience," become one's own. Persons, if they are not free of spatiotemporal extension (e.g., angels), will be subject to the challenge of integrating various experiences as their own. Sleep constitutes simply one example of such a challenge for integration.

An embodied self-consciousness, which achieves an integration in an experienced self-identity, can be understood without an appeal to the metaphysical presuppositions or the doctrine of potentiality required for those who hold that, since fetuses are potential persons, they should count as persons. The question is not whether to regard an entity that has never shown the capacities of a person, as if it were a person. The question is rather how to regard an entity that intermittently shows the full capacities of a moral agent. How should one regard that entity during periods of time when it is not showing those capacities, but when one holds it still has those capacities (i.e., its brain is fully intact) and will again in the future exercise them?

To begin with, there is a difference in kind in general secular morality between a body that *is* someone's body, and a body that *may become* someone's body. There is a difference in kind between knowing who is sleeping, in the case of an adult competent human, and knowing who a fetus will be. Once a person is a moral agent, a biography is gathered under that agency. With respect to a zygote, fetus, or even young infant, one does not yet know, at least within a general secular perspective, the person who will come to be "in" (or perhaps better, in, through, and with) that body.[32] With respect to a sleeping person, one knows whose body it is. One knows who is there. The person will again awaken, make judgments, and answer questions. The body with the full capacities of sensory motor integration that are the physical expression of a person's life is that person incarnate in the world. The body's capacities are the capacities of a particular person. One must distinguish between the potentiality to *become* a person and the potentialities *of* a person.

The point is that the very meaning of a spatiotemporally extended, sensibly intuiting person involves the spanning of, and the integration of, temporal extension. Our very experience of ourselves is as moral agents extended over time. Further, as an element of the practice of secular morality, the provision of moral authorization and its withholding presupposes moral agents as possessing an identity over time so that they can make agreements that continue to bind themselves and their interlocutors. This is not a consequentialist consideration. Rather, it is an acknowledgment of the reality of secular morality as it exists in contracts, the market, and the practices of limited democracy. In such practices whatever persons can unite under an "I self-consciously do this" (e.g., "I make this contract", "I do this act") is united to them as moral agents existing over time and in particular places. The existence of such persons in such practices is not set aside by temporal discontinuities across which their identity can reasonably be presumed to span by the "plausible" reporting of "I have done these acts."

Moral reality is social and has priority. Even scientific and metaphysical reality presupposes persons as entities (1) who can negotiate and agree regarding epistemic values and considerations and (2) who regard themselves as choosing among considerations and not as simply determined by causes. As a consequence, puzzles regarding personal identity are placed in terms of secular morality, which morality discloses the centrality of persons as those who establish the presuppositions for resolving such debates. Since the framing of all scientific and metaphysical accounts presupposes agreements to establish *ceteris paribus* conditions and the like, the practice of resolving controversies by agreement is always prior to any secular scientific or metaphysical puzzle regarding the status of those engaged in such controversies. All puzzles regarding the identity of persons with their pasts and with their futures[33] will need to be resolved, insofar as this is possible with moral authority, with and through agreements.

   This practice affirms the identity of human persons over time: individuals live in a world in which they experience themselves as moral agents over time and make agreements spanning their discontinuity. Problems for personal identity that arise from amnesia, split brains, and malfunctioning transporters on starships can be regarded either as TEYKU, deficient cases, or puzzles that can be resolved by agreement. One can envisage various science-fictional worlds in which persons flit in and out of existence and must fashion special practices to accommodate. So, too, one might think of how angels may be in agreement or disagreement, one with the other. However this might be, this is not our world as we experience it. Outside of and despite such puzzles, the practice of secular morality (e.g., secular morality with the centrality of the principle of permission) is the practice within which moral, metaphysical, and scientific issues arise and are negotiated. It carries with it the centrality of the spatiotemporally embodied negotiators that constitute it. It is they who over time must agree about the significance of any puzzles regarding personal identity and their bearing on contracts, market agreements, and assumptions of responsibility. In agreeing, they act over time with others who act and agree over time.

   Recognizing humans as spatiotemporally extended entities will mean regarding their intact embodiment as them, as long as that embodiment maintains the capacities that are the physical substrata of moral agents within the practice of secular morality. Humans, unlike angels in some accounts, do not live in the now of eternity. Humans as persons reach out of the present to the future, and the present of persons is found bound by past agreements and actions. As long as persons can unite their biographies across discontinuities of inattention and sleep under an "I have thought *X*" and "I have done *Y*," persons can treat themselves and think of themselves as extended over time. There will be revisions in their biographies on the basis of further empirical information (e.g., "Did I really do that? Well, it seems so."). But there will be no revision of the basic standpoint in terms of which biographies are revised in order to take account of persons as extended over time and across discontinuities of attention and consciousness. The standpoint for judging is one that regards itself as able to determine which pasts are truly its own and which are falsely ascribed.

The permission and agreements of humans necessarily span time and discontinuities in consciousness. Human moral agents are the kinds of entities that make agreements, including agreements that bind over time. If interruptions in attention or self-consciousness shattered the identity of persons, so that one could kill people as soon as they fell asleep without having this count as murder, the minimum moral fabric of the peaceable moral community would be set aside. Given the discontinuous nature of finite, spatiotemporal moral agents, if their usual discontinuities legitimated unconsented-to killings, this would make the moral community impossible. Or to restate the matter, if one allowed moral agents to exterminate without permission those innocent moral agents whose attention had temporarily waned, had become temporarily obtunded, or had fallen asleep, one would be allowing actions against the possibility of resolving moral controversies with the authority of permission, one would be acting against the possibility of a peaceable moral community. Since spatiotemporally extended persons fashion moral actions over time and across moments of attention and of sleep, they are the sort of entity that must be treated with respect (i.e., not used without their permission) even when they are inattentive or sleeping.

These considerations do not lead one to the position that one is morally obliged (i.e., in general secular moral terms) to bring moral agents into existence so as to continue actual moral communities through history. Such an argument would turn the moral community into one goal among many possible goals to be pursued. This would require an appeal to a particular concrete ranking of goals. Rather, what has been advanced is a sketch of conditions integral to the notion of a secular moral community of spatiotemporally extended persons. Insofar as we think of ourselves as moral agents, we must think of ourselves as acting across the discontinuities of self-consciousness that occur during sleep, anesthesia, and inattention. As long as our brains, our embodiments, remain intact, we can be perceived as existing over these discontinuities. This presumption of continuity is a condition for understanding ourselves within the practice of secular morality. One cannot respect other moral agents, while willing to destroy their unique place in the world, their embodiment. To will to destroy the embodiment of actual persons is to will to act against the very morality of mutual respect.

## Owning people, animals, and things

John Locke remarks, "it seems to some a very great difficulty how any one should ever come to have a property in any thing."[34] The difficulty is bringing things, objects, within a conceptual framework of possessions and possessors. Any particular system for speaking of possessors and possessions appears to be culturally relative and open to challenge by members of other communities with other conventions. One might think here of the conflict between the European immigrants to America and the various Indian tribes with regard to rights to the land and the use of the land. The resolution of the status of property claims is central to understanding moral justifications for the allocation of scarce resources, in particular, the allocation of scarce health care resources. One must understand who owns what and in what way in order to account for the rights of physicians, patients, and national and international political authorities when they allocate medical resources.

Some have held that property rights exist only within a particular civil society. Others such as Immanuel Kant hold that it is only within a civil society that full property rights are realized.[35] Still others such as William Blackstone (1723–80), while recognizing the right to private property, acknowledge the diversity of theories regarding the origin of property rights. Blackstone notes the view of Hugo Grotius that property rights are founded on a tacit assent of all mankind that the first occupant of a piece of territory should become the owner; in contrast, Locke holds that there is no such implied assent, but that possession derives from bodily labor transforming a mere thing into a possession.[36] As will become clear, I side with Locke, but in a Hegelian reinterpretation. Labor transforms an object from a mere object to an entity fashioned by the ideas and will of a person. By rendering the object a product, it is brought into the sphere of persons and their claims.

Hegel notes that we take possession of things (1) by directly grasping them physically, (2) by forming them, and (3) by marking them as our own. His paradigm example of possession is our possession of ourselves.[37] There is nothing we more fully grasp or use than ourselves. We render things ours by eating and devouring them, by incorporating them into ourselves. They become part of us, such that an action against them is an action against us as persons and therefore a violation of the morality of mutual respect. One's body, one's talents, and one's abilities are similarly primordially one's own. As Locke argues, "Every man has a property in his own person: this nobody has any right to but himself."[38] One's body must be respected as one's person, for the morality of mutual respect secures one's possession of one's self, and one's claims against others who would use one's body or one's talents without one's permission. Again, since spatiotemporally extended persons must occupy a space, to act against that space or place is to act against such persons themselves. Such unconsented-to interference would be an action against the very notion of mutual respect and the peaceable community.

The problem is how to account for other forms of ownership. This problem of justifying ownership is as much a problem for societies as for individuals. How does one or a society own tools or land? Owning other persons would appear to be more easily accounted for than the ownership of things. If others own themselves as we own ourselves, they can then convey title over themselves in whole or in part. Ownership rights in the services of other persons are based directly on permission, the morality of mutual respect. Respecting other persons includes respecting the right they have to agree to perform certain services and to enter into special relationships of obedience. Thus, one can understand the rights of the military to order its personnel (or at least those who have joined voluntarily) to submit to certain medical procedures. Indeed, various forms of indentured servitude, from joining the Marines or the French Foreign Legion, to entering a monastery, getting married, or, in some instances, becoming an intern in a hospital, can be understood as transferring to others in whole or in part rights one held over oneself. Certain special status relationships of being chattel can perhaps be understood in this way. Children, insofar as they remain unemancipated and fail to go out and support themselves on their own, by remaining in their parents' hands are in part owned (or, to recall the ancient Roman usage, they remain *in manu* or in parental *potestas*). In return for parental support, they can be seen as falling under the moral control and partial ownership of their parents. This holds only if the children or wards are persons in the strict sense, and can be regarded as having implicitly engaged in such an exchange of support for obedience. As a result, these considerations apply to the status of older children and adolescents, but not infants and very young children.

In short, indentured servitude provides the clearest example of notionally translucent ownership. One can own others insofar as they have freely transformed themselves into property. Their status as property is clearly understandable, because both owner and owned are persons, minds. That which is owned is not a thing in need of translation into conceptual terms in order to be appreciated as property. It is rather mind meeting mind to create a fabric of obligations. Again, examples of such indentured servitude abound. One might think here of the medical student who agrees to serve in the armed forces in return for financial support while studying medicine.

One also owns what one produces. One might think here of both animals and young children. Insofar as they are the products of the ingenuity or energies of persons, they can be possessions. There are, however, special obligations to animals by virtue of the morality of beneficence that do not exist with regard to things. Such considerations, as well as the fact that young children will become persons, limit the extent to which parents have ownership rights over their young children. However, these limits will be very weak, at least insofar as they can be made out in general secular terms, with regard to ownership rights in human zygotes, embryos, and fetuses that will not be allowed to develop into persons, or with regard to lower vertebrates, where there is very little sentience. For example, it would appear very plausible, within the bounds of general secular morality, that plants, microbes, and human zygotes can be fashioned as products, and be bought and sold as if they were simply things. In contrast, strong claims of ownership would cease, as children become persons and *sui juris,* self-possessing. At the point that an entity becomes self-conscious, the morality of permission or mutual respect would alienate the property rights of the parents over their children. New rights over the children could then come into being as the children submit to parental authority in exchange for parental support.

As to things, one need not hold that the matter itself is owned. Instead, one need claim only that the form imposed as an extension of the producer's self is a person's possession in a thing. As Hegel argues, in the ownership of things the right to the forbearance of others with respect to one's own body is extended to objects one has formed. Taking possession of objects is a process of fashioning them, forming them, transforming them in the image and likeness of one's ideas and according to one's will. It is a way of incorporating things within one's own will. In this fashion, one increases the sphere of one's embodiment and extends the border of one's rights to the forbearance of others. Things that are un-transformed by others one may freely transform for one's own purposes. Things on which one has impressed with one's ideas become property. Insofar as one does not abandon them, they may not be altered or changed by others without one's permission, except insofar as the others have some prior right in those objects. Insofar as animals are not self-conscious, and not able to regard themselves as under the moral law, they are in part things to be used, refashioned, or simply taken. As Gaius remarks in his *Institutes,* "if we capture a wild animal, a bird or a fish, what we so capture becomes ours forthwith and is held to remain ours so long as it is kept in our control."[39]

This approach offers an account of ownership. What I have suggested is that, insofar as an individual enters into a thing, refashions it, remolds it, and, to follow Locke's suggestion, mingles labor with the object, the object becomes a possession. As Locke characterizes this, "Whatsoever then he removes out of the state that nature hath provided, and left it in, he hath mixed his labour with, and joined to it something that is his own, and thereby makes it his property."[40] One's possessions would only reflect the outcomes of one's labor, or the labor of others received as gifts or in trade. Possession reflects the extension of one's own self or the selves of others. To seize, alter, or change without permission a substantial extension of a person is to act against that person. The morality of permission, of mutual respect, protects not only one's immediate embodiment but also the objects in which one embodies one's will and energies. Embodiment in this world does not stop at the edges of one's body, but is extended into other objects marked by one's will. Rights of ownership are derived from the funda-mental right not to be interfered with without one's permission. Once such a right is acquired, it may then be freely sold or otherwise transferred to others, just as persons may transfer rights over themselves.

This approach will go a good way toward accounting for the ownership of products. The nagging difficulty is what to say of the brute matter itself, the stuff out of which the products are fashioned. As untransformed, it would appear impossible to be owned by any particular person. At most, it would appear possible to speak of the rights of all to have equal access to that matter. Similar considerations have led individuals such as Thomas Paine,[41] Ogilvie,[42] and Baruch Brody,[43] to hold that taxes are justified as a collection of rent on the matter used in products. One may also be able to collect taxes on the basis of the so-called Lockean proviso. Locke qualifies the right of individuals to take possession of material through mixing their labor with it through the provision that there must still be "enough, and as good, left in common for others."[44] Taxes may then be collected as a payment due others for the extent to which an individual claiming a particular property through labor diminishes the opportunities of others to claim similar property through labor.

Such taxation should occur at an international level because objects cannot be fully possessed either by individuals or by particular groups of individuals (such as particular societies or states). Matter itself, the dimension of things that remains after the things are transformed into products, remains in common ownership. However, that common ownership is not the common ownership of a particular society or state, but of persons generally. This leads then to another difficulty. Taxes should not just be collected at an international level, but perhaps at an intergalactic level. However, those on other planets are plausibly due less since terrestrial use deprives them of little if anything on the basis of the Lockean proviso, unless intergalactic travel with ease becomes a reality. Such a tax would need to reflect a fair rent on such material, apart from considerations of its status as a product. This tax might also include special costs to others of the non-availability of the material for their use. Unquestionably, there would be much to clarify and to dispute with regard to setting tax rates. Nations would have no particular claim to being the proper tax collectors on such a general rent due on land. Here my view contrasts with that of Baruch Brody, who has argued for a negative income tax distributed on a national basis.[45] One would need to establish why nations would have a claim on the right to collect such a tax, since the tax involves at least the interests of all on the earth. This means that not only individuals and corporations need to pay this tax, but so, too, would governments. Since rent-tax concerns at least the rights of all on the earth, it would best be collected and distributed on an international basis.

Taxation on property in order to reclaim for all their element of ownership in that property will not produce communal goods. Such taxation as rent on property would lead to a duty on the part of the taxing authorities to provide payments to all individuals in a form somewhat similar to a negative income tax. A general taxing agency would lack authority to earmark those resources for particular projects, without the permission of those involved. Picking any particular project to support through such rent-tax would entail endorsing a particular concrete moral sense. The right to international negative income tax payments (and more basically the concerns expressed in the Lockean proviso) ground a right to protection from families that might aggressively reproduce in order to benefit from the international negative income tax (though one might note that individuals would not be due such payments until they become persons in the strict sense).

Reproduction, when it leads to compromising access to resources and the environment, affects the opportunities of others by creating new individuals with entitlements to the negative income tax collected on the rent of material generally. Such reproduction thus constitutes an action against the rights of others for which a tax can be levied to cover such costs. When individuals are not able to pay such a tax, it would be permissible, in general secular terms, to prevent their engaging in further reproduction.

Governments can come into being and gain revenue insofar as they are constituted as the free, common endeavor of their citizens. There is a major difficulty, however. Most, if not all, current governments are coercive beyond the scope that can be justified in general secular terms. Such coercion reaches not only to what individuals do with themselves and consenting others, but to the fruits of their talents and private resources. The question is the extent to which one can presuppose uncoerced consent sufficient to justify broad taxing authority. Since such authority cannot be derived from a particular canonical content-full understanding of justice, the common good, etc., it must be justified through permission. This is a matter to which we will turn shortly. Here it must be observed that there is a difficulty in understanding how governments can justify constraining their citizens toward particular endeavors, including the remittance of funds under the rubric of taxation. Such endeavors are usually redistributive, rather than being a collection of rent on the material of the earth. As a consequence, they require a justification of robust governmental authority. Indeed, the ownership of common funds by multinational corporations would appear to be morally much less suspect than the ownership of common resources by governments, in that governments are much more coercive than most, if not all, corporations, national or multinational. Corporations do not draft individuals into service. It is much easier to change jobs from corporation to corporation than to change citizenship. The consent of stockholders or workers, whether or not represented by unions, appears to be less overborne by threats of force in the case of corporations than in that of governments.

Insofar as one peaceably fashions corporations or governments, agreeing jointly to engage in particular common endeavors, one can produce commonly owned resources that need not be returned to the owners or participants. Common resources can also be produced through the sale by corporations and governments of goods and resources. In communities fully fashioned around thick and intact traditions and practices, persons may effectively cede all they own and themselves to the community as, for example, might occur when joining a monastery and placing oneself fully and absolutely under the authority of the abbot. Under such circumstances, private property ceases, as does the secular moral right to approach the black market (at least if forbidden by the abbot). In large-scale societies that compass numerous moral communities, such uncoerced transfers of authority and property will not occur, but such societies can still have corporate property. Societies in this special sense (which contrasts with communities tightly fashioned around a firm commitment to a common content-full moral vision) may come to possess property, but such corporate ownership will never approach the comprehensiveness of that available to certain communities (e.g., monasteries). In the case of both communities and societies, one must show how individuals joined together to give or produce corporate property. Communal or societal claims to property will always be more involved and tenuous than private claims, in that the cardinal principle of general secular morality is permission. Though private claims to real property are involved, private claims to talents, abilities, and services are straightforward and primordial. The view that communal or societal claims are primary stems from a confusion of the foundations of property rights with the need often in communal fashions to resolve disputes regarding property boundaries, etc. Still, there will be communal resources. Such resources need not be paid out in the form of dividends or negative income tax payments but can be used in various general welfare endeavors such as health care.

In the absence of strictly communal resources, one will only be able to provide a negative income tax payment as a return from rent-tax collections. In fact, as already noted, the land rent-tax (including that amount collected due to the Lockean proviso) would best be collected and distributed on an international basis, since it concerns at least the rights of all on the earth. Special funds for particular social groups and their projects would be available only insofar as one can trace the lineage of corporations or governments to peaceable agreements that produced the resources in question, and thus justify common ownership and common decisions about their use to provide health care, food for the poor, or art for general enjoyment.

There are then three forms of ownership: private, communal or social, and general. Things can be owned privately and communally, insofar as they are transformed into products. Even the use and care of rangeland can give it in part the character of a product, as can finding a precious stone. Its status is as the product of the labor and will of persons. However, since this transformation is never complete, a residual right is held by all persons individually. It is this last sense of ownership that I have termed general ownership.

Communal or societal ownership legitimately comes into existence only insofar as individuals enter into a joint endeavor with a view to creating a common fund for communal undertakings. This joining of resources can take place with moral friends in tightly knit communities or with moral strangers in large-scale societies. In all of this, both communities and large-scale societies gain their secular moral standing and authority from the permission or consent of the individuals who constitute them. The same thing can be said of their resources. To begin with, resources can come into the possession of individuals and associations only through coercion, profit, and charity (i.e., gifts). In the world as we see it, we find both robbers and taxmen taking resources through force, with the latter often having as little secular moral authority as the former. We find greed generating wealth and love providing alms. In the last two cases, in the absence of coercion, the transfer of resources does not face moral difficulties posed by all theft and much taxation. Given these qualifications, one can imagine states legitimately acquiring resources, indeed, wealth.

This is even more the case with respect to nongeographically located associations one can join and leave freely, such as corporations, religions, and unions. For example, an association into which one enters, or from which at majority one does not exit, may require that it be given the authority to tax one's income. One could imagine, for example, the Roman Catholics creating a worldwide taxing authority that would reach out to all members and across national boundaries. Thus, just as the German state collects taxes from members of the Roman Catholic Church on behalf of that entity, this practice could be established worldwide. Such associations in religious communities have a secular moral advantage insofar as (1) they are not geographically located so that those within their territory are not coerced either to join or to move, and (2) they can achieve thick consent around a common moral vision that all participants may be asked to endorse fully as a condition for membership.

In facing health care choices, given the character of property rights, private and general ownership rights will provide individuals with private funds through which they will be at liberty to purchase health care. Communally or socially supported positive rights to health care may come into existence only to the extent that common resources are available, and insofar as a common decision has been made to invest them in the creation of such rights. There should morally thus always be the opportunity to participate privately and communally (as well as socially) in the purchase of health care. Insofar as individuals privately own things, there will always be a right to purchase health care services on a fee-for-service basis and through private insurance, unless all physicians have surrendered their right to sell their services privately and all new physicians follow in their tracks—a material impossibility in the absence of coercion, which would void such agreements.

Finally, nongeographically localized associations should be able to create their own social systems, including health care systems. This conveys a number of advantages. First, the members of the association can clearly and fully give authority for the ways in which the resources are deployed. Second, they can avoid involvement in endeavors they find morally inappropriate and which members of the larger society may wish to undertake. Third, they can have the opportunity of creating a kind of personal law, a law that they carry with them across geographical boundaries. Such law not only could forbid particular activities on the properties owned by the association (e.g., no abortion to be allowed in Roman Catholic hospitals), but could permit visiting members with civil and criminal sanctions if they engaged in particular activities forbidden by the society (e.g., securing an abortion in a hospital not owned by the association).

*Endangered species, the Coliseum, and the bioethics of ecology*

The term bioethics was very likely coined by Van Rensselaer Potter with the goal of addressing broad issues in the relationship between morality and ecology.[46] In closing these brief reflections regarding ownership, it is important to notice that the problems of postmodernity and moral diversity touch home here as well. In the case of endangered species and wilderness areas, there is the problem of how properly to enjoy them and protect them. One might imagine setting them aside like a rare book locked in a vault in a library no one may visit. Yet this is only one among the many ways in which one might understand the proper appreciation of the environment. The management of the Temple Mount in Jerusalem, the pagan temples at Delphi, and the Coliseum at Rome confront similar questions. How does one allow unrestricted access to areas in which many different peoples claim profound interests? Are such areas best managed by allowing as many as much access as possible? Are such areas best managed by preserving them like rare objects, to be seen only on television? Should the Coliseum be maintained as it is, or perhaps restored as it once was? Or better yet, does the Coliseum cry out to be remodeled into a place for rodeos and livestock shows, Texas-style? Who can answer and how?

For that matter, how does one balance interest in various endangered species with concerns to protect human life and realize other human goods? There is no nonarbitrary way to understand how wildernesses should be protected, how endangered species should be preserved, or monuments maintained. We have over time and in different places had remarkably different understandings of the proper way in which to regard nature and artifacts. A suggestion from Hans-Martin Sass is useful here: our stewardship of such areas and objects should be regarded somewhat as our attitudes toward gardens.[47] Here, the diversity is instructive if one considers the differences among French gardens, English gardens, Japanese gardens, and American national parks. Each reflects a particular view of the proper relationship to nature.

Each view has important trade-offs. The attempt to preserve nature in a pristine fashion, in an imagined state before the intrusion of any humans, would likely lead to considerable losses of endangered species.[48] In order to preserve endangered species, one will often need to employ intrusive means. For example, it may be possible to protect certain endangered species only if one sells the rights for a certain number to be shot annually for sport. The income will increase interest in preserving the animals against the vicissitudes of nature and the intrusions of poachers. Unexpectedly for some, it may make perfect sense to affirm "Shoot an animal, save a species!" Or as provocatively, "Buy ivory, save an elephant!"[49] But are such means and attitudes toward the preservation of species acceptable? There are no universal answers.

Since there is no way to discover the correct answers regarding how to treat nature and important places, at least in general secular moral terms, the best that can be done is again to deploy the Lockean proviso and let various market and democratically driven forces set prices to opportunities and losses. For example, if it is not possible to establish uniform solutions about how endangered species or wilderness areas should be managed, it seems plausible to tax those who exploit them whenever that exploitation violates the Lockean proviso. When there is plenty of a species or plenty of a wilderness of a particular sort, the Lockean proviso will not be violated and there will be no ground for special taxation. Also, since governments will have in these or other contexts no greater right to own land than individuals, governments should be subject to a similar international wilderness land and endangered species tax. In such circumstances, if private enterprise outperforms governments in the preservation of wilderness and of species, there will be a major incentive for governments to sell out to private individuals and groups. In the end, one will need to acquiesce in a wide divergence of ecological bioethics.

*Ownership: a summary*

These reflections regarding ownership can be encapsulated in what one may term the principle of ownership. An account of ownership has been given that does not depend on a labor theory or a view of the usefulness of particular notions of property, but on persons as sources of permission and on objects as possessions insofar as they are extensions of persons. Since an appeal to the principle of permission is the only means to resolve moral controversies among moral strangers, it is only in terms of it that either individual or communal property, or entitlements in objects can be understood. This account consequently embeds ownership within the person as a source of authority through permission.

Because the only source of moral authority for moral strangers is permission, it follows that one may not use persons without their permission. But persons are not angelic powers who exist as geometrical points of no size. They exist embodied, extended in time and space, in the world. Thus, on the one hand, to act against a person's embodiment is to act against that person. On the other hand, persons can convey authority over themselves to others and in doing so convey authority over their bodies. This is to say that the foundational element of the principle of ownership (and indeed of the principle of political authority) is the principle of permission. The principle of ownership (as well as the principle of political authority) is a special expression of the principle of permission. In particular, the principle of ownership focuses on the circumstance that persons are not only in their bodies, but in that which they produce.

By holding, working, shaping, and producing objects, those objects are to various degrees made extensions of the persons who hold, work, shape, or produce them. Since such holding, working, shaping, and producing does not exhaust the being of objects, and in addition limits the opportunity of other persons to hold, work, shape, or produce them, one can recast the Lockean proviso so as to disclose a claim to compensation for the unavailability of owned objects. On the one hand, objects can take on the character of being an extension of a person. On the other hand, as one extends oneself into more and more objects, the opportunity of others who had as plausible an initial claim to these objects becomes restricted by those in possession. Hence an international property tax can be justified in terms of the unavailability of material incorporated into product and thus into property. The tax, though, may not be levied on the basis of the value of a product as product. For example, the tax is appropriate on the private or governmental ownership of freshwater lakes, but not of rare and expensive drugs made from common and easily available materials (even with rare materials the tax must reflect only the loss of opportunity costs, not the value added by their finding, refining, etc.).

The principle of ownership is central to understanding the roles of public and private funding of health care, as well as the rights of physicians to exempt themselves from the constraints of national health services. Owning private property, insofar as such private ownership exists, will always permit patients to buy around the established system. So, too, having the right to own one's talents will permit physicians to sell around the constraints of such systems. This can be tendentiously summarized as the basic right of persons to the black market.

---

PRINCIPLE III. THE PRINCIPLE OF OWNERSHIP

Ownership is derived from permission; it is constituted within the morality of mutual respect. One respects claims to ownership insofar as the entity owned has been brought within the sphere of the owner, such that violating that ownership would be a violation of the person of the owner. Ownership claims by societies are just as difficult to establish as those by individuals; indeed, they are more difficult in being more involved.

    i.  Things are owned insofar as they are the products of persons.

    ii.  Animals are owned insofar as they are fed and/or bred by persons, domesticated, and thus rendered like products, or insofar as they are captured. Such ownership rights are limited by the principles of beneficence and nonmalevolence. One may not use animals in ways that one recognizes as malevolent or against the goods one holds one should realize. As always, content-full visions of benevolence will take shape within communities of moral friends.

iii. Young children and human biological organisms are owned by the people who produce them. Ownership rights may be limited not only by the principle of beneficence, but by the circumstance that the young child (or embryo) will become a person.

iv. Persons own themselves. They own other persons insofar as they have agreed to be owned. Such ownership includes contracts for the provision of services and the provision of products, as well as special relationships such as being a member of an army.

A. There are three sorts of property: individual, communal (or societal), and general.

B. Ownership by implied contract: ownership of one's self, ownership rights in one's children and in one's products exist in terms of the morality of mutual respect, apart from any explicit rules. Explicit rules can give clarity and precision to these already existing entitlements. This form of ownership has similarities with what has been classically termed "natural modes of acquiring ownership."[50]

C. Ownership by explicit contract, or consent: such modes of ownership derive from formal, often stylized, procedures for agreeing to provide services or a product. One might think here of stock in a corporation or commodity futures. Though these forms of ownership may presuppose natural modes of ownership, these have been dramatically transformed through highly developed social understandings common to a group of individuals.

D. Justification of the principle: one cannot act against innocent persons in the absence of their permission without acting against the very notion of general secular moral authority and the notion of a secular peaceable community. An action against that property of another is an action against the owner and is a violation of the morality of permission or mutual respect, insofar as persons extend themselves into their possessions. That is, insofar as persons (1) extend themselves to objects by making those objects *theirs* by transforming them into products, (2) acquire rights to the person or body of others through the consent of those persons, or (3) have transferred to them rights in objects or persons, they have property rights that must be respected as a part of general secular morality.

E. Motivation for respect of the principle: one will be moved to respect the principle of ownership insofar as one is interested in the possibility of a peaceable community with common collaborative activities that have general secular moral authority. Moreover, insofar as one embraces the morality of beneficence and wills to others their good, one must will them as well to have that which is theirs. Therefore, the motivation for respecting property rights will be the motivation for respecting the principles of permission and beneficence. However, insofar as some have insufficient resources for their flourishing, there will be a conflict between the beneficent wish that none be deprived of what they own and the beneficent wish that all flourish. Since the principle of permission holds precedent, one should be moved to respect property rights even under such conditions of tension within the principle of beneficence (i.e., between giving to individuals their own property and giving to others what is necessary for life).

F. Public policy implications:

i. Ownership cannot be totally societal. In addition to there being individual private ownership, the things of the world also continue in part to be in the possession of all persons. Further, insofar as persons in particular communities and societies join in common endeavors, there is an opportunity to produce common resources.

ii.   Funds may be collected by taxation to be distributed to all persons on the basis of the common ownership of material in order to compensate all insofar as such possession by some fails to leave like material available for others to possess. Such taxes are best collected internationally and should be paid not only by individuals and corporations, but by governments as well.

iii.  Tax may also be collected as a charge for services.

iv.   There is a fundamental moral right over against societies and governments to participate in the black market. No secular polity has the right to forbid free individuals from exchanging their services or property for the services or property of other free individuals. This basic moral right justifies physicians in establishing private fee-for-service practices alongside any governmentally established health service.

G.  Maxim: Persons own themselves, what they make, and what other persons own and transfer to them; communities and societies have property insofar as persons fashion such communities and societies and then transfer funds to common ownership, or insofar as groups create common wealth. All have a right in the land and material; they must be compensated by owners for its unavailability to all. Therefore: Render to all that to which all have a right; refrain from taking that which belongs to others.

---

## States and their authority

The author of the Hippocratic text *The Law* remarks: "Medicine is the only art which our states have made subject to no penalty save that of dishonor."[51] Though there may have been no criminal sanctions, there were at least some civil remedies available in Greece for malpractice.[52] Currently, there is no question that the practice of medicine is controlled in nearly all important ways through law and regulation. Legal constraints exist with respect to the drugs physicians may prescribe or patients purchase. Heroin is available in the United Kingdom for the control of pain, but not in the United States even in the terminal stages of cancer.[53] The ability of physicians to provide abortion varies from country to country. There are civil remedies through which patients can bring suits against physicians. The practice of medicine now, unlike the time of ancient Greece, is restricted to those licensed by the state. Indeed, even the purchase by hospitals of expensive medical devices, as well as the decision whether to treat defective newborns, has in various fashions been touched by law and governmental regulation. State authority is so ubiquitous and commonplace that its justification is rarely if ever brought into question other than in a piecemeal fashion.

To understand the position of those who live under heavily regulating governments, physicians, other health care workers, and patients must raise fundamental philosophical questions regarding the moral authority of the state. To what extent do states and their representatives have moral authority to regulate the character of health care? Is there any secular moral force to the mass of governmental regulation of health care? Or are violations of law or state regulations at most imprudent, considering the substantial risk of being discovered and punished? Aside from the obvious sanctions of criminal and civil punishment, does any secular moral blameworthiness attach to those who violate the law? May their actions be condemned as immoral? A decent intellectual answer to these very important questions can be secured only by examining the justification of state authority.

Do states possess any authority not possessed by individuals? If states derive their authority directly from the foundations of moral law, they will in fact have no authority beyond that possessed by any particular individual or group of individuals. In that case, states may do only what any individual may do to secure the mutual respect of persons, to support the discharge of obligations of beneficence, and to protect the property rights of individuals and communities. One can at least in part determine the moral authority of any moral regulation by retracing it to the three cardinal principles of secular morality (i.e., permission, beneficence, and ownership). If the regulation failed to show such a lineage, then it may be prudent to obey the rule, but not morally obligatory in secular morality. But what of the wide range of contemporary state interventions?

In bioethics and health care policy, such questions are far from academic. The state dramatically regulates the character of health care. For example, may a state determine hospital charges, even if individuals and particular health insurance groups would be willing to pay more than the statutory established amount. Would it be immoral to accept extra funds under the table for better services just because there is a law against such a practice? What if a government required hospitals to condition physicians' admitting privileges on their accepting only those payments established by governmental policy? Such questions lead us to reviewing the ways in which one might forward an intellectual justification for the moral authority of the state. I will examine ways in which authority for the state has been justified. This review, though somewhat arbitrary and procrustean, allows one to appreciate major justifications for state authority, the strength of their rationales, and the consequence limits on the secular moral authority of the state.

First, one might consider the argument that the authority of the sovereign comes from God. This view has been advanced in Christianity, often citing passages from St. Paul such as "the powers that be are ordained of God" (Romans 13:1). This account was developed in the Western Middle Ages into a doctrine of the two authorities, that of the pope of Rome and that of royal power, with the authority of royal power (in particular, the authority of the Western emperor) coming from God through the pope. One might think here of the

contentions of Innocent III in his October 30, 1198, "Sicut universitatis condi-
tor," where he speaks of the two luminaries in the firmament of authority, the
*pontificalis auctoritas* and the *regalis potestas.*[54] This view of the standing of
secular authority received an interesting articulation in the Council of Constance
of July 6, 1415. Jean Petit, master of the University of Paris, on March 3, 1408,
defended the thesis that it was legitimate to kill a tyrant. The subject of this
contention was the duke of Burgundy, who had killed the duke of Orleans on
November 23, 1407. The council condemned as an error the claim of a right to
kill tyrants.[55] This doctrine of the sovereign ruling by *jure divino* was strongly
contested in the seventeenth and eighteenth centuries.[56] In any event, the doctrine
of the divine right of sovereigns is untenable in secular pluralist contexts. The
premises needed to secure the notion of such a divine right depend on particular
cultural and religious suppositions, which are neither agreed to by all nor open to
a general secular rational justification.

One might hope to establish the authority of a government by showing that it is
in fact acting to achieve the morally canonical concrete understanding of the good
life and moral obligations. One might attempt to justify this view of the good life
and of moral obligations by an appeal to intuitions, case analyses, consequences,
the choice of unbiased observers, the nature of rational moral choice, a notion of
rational choice of proper game-theoretic resolutions of controversies, the character of reality, or the proper role of middle-level principles. If one could by sound
argument establish an account as binding on all, that account, and the state
interventions it would support, would have the authority of reason, the use of
force on its behalf would have rational warrant, and such coercive power would
not act in an alien way but restore us to our proper selves. As chapters 2 and 3
have already shown, it is impossible to establish a particular canonical concrete
secular view of the moral life or morality.

A third option would be to attempt to justify governmental authority by an
appeal to a hypothetical contract (a special variant of the last approach). One
might envisage an intellectual construct somewhat similar to John Rawls's original position,[57] in which he invites us to imagine ourselves establishing general
moral rules as if we were individuals ignorant of our particular advantages in
society. According to Rawls, what we would rationally choose under those
circumstances should count as the basic rules of societal justice. One could then
use those fundamental rules to guide an actual constitutional convention and
legislatures in developing actual laws.[58] The problem here is as before. One must
impute to the hypothetical contractors a particular moral sense in order for them
to rank some primary social goods (e.g., liberty) higher than others. As a consequence, the device of appealing to hypothetical contractors will not authoritatively deliver a canonical concrete and universal understanding of the principles
of justice and of other principles of morality so as to justify the modern state with
its wide range of laws and regulations governing health care. All appeals to

ahistorical consent or ahistorical contracts fail in requiring the acceptance of one among many content-full views of the proper character of such consent or contracts.

To derive political authority, appeal has also been made to the notion of an actual past originary agreement of all to the conventions of government in general or to a particular constitution. One might think here of the political arguments of individuals such as Jean Jacques Rousseau, Thomas Hobbes, and John Locke. Indeed, these philosophical considerations direct many of the presuppositions of American constitutional law, which presumes that the actions of individuals between 1787 and 1790 in adopting the current American Constitution bound all Americans in the future to that constitution and to its processes for enacting, enforcing, and interpreting laws to its means for amendment.[59] Such a view is at least as metaphysical as the appeal to the divine right of sovereigns. One may agree that once all have subscribed to a particular constitution, all those who had indeed agreed are then bound. However, such was surely not the case with the American Constitution of 1789 (which provided for means of adoption in violation of the Articles of Confederacy), or for that matter any constitution written for any large-scale state. Moreover, such an agreement among long-dead persons will not of itself bind current generations. At least, one would need to show why the dead should rule the living. Such doubts would seem to return us to the clash of asserted right with asserted right. One might think here of Blackstone's characterization of the law that binds nations, namely, the law of arms, where ''the only tribunal to which the complaints can appeal is that of the God of battles.''[60]

The prospect of such conflicts leading to civil and intestine wars introduces the fifth possible justification for the authority of government, namely, that of prudence. Consider that one is living in a village regularly attacked by marauding groups who murder, rape, and pillage. After years of such uncontrollable, wanton carnage, the village is approached by a warlord who agrees to protect the village from the roving bands as long as he and his men are paid a tenth of the crops per year, can draft for two years' service a tenth of the women for their concubines and a tenth of the men for their army, and can establish a village health service in which all physicians must participate for a salary, while forgoing all fee-for-service practice. In addition, the warlord's men will aid in protecting members of the village against any who may murder, rape, or pillage the villagers, other than on the orders of the warlord. The warlord adds that if they do not agree, he and his men will themselves begin pillaging at once. If the losses of life, liberty, and property are likely to be much less under the rule of the warlord than under local independence, agreement to the authority of the warlord may be a prudent arrangement. The justification for the authority of the warlord and his men is that of prudence. In the absence of the warlord's power and the uniformity of his administration, there will be more pillage, which will bring much greater costs to all. Here one might think of Hobbes's remark on the state of nature where "the life of man [is] solitary, poore, nasty, brutish, and short."[61] It is for considerations such as these that Hobbes holds that men and women fashion the mortal god, the leviathan, a government, a commonwealth, a civitas.[62]

Hobbes wishes the authority of the commonwealth to be more than one based simply on prudence. He sees the authority of a government arising out of the following explicit or implicit agreement: "I authorise and give up my Right of Governing my selfe to this Man, or to this Assembly of men, on this condition, that thou give up thy Right to him, and Authorise all his Actions in like manner."[63] He defines the essence of the commonwealth as "One Person, of whose acts a great Multitude, by mutuall Covenants one with another, have made themselves every one the Author, to the end he may use the strength and means of them all, as he shall think expedient, for their Peace and common Defence."[64] The difficulty is that everyone has *not* in fact agreed. Not all, as Hobbes alleges, enter into "the Congregation of them that were assembled," having agreed to be bound by whatever the majority decides.[65] Many may simply respond that the commonwealth may go its way peacefully, as they will go their way peacefully. Such dissenters may include both individuals who were there as the original compact was framed, as well as children born of the original consenters. Unless one can develop a somewhat metaphysical doctrine of hereditary consent (perhaps on the model of the old doctrines regarding hereditary slavery),[66] those who are born since the covenant are not a party to it unless they, too, agree. Those who might challenge such dissenters with the maxim "Consent to the commonwealth or leave it" must be prepared for the dissenters' rejoinder, "Why shouldn't the commonwealth leave us alone? Why should we be the ones forced to leave?" There appears to be no effective retort available to the commonwealth, since it is impossible to establish a commonwealth's claim to political boundaries without exclaves.[67] A commonwealth may surely exclude dissenters from welfare rights and the protection of civil rights. But dissenters may claim a repayment of taxes collected by coercion and proceed to hire a security force with the funds.

The dissenters can assert that they hold certain values dearer even than certain forms of personal safety, and that they will not agree to the authority of leviathan in general or in certain areas. Such dissenters, individuals who have not freely committed themselves to obey the laws and regulations of the commonwealth, when they find themselves in a commonwealth may with moral justification refuse to participate not only in those endeavors of the commonwealth they recognize to be immoral, but also in those to which they do not wish to give their energies.

There is a conflict between the desire of those who govern to have authority and of those whom they wish to govern to be governed as little as necessary, and in any event only insofar as they consent. The coercive force of rulers and how it can be distinguished from that of robbers and pirates is a classical theme, which reemerges here in the context of health care policy. How is the intrusion, regulation, and taxation visited by governments to be distinguished from that imposed by various illegitimately coercing groups, especially if there is no secular canonical moral vision? This question is posed by Augustine of Hippo when treating the theme borrowed from Cicero[68] of Alexander the Great's encounter with a pirate. "When the king asked him [the pirate] what he was thinking of, that he should molest the sea, he said with defiant independence: 'The same as you when you molest the world! Since I do this with a little ship I am called a pirate. You do it with a great fleet and are called an emperor.'"[69] If the authority of government is not simply to be respect given to superior force, a general justification must be forthcoming.

One is then brought to the final source for the moral authority of government, namely, the actual consent of the citizens to the actions of the government. This condition is not as difficult to meet as one might at first suspect. Since peaceable individuals may at any time defend other innocents against the use of force, so too may governments act to protect the innocent from such crimes as murder, rape, and robbery. Since it is a morally praiseworthy act to aid individuals in the honoring of contracts to which all parties have agreed, so too it is morally permitted for governments to enforce contracts that citizens record as binding among them. All of these actions of government have undisputed secular moral authority, for all peaceable individuals involved have consented to them. Beyond that, property held in common can be distributed in whatever way those who fashioned the common ownership stipulated. In this fashion, original constitutions can bind descendants who come to participate in a commonwealth to distribute such property through a democratic process. To become a citizen is to have a share in a limited corporate undertaking. Being a citizen becomes equivalent to being a shareholder. In short, within the constraints of actual consent of all those involved, one can still fashion a government with a wide range of substantial capacities and authorities. Unconsented force can be forbidden, contracts enforced, and health care provided as a welfare right out of commonly held resources. It is simply that such state secular moral authority will not extend to the control of the consensual action of free individuals, including their use of their private property.

There will be issues to be settled that cannot be resolved by the agreement of all. Property boundary lines must be established, punishments for crimes determined, the jurisdiction of courts specified, and a series of determinations in gray areas set by stipulation. Here, when moral strangers meet, there are not sufficient moral premises for sound rational arguments to be conclusive. Nor will there be a sufficient communality of understandings so that an explicit agreement of all can resolve matters. In such cases, one will need to do the best one can and resolve controversies by means that involve the least coercion and the greatest amount of consent. The procedures best adapted to this are market mechanisms because these reflect the results of numerous acts of consent and do not incorporate a particular moral vision but the result of individuals acting with each other out of divergent moral understandings. Where such are not sufficient, robustly limited democratic mechanisms, limited by eschewing any goal but the stipulation of points of unclarity, will need to be employed. These democratic mechanisms will be morally limited by the authority of individuals to act freely with themselves, their property, and consenting others. Justifiable governmental form is characterized more by its authority being limited than by its being democratic. The plurality of moralities, bioethics, and health care policies requires a government that maximally encompasses peaceable diversity.

Content-full authority thus passes naturally to free will associations while government is best international, fundamentally limited, and evacuated of content-full moral goals. Geographically located governments of any size pay the price of including a plurality of moral communities, whereas the governance of consensual, nongeographically located communities can draw authority to content-full commitments on the part of those who join.

This short review of why arguments to establish much of the strong moral authority claimed by states and by governmental health care policy fail recapitulates the examinations in chapter 2 as to why arguments to establish a canonical content-full secular morality or bioethics fail. If all do not convert to the same ideology or religion, then one will either have to appeal to the authority of reason or agreement. If one is not to establish governmental authority by an appeal to God, the ground of all being and authority, then one can appeal to rational argument as the source of authority in resolving controversies among rational individuals regarding what one ought to do and how governments should regulate the citizens, here, in particular, their health care. However, as chapter 2 shows, a canonical content-full secular moral understanding and bioethics cannot be established by appeals to intuition, casuistry, the calculation of consequences, the invocation of ideal observers or unbiased contractors, the nature of rational moral choice, game-theoretical understandings, the character of nature, or the role of middle-level principles. Nor will appeals to the existence of overlapping consensus or contingent moral convictions establish the rational canonical normativity of a particular secular morality, bioethics, or understanding of governmental health care regulation. All such appeals crucially presuppose a particular guiding moral sense, thin theory of the good, or moral understanding. Each at its root presupposes that which it is to establish.

### The limited moral authority of the secular state

Attempts to justify an all-encompassing state fail. They go aground on the inability to establish the moral authority of the state by invoking divine authority, the authority of reason expressed in a canonical vision of secular moral authority, or the agreements of the dead to bind the living. Appeals to hypothetical contractors or to prudence will not succeed outside of a canonical moral vision, which gives content to direct the contractors and authority to make prudential choices. As we have seen in chapter 2, such secular canonical moral understandings are not available. Attempts to establish the state as the defender of a canonical moral vision, understanding of justice, or ideology fail in the face of the plurality of moral visions and the diversity of moral communities among which there is no canonical basis for content-full choice. As a consequence, large-scale pluralist states have limited moral authority to impose or establish all-encompassing content-full health care policy. As a consequence, citizens need not, indeed in general secular terms ought not, aid in impeding by the use of state force citizens from buying or selling better basic or luxury health care. They must refrain from the use of state force against individuals "guilty" of victimless crimes, no matter how immoral they recognize such crimes to be (i.e., crimes to which all those involved have agreed freely to participate: the sale of pornography, the conduct of prostitution, the sale of heroin and marijuana, or the provision of better basic health care in contravention of a national health care system). The unquenchable markets for pornography, prostitution, drugs, and better private health care must be tolerated because of the basic human right to the black market—a right that expresses the limits of plausible state authority.

Consider a physician living in a country with a mandatory single-payer health care system with controlled access to diagnostic and therapeutic services, where private health care services are forbidden, who is asked by a patient for an examination to rule out the presence of cancer. The patient wishes to avoid the usual wait within the governmentally controlled universal system in order not to prolong anxiety and to be able to decide whether to go abroad for treatment. If the physician can perform the examination after hours and on equipment smuggled in from abroad, is this permissible? May the physician accept payment for the services?

In general secular moral terms, the physician would be morally free, except for considerations of prudence, to perform the treatment and even to demand payment, unless the physician had agreed explicitly, freely, and without coercion to give up that right to the state. However, the physician as a prudent individual might also be concerned about being caught, fined, and imprisoned. The physician might in addition be concerned that if a general practice of disobeying laws were accepted, the fabric of society might weaken, leading to the general injury of all. But if physicians thought they could usually act without detection and without such consequences outweighing benefits, there would be no general secular grounds for holding them to have acted immorally.

Some may find these conclusions perturbing. They indicate that the moral position of those who would attempt to forbid a private tier of health care is, in secular morality, considerably more dubious than the secular moral standing of whores and whoremongers. On reflection, this should not be too surprising. As this chapter has shown, the principle of permission is central to the intellectual standing of ethics itself. Insofar as whores and whoremongers can show that those involved in prostitution are engaged in it freely, the lineage of secular moral authority for their action can be clearly demonstrated. Prostitutes can explain what they are doing with their clients in terms of mutual agreements. Governmental officials who would forbid the sale of private health insurance and private health care are not so advantaged. They must presuppose a view of governmental authority impossible to justify in general secular terms. They must show that governmental authority is so all-encompassing that individuals may not establish a private health care system with the resources they have remaining after paying their taxes. Such requires a view that the goods and services of individuals are totally at the disposal or control of the community. The more such a claim appears implausible, the weaker the general secular moral authority of the state becomes.

One is left, then, with the preliminary conclusion that in general secular moral terms it is prudent to obey all (most? some?) of the rules and regulations of one's government, but the general moral authority of governments to fashion such rules and regulations is not as strong as the moral authority of multinational corporations such as IBM, Dow Chemical, or Exxon to fashion rules for their workers, or of unions for their members, presuming that the employees and union members have joined without coercion. Governments are morally suspect, for they traditionally use force to coerce those in their territory to accept their authority. It is very difficult to show that individuals have agreed to the authority of the commonwealth within which they reside, absent threats of coercion. (Who reading this volume, for instance, has freely agreed that their government may make it impossible for them to purchase heroin to control the pain of terminal cancer, as is forbidden in the United States?) What one would never tolerate from multinational corporations or unions is accepted as a matter of course when done by governments. There is no evidence, for example, that Dow Chemical has ever drafted individuals to serve in its security forces.

These considerations show severe limitations on the authority of the government (i.e., geographically located governments) in regulating the practice of health care outside of governmentally owned facilities. As a moral test, one might ask oneself under what circumstances Exxon or Dow Chemical security forces may control health care with moral authority in order to disclose the moral limits of state force in the regulation of health care. Governments will be justified in protecting patients and health care workers from coercion, fraud, and breach of contract. In addition, regulations may be imposed on the use of governmental funds and properties through majority vote. But individuals will continue to possess moral rights to do with themselves and consenting others and their resources as they and those consenting others decide. In doubt one should refrain from using persons and their property, including their talents and services, without their permission. Even if communal property and rights were substantial, the existence of some private resources (e.g., rights to one's own services and talents) and the right to contract with willing others would fundamentally limit governmental authority and the secular moral authority of governmental health care policy.

## Toward utopia

Were these understandings to shape public policy, they would lead to radical changes in tax laws, in the ways in which the free consensual acts of individuals are controlled, and in the government's role in the regulation of health care. I will not explore the radical implications of these reflections at length here. It is enough to note that current arrangements would be dramatically altered. With the advent of a general, worldwide, peacekeeping authority limited by the morality of mutual respect (which is to say, with the coming of the secular millennium), one could be assured of the possibility of individuals freely joining in various associations, which need not be limited to any particular geographical area. One might think here of the ways in which individuals of different faiths may proceed to gain a divorce in Israel, on the basis of the rules of their particular religious groups. In such associations, individuals could pursue their own views of the good life. Each association could in its own way provide a level and kind of health care in accord with its guiding view of the good life. Such associations would tax their members. Some associations (e.g., religions) would establish a thick set of regulations and canons. The result would likely be a world in which individuals would belong in different ways to different associations. As a consequence, individuals could have complex entitlements to health care and other support.

Were this a volume focused primarily on political theory rather than bioethics, one would need to explore in detail the extent to which states might properly continue to perform some of the functions we now associate with them. For instance, there may be no justification for states to have a monopoly on the enforcement of justice. There are, in fact, arguments to support the efficiency of the private enforcement of justice in the historical example of Iceland, where from the tenth to the thirteenth centuries the enforcement of justice was a private matter.[70] One might still envisage a need for the police of the general secular pluralist peaceable society to monitor the activities of private police forces as an overseer of last resort. To this proposal there will be the reaction that the market is likely to produce police forces able to perform this function just as well or better within constraints set by national or international law courts. One may need also to consider the balance of powers between private and public policy forces, as well as the arrangement of courts for the trial of public crimes. In a world where true toleration is given for the diversity of human beliefs and for the diversity of human communities likely to be formed, there will be numerous special legal systems developed to govern rights and obligations within particular corporations, associations, and communities. One might foresee such an arrangement somewhat on the model of the relationship that once obtained between civil and canon law, save for the fact that there will be numerous genres of canon law. There will be the problem of whether one may establish a single set of courts for civil law. Perhaps the general secular pluralist state could at most impose a form of arbitration on individuals in the process of selecting a particular genre of civil courts, which arbitration process and which courts would need to be in accord with the principle of permission. These are complex and important matters that will need to be treated elsewhere than in this volume.

The realization of such possibilities must at this time be but a dream, a hope: the allure of a possible utopia of free individuals in free associations. Still, this vision realizes two of the goals often sought from government. First, it offers the impartial protection of citizens. The international police force would dispassionately protect persons from murder, robbery, and other unauthorized touchings of themselves or their property. It would protect recorded contracts and distribute to all their equal share in the revenues from the general land rent or tax on material. However, it would have no view of the good life, it would enforce no concrete sense of morality, it would provide no welfare rights such as a right to health care. For special welfare rights, one would have to appeal to particular corporate entities such as individual states, associations such as the AFL-CIO, or corporations such as IBM and Exxon. Such may hold property in common for their members and through some preestablished procedure decide how to use it and the income it produces. Finally, individuals could belong to particular, closely knit communities sharing well-articulated concrete views of the good life—communities that may not be restricted to particular geographical areas. Under such circumstances there may be the possibility for numerous objects of patriotic dedication. The polytheistic metaphor may find a secular expression in political life.

Although these visions are fantasies, they are instructive in reminding us that states possess no special secular moral status. States are no more legitimate as rule makers than are multinational corporations, unions, or other large organizations. In fact, as has been noted, their secular moral legitimacy is less secure. One might observe, since there is much greater danger both to individuals and to the world at large from states claiming encompassing sovereignty than from corporations, unions, religions, or similar voluntarily constituted bodies, the idea of the sovereign state with strong authority over the person and property of its citizens is one whose time should pass. These visions should help to remind us of the need to inspect the claims for moral authority advanced by particular groups of rule makers. The absence of secular moral legitimacy should not necessarily inspire a physician or nurse to violate the rules (including local, state, and national laws). Obeying the rules may be prudent not only for nurses and physicians, but for their professions generally, as well as the patients under their care. Still, there may be a certain moral satisfaction from knowing whether the order within which one must practice is one ordained through morality, or rather accepted out of expediency.

This reassessment of the state, given the failure to ground content-full claims regarding morality and political authority in an appeal to reason, does not despoil the state of meaning and significance. The state is precisely that social structure in which one can understand a moral authority binding persons and communities with different moral visions and through which general rights to forbearance can be secured and protected. The state is a way of achieving social organization that is not simply another community.[71] One among the many Enlightenment errors is to try to discover in reason a canonical basis for authoritative, large-scale, secular communities. This hope has been shown to be vain. The state is rather a social structure that can compass a diversity of communities protecting both the rights of those communities and the individuals who are its members. When one thinks of the state as a community, one is tempted to impose a particular ideological rectitude, political correctness, or canonical content-full understanding of the moral life. The state is precisely that structure that encompasses numerous communities with diverse moralities and understandings of the good life. The state may enforce recorded contracts and provide for certain welfare rights. But it does this in a transmoral fashion. Where moralities are diverse, the state draws its authority not from what it does, but from the permission of those who participate.

The failure to discover a canonical, content-full moral vision through an appeal to sound rational argument, the persistence of a diversity of moral communities, and the ability peaceably to compass such communities in an authoritative, large-scale social structure require a limited state. To have secular moral authority or legitimacy for individual and communal action, the state must leave moral spaces. Such spaces can be understood as marked or bordered by rights to privacy. They are the social environments within which different communities can act on diverse understandings of the good. They are moral environments into which the state may not intrude because it possesses neither the authority nor the canonical moral vision to legitimate or instruct such action. It is within these spaces, spaces left by the failure of secular rational thought to establish a canonical content, that diverse health care policies may develop and take shape.

---

PRINCIPLE IV. THE PRINCIPLE OF POLITICAL AUTHORITY

Morally justified political authority is derived from the consent of the governed, not from a canonical content-full understanding of the good life or moral obligations, including commitments to beneficence; the actual significance of such views or commitments must be framed by common agreement. The character of consent to an organization's authority will differ, for example, if one compares a territorial state such as Texas with a multinational corporation such as IBM. Political or corporate entities possess authority to:

    i. Protect the innocent from unconsented-to force (e.g., against being subjects of medical experimentation without their consent, or from having their free access to private health care impeded);

    ii. Enforce contracts (e.g., the commitment to confidentiality on the part of physicians);

    iii. Develop welfare rights through the use of common resources (e.g., health care welfare rights);

    iv. Clarify boundaries and establish procedures to resolve disputes when such cannot be accomplished through market mechanisms and then only while eschewing any content-full understanding of morality.

A. Authority from implied consent: the principle of permission, the notion of the peaceable community presumes acquiescence in the protection of the innocent from unconsented-to force (e.g., using patients for goals to which they have not consented).

B. Authority from explicit consent: Particular individuals, through participating in a community, can fashion a web of explicit agreements through which authority is transferred to a political entity in order to administer common endeavors and resources. In this fashion, states and corporations create specific health care rights for their members.

C. Justification of the principle: Political authority receives primary moral justification in terms of the principle of permission, the morality of mutual respect. It receives justification as well in terms of the principle of beneficence. However, such authority must always be placed within the constraints of the principle of permission, in that the principle of beneficence is specified through mutual consent.

D. Motivation for respecting political authority: To act contrary to legitimate political authority is to lose grounds for protest against punitive and defensive force. The motivation for respect is thus drawn in part from the considerations that underlie the principle of permission, the morality of mutual respect. In addition, corporate entities provide the basis for individuals to pursue, in common, goods that would be impossible to achieve, were they to act individually. One might think here of how Plato remarks that an ample city is requisite for the luxuries of life (*Republic,* 2.373). Issues of beneficence, of achieving a particular view of the good, will thus further motivate individuals to create special corporate endeavors. Content-full visions of beneficence are to be found only in communities of moral friends or in special stipulations made through the agreement of moral strangers. Finally, considerations of expedience and prudence may as well bring acquiescence in the laws and rules of government.

E. Public policy implications: The authority of governments is suspect, insofar as they

    i. Restrict the choice of free individuals without their consent (e.g., attempts to forbid the sale of human organs or private health care insurance);

    ii. Regulate the free exchange of goods and services, beyond protecting against such evils as fraud, coercion, or the violation of contracts; however,

    iii.   Political authority is properly exercised over commonly held land and other possessions, according to the rules established by the participants in the corporate endeavor.

F. Maxim: Though respect of governmental rules and laws regarding health care is prudent, one is morally blameworthy in general secular moral terms only if one acts against legitimate moral authority. Therefore: Obey laws when one must; feel guilty about infractions when one should.

---

## A postmodern reflection on property, states, and health care policy

We are left with an understanding of ownership, state authority, the authority of public policy, and the legitimacy of health care policy quite different from that born of the rationalist assumptions of the modern age, of the Enlightenment. In the absence of a canonical content-full morality or a universal moral narrative, it is as difficult, if not more difficult, to establish communal claims to ownership than to establish individual claims. Moreover, neither individual nor communal claims can be shown in general secular terms to be exhaustive. All persons are left with a general claim to the use of the earth and of material resources. This residual claim is the basis for an international land tax, which all must pay, individuals, corporations, and states alike, with the proceeds paid out as a negative income tax. This state of affairs is not endorsed because it is desirable, useful, or valuable. It is the most that can be made out within general secular morality.

Similarly, the state and its authority must be radically reconsidered in the face of numerous moralities and competing moral narratives. In particular, unlike corporations, religious associations, unions, and other free-will communities, geographically located states cannot justify their authority to impose a particular morality. Given the collapse of the Enlightenment project and against the diversity of moral visions, the authority of large-scale social institutions to govern depends on the plausibility of their claim that they act with the permission of those whom they rule. Despite the collapse of the Enlightenment project and the diversity of moral visions, it is possible to defend against, and to punish, the unconsented-to use of others. The state can enforce recorded contracts and create refusable welfare rights. Gray areas, unclear boundaries, and unavoidable puzzles will remain. Insofar as these can be resolved by market mechanisms, this is to be preferred, for these mechanisms draw authority from the permission of all those who participate. When such solutions are not feasible, boundaries must be clarified, courts established, and punishments determined by democratic decision. Democratic choices provide the secular version of Elijah's service in the face of TEYKU controversies. Where a decision has to be made and the spontaneous order of the market will not authoritatively select among choices, one should attempt to enlist as many as possible in "flipping the coin" in the selection among alternatives.

Against this continued role for democratic decision making, communal and individual rights to privacy loom large, and the general secular authority of large-scale states is radically limited. Given the limits of general secular moral authority, particular nongeographically located communities may organize social structures and sustain special civil rights and welfare rights, including rights to health care. This unavoidable diversity of moral visions may organize and take communal shape. This is not something that is endorsed because it is good, valuable, or desirable. Instead, one finds what can be saved in the face of diversity, relativism, and threatening nihilism. Some of the hopes of the Enlightenment can be realized. But that which is salvaged has no content and is but a set of procedures for limited collaboration (e.g., consent, contract, the free market, and limited democracies). The very limitations we face give moral space and opportunity for virtue and character.

## Notes

1. It should be noted that persons, when resolving moral controversies, need be neither moral nor metaphysical friends. They can engage in the practice of resolving moral controversies, insofar as they meet as moral strangers, while disagreeing regarding the content of the moral life. So, too, in science *ceteris paribus* conditions can be established and other agreements can be made so that science can be engaged in as a means of intersubjectively resolving empirical disputes without deep-level metaphysical agreement. Persons can engage in the practice of empirical science while being metaphysical strangers.
2. Kant, *Grundlegung zur Metaphysik der Sitten,* AK IV 438.
3. Ibid., AK IV 452.
4. Ibid., AK IV 453; *Foundations of the Metaphysics of Morals,* trans. L. W. Beck (Indianapolis: Bobbs-Merrill, 1976), p. 72.
5. For contemporary exploration of puzzles regarding freedom and the reduction of freedom to neurological processes, see Patricia Churchland, *Neurophilosophy* (Cambridge, Mass.: MIT Press, 1986).
6. *Grundlegung,* AK IV 452.
7. This point is explored at great length by Kant in his treatment of the third antinomy in the *Critique of Pure Reason.* The third antinomy presents the unavoidable contrast between the deterministic perspective and the moral perspective. This contrast or tension cannot be resolved, as Kant argues, in terms of one of the particular perspectives alone. This leads, as a consequence, to holding on the one hand that all human actions are in principle predictable (*Kritik der reinen Vernunft,* 2d ed., 1787, p. 578, B578), while on the other holding that we must think of ourselves as free, though we cannot prove that we are free.

8. Ramsey was reluctant to allow experimentation on fetuses and children because they cannot consent. Such a line of argument presumes that fetuses can justifiably be the object of such respect. Ramsey also objects to the use of children in research not aimed at their benefit, because such would entail using that individual "without his will." However, there is no will to respect in the case of infants. Paul Ramsey, *The Patient as Person* (New Haven, Conn.: Yale University Press, 1970), p. 35.

9. Dr. Jerome Lejeune, in testimony to the United States Senate, stated: "But now we can say, unequivocally, that the question of when life begins is no longer a question for theological or philosophical dispute. It is an established scientific fact. Theologians and philosophers may go on to debate the meaning of life or the purpose of life, but it is an established fact that all life, including human life, begins at the moment of conception." Testimony by Dr. Jerome Lejeune on the Human Life Bill: Hearings before the Subcommittee on Separation of Powers of the Committee of the Judiciary, 97th Congress (Washington, D.C.: U.S. Government Printing Office, 1982), vol. 1, p. 13.

10. With the issue of abortion one finds revealed the immense gulf between what can be established in general secular moral terms and what can be appreciated properly in terms of canonical content. It is important to note that Christianity did not traditionally use arguments such as those developed in the Western Middle Ages to determine when abortion should count as murder. Abortion as well as infanticide is simply understood as wrong. "Thou shalt not procure abortion, nor commit infanticide." The Didache in *The Apostolic Fathers,* trans. Kirsopp Lake (Cambridge, Mass.: Harvard University Press, 1965), vol. 1, pp. 313, 315, III, 5. Nor is a distinction made in terms of the development of the embryo. Destruction at any time counts as murder. Council in Trullo, Canon XCI. This reflects the original Christian view that life must be respected from conception.

11. Thomas Aquinas distinguishes between the status of the early and late fetus in *Summa Theologica* 1, 118, art. 2. He also opines in his commentary on Aristotle that Aristotle shows moral sensitivity in favoring the use of early abortion rather than infanticide or late abortion. Such early abortion was not held to be murder. *Aristoteles Stagiritae: Politicorum seu de Rebus Civilibus,* Book 7, Lectio 12, in O*pera Omnia* (Paris: Vives, 1875), vol. 26, p. 484. This issue is also discussed by Aquinas in *Summa Theologica* 2-2, 64, art. 8. See also *Commentum in Quartum Librum Sententiarium Magistri Petri Lombardi,* Distinctio 31, Expositio Textus, in *Opera Omnia,* vol. 11, p. 127.

12. A good overview of the history of abortion in Roman Catholic canon law is provided by John T. Noonan, Jr., "An Almost Absolute Value in History," in John T. Noonan, Jr. (ed.), *The Morality of Abortion* (Cambridge, Mass.: Harvard University Press, 1971). The view of the Roman Catholic church developed under a number of influences. The Septuagint translation of Exodus 21:22 was taken to suggest that there is a moral difference between formed and unformed embryos, between ensouled and unensouled embryos. This scriptural distinction is similar to one drawn by Aristotle, between the fetus before and after it possessed an animal soul. *De Generatione Animalium* 2.3.736a–b and *Historia Animalium* 7.3.583b. Theological and philosophical reflections on the bases of these and other considerations led to the develop-

ment in Roman Catholic theology of the dispute between those who favored mediate animation (the soul entering some time after the conception of the body) and those favoring immediate animation (the soul entering at the time of the conception of the body). J. Donceel, "Abortion: Mediate v. Immediate Animation," *Continuum 5* (Spring 1967): 167–71, and "Immediate Animation and Delayed Hominization," *Theological Studies* 13 (Mar. 1970): 76–105. See also Canon Henry de Dorlodot, "A Vindication of the Mediate Animation Theory," in E. C. Messenger (ed.), *Theology and Evolution* (London: Sands, 1952), pp. 259–83. A twelfth-century canon law case entered Roman Catholic canon law in the thirteenth century, setting a precedent that recognized the difference between the crime of murder and the act of destroying an unformed (i.e., unensouled) fetus. *Corpus Juris Canonici Emendatum et Notis Illustratum cum Glossae: decretalium d. Gregorii Papae Noni Compilatio* (Rome, 1585), *Glossa ordinaria* at book 5, title 12, chap. 20, p. 1713.

The change in Roman Catholic treatment of early abortion was influenced, it would appear, by the setting of the dates for celebrating the Immaculate Conception of the Blessed Virgin Mary (Dec. 8) as nine months prior to the date for celebrating her birth (Sept. 8).

This is not to suggest that there were not individuals who held that early abortion should be considered equivalent to acts of murder. See, for example, Pope Sixtus V, *Contra procurantes, Consulentes, et Consentientes, quorunque modo Abortum Constitutio* (Florence: Georgius Marescottus, 1888). Pope Sixtus V for three years (1588–91) made early abortion equivalent to taking the life of a person.

13. For an excellent study of the significance of the Roman Catholic sin of contraception and its relation to the sin of abortion, see John T. Noonan, Jr., *Contraception* (Cambridge, Mass.: Harvard University Press, 1965). See also, for a helpful treatment of current Catholic viewpoints in this matter, James J. McCartney, "Some Roman Catholic Concepts of Person and Their Implications for the Ontological Status of the Unborn," in W. B. Bondeson et al. (eds.), *Abortion and the Status of the Fetus* (Dordrecht: Reidel, 1983), pp. 313–23.

14. It is important to note that, though the Roman Church did not hold early abortion to be murder, the act of abortion prior to "ensoulment" was still recognized as gravely evil.

15. S. I. Benn, "Abortion, Infanticide, and Respect for Persons," in Joel Feinberg (ed.), *The Problem of Abortion* (Belmont, Calif.: Wadsworth, 1973), pp. 92–104.

16. The distinction between pain and suffering is explored by George Pitcher, "Pain and Unpleasantness," pp. 181–96; David Bakan, "Pain—The Existential Symptom," pp. 197–207; Bernard Tursky, "The Evaluation of Pain Response: A Need for Improved Measures," pp. 209–19; and Jerome A. Shaffer, "Pain and Suffering," pp. 221–33, in S. F. Spicker and H. T. Engelhardt, Jr. (eds.), *Philosophical Dimensions of the Neuro-Medical Sciences* (Dordrecht: Reidel, 1976).

17. Robert Nozick, *Anarchy, State, and Utopia* (New York: Basic Books, 1974), p. 39.

18. Ibid.

19. Kant employs at least six different senses of persons, the ego, or the subject. The first is the transcendental ego, the logical form of the spontaneity of the intellect, whose functions of judgment are the categories (*Critique of Pure Reason*, B137, 140, 143).

It is this transcendental ego that accompanies any and all judgments (*Critique of Pure Reason*, B406, 419). There is, second, the consciousness of the bare fact that one exists (*Critique of Pure Reason*, B156). This fact cannot be captured as true knowledge (*Critique of Pure Reason*, A346 = B404) but can be apprehended as an intellectual representation or thought (*Critique of Pure Reason*, B158). There is also, third, the empirical ego, which is the subject as it appears to itself in inner sense, but not as an object (*Critique of Pure Reason*, B278, A347 = B405, A381f.). The fourth sense, that of the ego of rational psychology, is the false hypostatization of the logical function I think (*Critique of Pure Reason*, A403f.). The fifth sense, that of the noumenal ego, is that of the person as a moral agent, through which we think our actions, but concerning which there is no theoretical knowledge, since the subject cannot be given in experience (*Critique of Pure Reason*, A538–40 = B566–68). It is this sense that is important to the reflections in this book about persons as moral agents. It is persons in this sense who exist as the constituting sources of the moral world. The last sense in which Kant treats of the subject or person is as a psychological idea read into experience through a regulative use of the idea giving a further unity to our knowledge of persons. *Critique of Pure Reason*, A665 = B693, A671–74 = B699–702, A682–84 = B710–12. Kant suffers from a need for a general category of subject. An account of such a category must be approached through a more expanded categorial account. See H. T. Engelhardt Jr., *Mind–Body: A Categorial Relation* (The Hague: Martinus Nijhoff, 1973).

20. *Metaphysik der Sitten,* AK IV 223; *The Metaphysical Principles of Virtue: Part II of the Metaphysics of Morals,* trans. James Ellington (Indianapolis: Bobbs-Merrill, 1964), p. 23. For an attempt to develop a general Kantian bioethics, see Mats G. Hansson, *Human Dignity and Animal Well-being: A Kantian Contribution to Biomedical Ethics* (Uppsala: Almqvist & Wiksell, 1991).

21. Immanuel Kant, *Lectures on Ethics,* trans. Louis Infield (Indianapolis: Hackett, 1979), p. 240.

22. Ibid. Kant argues that one should keep an old dog until it dies, for "such action helps to support us in our duties towards human beings, where they are bounden duties." Ibid. However, if the man shoots his dog, according to Kant, he does not fail in his duty to the dog, "but his act is inhuman and damages in himself that humanity which it is his duty to show towards mankind." The dog owner has no duty to the dog, but a duty to humanity regarding the dog. In my arguments I have indicated that the dog owner in addition has a duty of beneficence to the dog. I agree with Kant that the purposes of humans can outweigh the considerations of beneficence to animals. "Vivisectionists, who use living animals for their experiments, certainly act cruelly, although their aim is praiseworthy, and they can justify their cruelty, since animals must be regarded as man's instruments, but any such cruelty for sport cannot be justified." Ibid., pp. 240–41. General secular morality does not preclude the use of animals for purposes of sport. As an example, consider the report of a gun club using live pigeons for target practice. Olive Talley, "Gun Club Again Using Live Pigeons," *Houston Chronicle* (Feb. 16, 1985), sec. 1, p. 32.

23. What I raise here is the moral equivalent of some of the arguments that have been advanced in support of tort-for-wrongful-life suits. Within secular morality if one

initiates a pregnancy, intentionally damages the fetus, and then fails to abort the fetus over which one has authority, one can then become the author of a harm that could have been prevented had one in a timely fashion had the fetus aborted. For an overview of the issues raised by tort-for-wrongful-life cases, see Angela Holder, "Is Existence Ever an Injury?: The Wrongful Life Cases," in S. F. Spicker et al. (eds.), *The Law–Medicine Relation: A Philosophical Exploration* (Dordrecht: Reidel, 1981), pp. 225–39.

24. Richard H. Feen, "Abortion and Exposure in Ancient Greece: Assessing the Status of the Fetus and 'Newborn' from Classical Sources," in Bondeson et al. (eds.), *Abortion and the Status of the Fetus*, pp. 283–300. In Viking law the child could not be exposed once it had been given suck. P. G. Foote and D. M. Wilson, *The Viking Achievement* (London: Sidgwick & Jackson, 1980), p. 115.

25. This point is noted in *Kitzur Shulhan Arukh*, by Rabbi Solomon Ganzfried (the standard condensed version of the code of Jewish religious law, entitled *Shulhan Arukh*, compiled by Joseph Karo [1488–1575], sec. 203, par. 3): "if an infant dies within the first 30 days of its life, or even on the 30th day of its life, and even if there has been growth of its hair and nails, you do not follow any of the observances of mourning, because it is as if there had been a miscarriage" (adapted and translated by Professor Isaac Franck).

26. One might think here of the suggestions by Raymond S. Duff and A. G. M. Campbell regarding the ways in which parents may be assisted in making choices regarding when to refuse treatment for their severely defective newborn. "Moral and Ethical Dilemmas in the Special Care Nursery," *New England Journal of Medicine* 289 (Oct. 25, 1973): 890–94. See also Anthony Shaw, "Dilemmas of Informed Consent in Children," *New England Journal of Medicine* 289 (Oct. 25, 1973): 885–90.

27. The U.S. government attempted to stop parents or physicians from discriminating against neonates in treatment choices on the basis of physical and mental disability. The issues raised by such interferences are discussed in chapter 6.

28. Gary E. Jones, "Engelhardt on the Abortion and Euthanasia of Defective Infants," *Linacre Quarterly* 50 (May 1983): 172–81.

29. Engelhardt, *Mind–Body: A Categorial Relation*.

30. Alfred Schutz and Thomas Luckmann, *The Structures of the Life-World*, trans. R. M. Zaner and H. T. Engelhardt, Jr. (Evanston, Ill.: Northwestern University Press, 1973), p. 47.

31. John Hughlings Jackson (1835–1902), the father of modern neurology, examined this issue. See, in particular, "Evolution and Dissolution of Nervous System," in *Selected Writings of John Hughlings Jackson*, ed. James Taylor (New York: Basic Books, 1958), vol. 2, pp. 45–75; reproduced from the initial publication of the Croonian lectures delivered at the Royal College of Physicians, Mar. 1884, and published originally as "Evolution and Dissolution of the Nervous System," *British Medical Journal* 1 (1884): 591–93, 660–63; "Evolution and Dissolution of the Nervous System," *Medical Times and Gazette* 1 (1884): 411–13, 445–58, 485–87; and "Evolution and Dissolution of the Nervous System," *Lancet* 1 (1884): 555–58, 649–52, 739–44. See also H. T. Engelhardt, Jr., "John Hughlings Jackson and the Mind–Body Relation," *Bulletin of the History of Medicine* 49 (Summer 1975): 137–51.

32. Orthodox Christians recognize individuals as existing from their conception, as is shown by their celebration of the Feasts of the Conception of John the Baptist (Sept. 23) and the Virgin Mary (Dec. 9).

33. For an example of such metaphysical worries, see Derek Parfit, *Reasons and Persons* (Oxford: Clarendon Press, 1984).

34. John Locke, *The Treatises of Government, in the Former, the False Principles and Foundation of Sir Robert Filmer, and His Followers, Are Detected and Overthrown; the Latter, Is an Essay concerning the True Origin, Extent, and End, of Civil Government,* book 2, chap. 5, sec. 25.

35. Kant, *Metaphysik der Sitten,* AK IV 245–58. For Kant, one owns external property in a state of nature in anticipation of a civil society.

36. William Blackstone, *Commentaries on the Laws of England,* ed. St. George Tucker (New York: Augustus and Kelly, 1969), book 2, chap. 1, pp. 8–9, vol 3, p. 8.

37. Hegel, *Hegel's Philosophy of Right,* trans. T. M. Knox (London: Oxford University Press, 1965), sec. 54.

38. Locke, *Treatises of Government,* book 2, chap. 5, 27.

39. Gaius, *The Institutes of Gaius,* trans. F. de Zulueta (Oxford: Clarendon Press, 1946), part 1, sec. 67, p. 83.

40. Locke, *Treatises of Government,* no. 27.

41. Thomas Paine, *Agrarian Justice* (London: T. G. Ballard, 1798).

42. W. Ogilvie, *Essay on the Right of Property in Land* (London: J. Walter, 1781).

43. Baruch Brody, "Health Care for the Haves and Have Nots: Toward a Just Basis of Distribution," in Earl E. Shelp (ed.), *Justice and Health Care* (Dordrecht: Reidel, 1981), pp. 151–59.

44. Locke, *Treatises of Government,* book 2, chap. 5, no. 27. This notion of the right of all to the rent on things generally does not give any person any specific right to any specific bit of land. Insofar as individuals come to work or transform particular land, they have a right not to be disturbed by others, for example, walking through their houses late at night, claiming that all land belongs to all. Such an intrusion would violate their actualized claim to that land, insofar as they have transformed it by their activities. What others have is a right to be compensated for the inconvenience of having to walk around private property and to use public parks for picnics instead of the lawns in front of private houses. The Lockean proviso is a principle of compensation for inconvenience, as well as forgone opportunities for profit. The person who has transformed land, or properly come into possession of transformed land, has a right that conflicts with the rights of those who might have wished to be able to possess that land themselves. The latter do not own that land but have a right to be compensated for the opportunities lost.

The answer to how much rent to charge cannot be discovered but must be created. The best mode for creation is the one with maximal authority. That is, it should occur through some democratic process. This does not return us to an ownership of all by all. First, the rent may be collected only on land and raw materials. Second, the amount of the rent cannot be determined on the basis of redistributive goals. Indeed, the whole notion of the rent on the land would lead to something very close to an international property tax paid out as an international payment due to all.

45. Brody, "Health Care for the Haves and Have Nots," pp. 151–59.
46. Van Rensselaer Potter, *Bioethics, Bridge to the Future* (Englewood Cliffs, N.J.: Prentice-Hall, 1971), and *Global Bioethics* (East Lansing: Michigan State University Press, 1988).
47. Hans-Martin Sass, "Mensch und Landschaft: der anthropologische Ansatz einer Umweltphilosophie," in *Landschaft und Mensch,* ed. Humboldt-Gesellschaft (Mannheim: Humboldt-Gesellschaft, 1981), pp. 293–322.
48. Alston Chase, *Playing God in Yellowstone* (Boston: Atlantic Monthly Press, 1986).
49. National Center for Policy Analysis, *Progressive Environmentalism* (Bozeman, Mont.: Political Economy Research Center, 1991). See, also, Robert K. Davis, Steve H. Hanke, and Frank Mitchell, "Conventional and Unconventional Approaches to Wildlife Exploitation," in *Transactions of the Thirty-eighth North American Wildlife and Natural Resources Conference* (Washington, D.C.: Wildlife Management Institute, 1973), pp. 75–89; and Randy Simmons and Urs Kreuter, "Herd Mentality: Banning Ivory Sales Is No Way to Save the Elephants," *Policy Review* 50 (Fall 1989): 46–49.
50. Gaius, *The Institutes of Gaius,* part 2, pp. 75–80.
51. Hippocrates, *Law in Hippocrates,* trans. W. H. S. Jones (Cambridge, Mass.: Harvard University Press, 1959), vol. 2, p. 263.
52. The character of "malpractice suits" in both ancient Greece and Rome has been explored at length by Darrel Amundsen, "The Liability of the Physician in Roman Law," in H. Karplus (ed.), *International Symposium on Society Medicine and Law* (New York: Elsevier, 1973), pp. 17–30; "The Liability of the Physician in Classical Greek Legal Theory and Practice," *Journal of the History of Medicine and Allied Sciences* 32 (Apr. 1977): 172–203; "Physician, Patient and Malpractice: An Historical Perspective", in Spicker et al., *The Law-Medicine Relation,* pp. 255–58.
53. Marcia Angell, "Should Heroin Be Legalized for the Treatment of Pain?" *New England Journal of Medicine* 311 (Aug. 23, 1984): 529–30; and Edward N. Brandt, Jr., "Compassionate Pain Relief: Is Heroin the Answer?" *New England Journal of Medicine* 311 (Aug. 23, 1984): 530–32.

From both libertarian and utilitarian perspectives, one might ask why any access to drugs should be forbidden. Which is more dangerous to individuals, the risk of being addicted to a dangerous drug or that of being involuntarily subjected to drug-related crimes? Under current circumstances, addicts steal property to sell it at a fraction of its worth in order to buy drugs priced at many times their value. Because drugs are illegal, there is a booming illicit drug industry whose profits are in the billions. This trade is then taken to justify specially directed police forces and terrifying intrusive laws, whose interventions succeed in maintaining the high prices of illicit drugs and therefore supporting the continued great incentives for illegal sales.
54. Pope Innocent III, "'Sicut universitatis' ad Acerbum consulem Florentinum, 30 October 1198," in H. Denzinger (ed.), *Enchiridion Symbolorum,* 33d ed. (Rome: Herder, 1965), p. 244.
55. See "Erronea propositio de tyrannicidio," in *Enchiridion Symbolorum,* p. 326.
56. Blackstone, *Commentaries,* vol. 2, book 1, pp. 191–92.

57. John Rawls, *A Theory of Justice* (Cambridge, Mass.: Harvard University Press, 1971), pp. 62–63, 136–42, 302–3.

58. Ibid., pp. 195–201, 221–34.

59. One must observe that there has been a considerable dispute in the history of America regarding the significance of the original consent to the American Constitution of 1789. Though this dispute peaked during the War Between the States, its origins can be found already well articulated in the resolutions of the Kentucky legislature endorsing nullification and the general assembly of Virginia endorsing interposition during the time of John Adams's restrictions of civil liberties. See the Resolution of the Kentucky Legislature in the House of Representatives, Nov. 14, 1799, and the General Assembly of Virginia in the House of Delegates, Jan. 7, 1800, reprinted in *We the States* (Richmond, Va.: William Byrd Press, 1964), pp. 155–59.

60. Blackstone, *Commentaries*, vol. 2, book 1, part 2, p. 193.

61. Thomas Hobbes, *Leviathan, or the Matter, Forms, & Power of a Common-wealth Ecclesiastical and Civill* (London: Andrew Crooke, 1651), part 1, chap. 13, p. 62.

62. Ibid., part 2, chap. 17, p. 87.

63. Ibid. Hobbes can also be interpreted as appealing not to a contract but to a rational, game-theoretic resolution of problems of both enforcement, coordination, and free riders. Some of the difficulties with such game-theoretic resolutions have been explored in chapter 2.

64. Ibid., p. 88.

65. Ibid., part 2, chap. 18, p. 90.

66. One might recall here the defense of slavery given by Hugo Grotius in his *De jure belli ac pacis*. He argues that morally justified hereditary slavery comes into existence when a person is captured in a war and not killed. In forgoing the right to kill the captive, the captive taker gains the right to the children born of the slave *ad indefinitum*. See book 3, chap. 7, especially sec. 1–5. These considerations were in fact endorsed by Western Christian theologians of the time, though Christians were held to be bound to forbear from taking Christians as slaves. See book 3, chap. 7, sec. 9.

One should note that, even if slaves were not persons before the law, the very theory of slavery still presumed that they were moral persons. This was the case even despite special rationalizations that underscored the moral and psychological infirmities or disabilities of slaves in order to make the peculiar institution more acceptable. One might note, for instance, that in both Tennessee and Texas before the War Between the States slaves were held to be in a position analogous to that of individuals in Norman villenage, conferring upon slaves a certain standing before the law. A. E. Keir Nash, "Texas Justice in the Age of Slavery: Appeals concerning Blacks and the Antebellum State Supreme Court," *Houston Law Review* 8 (1971): 438–56.

67. A rejoinder would require establishing in general secular terms a partial canonical content-full moral vision as long as consent is not forthcoming and those in the exclave are peaceable.

68. "XIV. . . . for when he was asked what wickedness drove him to harass the sea with his one pirate galley, he replied: 'The same wickedness that drives you to harass the whole world.'" Marcus Tullius Cicero, *The Republic* 3.14.24.

69. Augustine of Hippo, *City of God*, trans. George McCracken et al. (Cambridge, Mass.: Harvard University Press, 1957), 4.4.25.

70. David Friedman, "Efficient Institutions for the Private Enforcement of Law," *Journal of Legal Studies* 13 (June 1984): 379–97; "Private Creation and Enforcement of Law: A Historical Case," *Journal of Legal Studies* 8 (Mar. 1979): 399–415. The Icelandic experience developed out of the same general pagan Teutonic roots that gave rise to much of Anglo–Saxon law. For a study of the Icelandic legal and social system, see P. B. Foote and D. M. Wilson, *The Viking Achievement* (London: Sidgwick & Jackson, 1970). Original material concerning old Icelandic law and customs can be found in the Njals Saga and in the Gragas, the earliest compilation of Icelandic law.

71. H. T. Engelhardt, Jr., "Sittlichkeit and Post-Modernity: An Hegelian Reconsideration of the State," in H. T. Engelhardt, Jr., and T. Pinkard (eds.), *Hegel Reconsidered: Beyond Metaphysics and the Authoritarian State* (Dordrecht: Kluwer, 1994), pp. 211–24.

# 5

## The Languages of Medicalization

### Shaping reality

Medicine medicalizes reality. It creates a world. It translates sets of problems into its own terms. Medicine molds the ways in which the world of experience takes shape; it conditions reality for us. The difficulties people have are then appreciated as illnesses, diseases, deformities, and medical abnormalities, rather than as innocent vexations, normal pains, or possession by the devil. Medical problems are clusters of phenomena seen as amenable to medical assessment, explanation, and up to a point, alleviation or cure. Here one finds clusters of difficulties often termed diseases, sicknesses, illnesses, deformities, disabilities, and disfigurements, which are beyond the immediate control of the individuals afflicted, and which are presumed to have a basis in physiological, anatomical, or psychological causal matrices. Their sense, significance, and reality are cast in terms of the social and intellectual institutions of medicine. In being seen as medical problems, they are usually characterized as circumstances that deviate from physiological or psychological ideals regarding proper levels of function, freedom from pain, and achievement of expected human form and grace. An ache or pain thus becomes a medical disorder. In addition, since medicine is a social institution, the pains, deformities, and dysfunctions are given a social valence.

Consider the transformation of experienced reality accomplished by the diagnosis of heart disease. A slight shortness of breath or the swelling of ankles after a long day of work becomes a sign of disease. Sleeping on two pillows is no longer

189

an innocent occurrence, but a possible stigma of a deadly disease. The individual's view of life is changed by a set of expectations regarding the dangerousness of heart disease and the possibility of an early death. New relations are likely to develop with physicians and other health care personnel. New rituals are imposed with a force and character comparable to those of a religion. One must now regularly take medication and conform to a new diet in order to lower salt and cholesterol intake. What were previously innocent undertakings, such as eating, exercise, and recreation, now become serious matters of health, if not of life and death. Cigarette smoking will now clearly appear as dangerous. The individual may even worry that sexual intercourse could lead to death. The social circumstances of the individual will be transformed by the expectations of others as they learn of the diagnosis. Friends will wonder whether John can go on the ski trip, after all. Is it likely to be too much for him? If he is a pilot for an airline, he may no longer be able to continue in his job. Insurance companies are likely to issue insurance now only at a markedly increased premium. In short, a major transformation of experienced reality will have taken place.

Such is not unexpected. The world in which we live is not furnitured by uninterpreted facts. We see the things around us in terms of social and theoretical expectations. We are taught early how to explain the occurrences of our world. Within the generally dominant scientific world view, we take for granted that a set of complex, etiologic forces directs the production of illness and disease. Individuals in other cultures, or our antecedents in our own culture, untutored by our current scientific world view, do not or did not see illness as the result of infectious agents, genetic flaws, or endocrinological abnormalities. We, however, do. Our world is structured by a special set of assumptions about the rule-governed character of our experience. These scientific and metaphysical presuppositions fashion for us our everyday expectations. They give shape to our lifeworld. In addition, the particular character of our social institutions invests occurrences with social significance. The current arrangement among dentists, surgeons, physicians, and psychiatrists is the result of a set of past historical forces in great proportion peculiar to our particular culture, but which contributes to the appreciated significance of a toothache, appendicitis, heart disease, or schizophrenia.

We see the world through our social, scientific, and value expectations. The medical facts with which bioethics deals are not timeless truths, but data given through the formative expectations of our history and culture. Recognizing a state of affairs as heart disease, cancer, depression, homosexuality, or tuberculosis is a rich and complex process. All knowledge is historically and culturally conditioned, and the influence of history and culture is often, as we shall see, particularly marked in medicine. This is not to say that investigators do not attempt to know, timelessly unconstrained by social and cultural forces. In endeavoring to know truly, one attempts to understand the world as it would be seen from

God's eye, from the viewpoint of dispassionate, scientific observers or investigators, so that the findings could be shared with other investigators, even those outside our culture—in principle, even with alien investigators on planets circling distant stars.

The goal of undistorted knowledge is a heuristic. It directs us as knowers, as scientists, toward the truth. As Charles S. Peirce (1839–1914), the founder of pragmatism, observed, "Finally, as what anything really is, is what it may finally come to be known to be in the ideal state of complete information, so that reality depends on the ultimate decision of the community; so thought is what it is, only by virtue of its addressing a future thought which is in its value as thought identical with it, though more developed."[1] Peirce is suggesting that it is impossible to speak of reality apart from possible knowers of reality. Any concept we can have of reality is that of a reality that is experienced, even if experienced by ideal observers. To speak of the nature of reality or of medical facts undistorted by historical and cultural contexts is to speak of a view that would be possessed by knowers in full possession of all information and unmoved by assumptions not grounded in reality. The interest in knowing reality as it would be known from no particular perspective sets knowers on a journey from their unrecognized assumptions toward an ever more complete overcoming of those particular assumptions through a recognition of them and through endeavors to compensate for them in order to achieve a greater capacity to describe reality, unconditioned by the idiosyncrasies of one's cultural context. One seeks a view of reality that can be shared with moral and metaphysical strangers. In pursuing the ideal of Peirce's community of perfectly advantaged scientists, one is able to distinguish between better and worse portrayals of reality by reference to an ideal, which one need not claim can actually be achieved. The ideal is ingredient in the very practice of science, in the very endeavor of science as a cultural undertaking directed toward intersubjectivity in knowledge claims secured by and regarding an external reality. In naming, classifying, grading, staging, and explaining diseases, we would hope to do these tasks, as would be done by a community of ideal investigators responding to an external reality. Again, we never reach this goal. All descriptions of reality are from a particular perspective.

Although there has been much recent attention to the historically and culturally conditioned character of knowledge, the roots of this appreciation are deep. Indeed, from Giambattista Vico (1668–1744) through G. W. F. Hegel (1777–1831) and Wilhelm Dilthey (1833–1911) to the present, there has been an ever-increasing appreciation of the extent to which our construals of reality exist within the embrace of cultural expectations. The recent development of these insights by Ludwik Fleck (1896–1961)[2] and Thomas Kuhn[3] has led to a better understanding of the role of historical and cultural forces in science generally and in medicine in particular.[4] As Fleck has shown, medicine is a promising arena in which to explore the role of values and goals in scientific knowledge claims. In medicine, concerns to know truly and to intervene efficiently intertwine.[5] The role of social values is often outrageously salient.

Consider, for example, the following case history provided in Isaac Baker Brown's *On the Curability of Certain Forms of Insanity, Epilepsy, Catalepsy, and Hysteria in Females*.[6] The volume from which the case is taken is a classic in the literature that focused during the eighteenth and nineteenth centuries on the "disease" of masturbation.[7] Individuals were thought in that period to die from masturbation[8] and autopsy findings substantiated the effects of self-abuse on the spinal cord.[9] Against this background, Dr. Brown recommended that, in order to treat female masturbators, the clitoris be excised to terminate the "long continued peripheral excitement, causing frequent and increasing losses of nerve force."[10] By experience he found that the best approach was, after placing the patient "completely under the influence of chloroform, [to have] the clitoris freely excised by scissors or knife—I always prefer the scissors."[11] It is in terms of these assumptions that Dr. Brown published a number of cases to demonstrate the success of his therapeutic interventions. Consider as an example case number thirty-one of the some forty-eight cases included in his volume.

Case XXXI. Cataleptic Fits—Two Years' Illness—Operation—Cure.M.N., aet. 17; admitted into the London Surgical Home September 4, 1861.

History.—Was perfectly well up to the age of fifteen, when she went to a boarding school in the West of England. In the course of three or four months she became subject to all symptoms of hysteria, and from that time gradually got worse, having fits, at first mild in character and of rare occurrence, but gradually more severe and frequent, till she became a confirmed cataleptic. For several months before admission, she had been attacked with as many as four or five fits a day, and during the whole journey from the North of England to London she was unconscious and rigidly cataleptic. She was seen immediately on arrival, and there was no doubt that it was a genuine case of this disease. So sensitive was she, that if any one merely touched her bed, or walked across the room, she would immediately be thrown into the cataleptic state.

Before making any personal examination, Mr. Brown ascertained both from her mother and herself, that she had long indulged in self-excitation of the clitoris, having first been taught by a school-fellow. The commencement of her illness corresponded exactly with the origin of its cause; in fact, cause and effect were here so perfectly manifested, that it hardly wanted anything more than the history to enable one to form a correct diagnosis. All the other symptoms attending these cases were, however, well marked.

The next day after admission she was operated upon, and from that date she never had a fit. She remained in the Home for several weeks. Five weeks after operation, she walked all over Westminster Abbey, whereas for quite a year and a half before treatment, she had been incapable of the slightest exertion.[12]

The young woman was successfully diagnosed and treated. Social and cultural expectations had shaped the process of observation. It had structured the psychology of discovery.

One need not go to the nineteenth century to encounter the obvious intrusions of social values. The recent history of homosexuality has seen it develop from an instance of sociopathic personality disturbance in the first *Diagnostic and Statistical Manual of the American Psychiatric Association* (DSM-I),[13] to a personality disorder in *DSM-II,*[14] and to an instance of psychosocial dysfunction in *DSM-III* under the taxon ego-dystonic homosexuality,[15] and then to an instance in *DMS-III-R* of sexual dysfunction under the obscure taxon sexual disorder not otherwise specified, in a way that would include heterosexuals' "persistent and marked distress about their sexual orientation."[16] In *DSM-IV*, homosexuality remains under the same rubric as in *DSM-III-R*.[17] In short, it is now a mental disorder only if the individual has a persistent concern to change sexual orientation. This shift in the medical understanding of homosexuality was tied to changes in ideas of sexuality, the notion of perversion, and views regarding the proper bounds of disease language. Similar controversies have been directed to the classification of disorders such as Late Luteal Phase Dysphoric Disorder (commonly called premenstrual stress syndrome), Sadistic Personality Disorder, and Self-defeating Personality Disorder.[18] The fashioning of classifications for psychiatric disorders reveals the ways in which values and expectations legitimate particular classifications of disease.[19] What is at stake are not simply ways in which the psychology of discovery has been directed by background expectations, but the role of moral and metaphysical understanding and how they are sustained and directed by different communities.

The difficulties in becoming clear regarding what should count as a disease are not restricted to psychiatry or to sexuality. One might think of the fashionable nineteenth-century disease of chlorosis, "impoverishment of the blood, constipation, dyspepsia, palpitation, and menstrual derangements and irregularities."[20] Reputable physicians from Thomas Sydenham (1624–89) in the seventeenth century to numerous physicians in the nineteenth century described women as in fact turning green from the disease. The past is replete with views and experiences of illness at odds with our current understandings. Among such one might also include the ways in which fevers were considered diseases, not just symptoms, through the eighteenth century.[21] The more one moves to the past, the more the landscape of disease departs from the one to which we are accustomed.

In fact, the further one retreats into the past, the more difficult it is to recognize diseases with which we are familiar. Physicians then did not have the same concerns as we do. As a result, they described illnesses in somewhat different fashions. Their views of the line between what should count as noise and information were fashioned in terms of presuppositions often quite unlike ours. Consequently it is often difficult to understand what diseases they were in fact describing. Consider a case given in the Hippocratic corpus.

In Meliboea a youth took to his bed after being for a long time heated by drunkenness and sexual indulgence. He had shivering fits, nausea, sleeplessness, but no thirst.

First day. Copious, solid stool passed in abundance of fluid, and on the following days the excreta were copious, watery and of a greenish yellow. Urine thin, scanty and of no colour; respiration rare and large with long intervals; tensions, soft underneath, of the hypochondrium, extending out to either side; continual throbbing throughout of the epigastrium; urine oily.

Tenth day. Delirious but quiet, for he was orderly and silent; skin dry and tense; stools either copious and thin or bilious and greasy.

Fourteenth day. General exacerbation; delirious with much wandering talk.

Twentieth day. Wildly out of his mind; much tossing; urine suppressed; slight quantities of drink were retained.

Twenty-fourth day. Death.[22]

Though we might have a number of suppositions regarding the nature of the disease, it is difficult to advance any particular diagnosis with assurance. This is not simply because Hippocrates fails to provide us with laboratory data; he also does not provide us with the sort of physical examination we would undertake, were we faced with the same case and the need to make a diagnosis in the absence of any laboratory findings. We would also provide a more complete past history, filled out in terms of our presuppositions regarding the youth's fatal illness.

We also readily recognize some constellations of findings in the descriptions of past physicians. One might think here of the famous Hippocratic description of mumps with orchitis.

Many had swellings beside one ear, or both ears, in most cases unattended with fever, so that confinement to bed was unnecessary. In some cases there was slight heat, but in all the swellings subsided without causing harm; in no case was there suppuration such as attends swellings of other origin. This was the character of them: flabby, big, spreading, with neither inflammation nor pain; in every case they disappeared without a sign. The sufferers were youths, young men, and men in their prime, usually those who frequented the wrestling school and gymnasia. Few women were attacked. Many had dry coughs which brought up nothing when they coughed, but their voices were hoarse. Soon after though in some cases after some time, painful inflammations occurred either in one testicle or in both, sometimes accompanied with fever, in other cases not. Usually they caused much suffering. In other respects the people had no ailments requiring medical assistance.[23]

Is mumps more of a contextless, naked fact than the disease that killed the youth from Meliboea? How does one determine what is really the case in medicine? How does one protect against the errors of physicians such as Baker Brown and properly build a science of medicine on data such as the Hippocratic description of mumps?

These are practical, not just theoretical questions, because medicine's theories lead to actual interventions, as occurred with the clitoridectomies of the nineteenth century. In fact, simply regarding a phenomenon as a medical problem can alter the character of societal expectations. For example, to see the process of giving birth as freighted with medical risks requiring medical interventions from episiotomies to cesarean sections is to change the meaning of giving birth and alter the socially supported rights of expectant mothers and fathers vis-à-vis physicians. As Ivan Illich has argued, the medicalization of life is ubiquitous and can be devastating.[24] Seeing an element of life as a medical problem raises more than issues of scientific medicine. The medicalization of reality raises issues of public policy and of ethics. What one classifies as a disease and how it is classified as a disease has an immediate impact on persons' lives and on society in general. In examining a Pap smear, a decision must be made regarding how many cells with deviant changes of what character must be present before the smear is read as indicating cancer. To be too liberal in classifying cells as cancerous will lead to unnecessary operations. To be too conservative in the classification will lead women to receiving treatment too late for successful cure. How one in part discovers and in part creates lines between cancerous, noncancerous, and precancerous findings is of considerable moment for individuals concerned to keep their bodies intact while avoiding cancer, and for societies interested in containing medical costs and maximizing benefits for their members.[25] How one fashions such classifications will have implications for morbidity, mortality, and financial costs.

In both strong and weak senses, medicine creates a socially accepted reality. Through denominating a problem a medical problem, expectations are created and personal destinies influenced. They are obviously strong senses of fashioning reality in the case of classifications embedded in legally enforced medical viewpoints. Here one might think of the vote by the American Psychiatric Association whether to classify homosexuality as a disease.[26] The medical regard of homosexuality as a disease was integrated within the legal proscription of homosexual activities. Somewhat less socially enforced are the particular stagings of cancer, which lead to particular levels of treatment.[27] Such systems for staging reflect decisions made by communities of physicians regarding the most appropriate and useful ways to characterize an area of reality. The acceptance of a particular staging system involves agreeing to see and react to reality in a disciplined and coordinated fashion. The difference between a stage I and a stage II cancer will be expressed in the differences between limited surgical procedures and more extensive interventions with chemotherapy and/or radiation along with a less optimal prognosis. This is a point to which we will return after an examination of the character of medical accounts of reality.

Medical reality is the result of a complex interplay of evaluative, descriptive, explanatory, and social labeling interests. The ways in which we speak of, react to, and experience medical reality are shaped and directed by these interests. These four clusters of concerns I will synoptically call the four languages of medicine. However, they are more than languages. They represent four conceptual dimensions, within which clinical problems are regarded. They are modes of medicalization. "Language," however, provides a useful metaphor by suggesting that each mode has its own grammar or rules for constructing meaning. There are four different clusters of "syntactical" and "semantical" constraints that shape the ways we speak of, understand, and experience medical reality.

### The four languages of medicine

The experienced reality with which medicine deals is shaped by (1) evaluative assumptions regarding which functions, pains, and deformities are normal in the sense of proper and acceptable; (2) views of how descriptions are to be given; (3) causal explanatory models; and (4) social expectations regarding individual ills or particular forms of sickness. The more we share assumptions with those who frame an account of a disease, the easier it is to recognize the diseases they portray and to agree with their characterizations offered of medical reality. The more the assumptions differ, the less the accounts will be intersubjective.

Consider the differences between current classifications of pain and those of the eighteenth century. In the twentieth century, pains are regarded, for the most part, as symptoms of diseases, rather than as diseases in their own right. Pains do not appear among the major classes of disease in the current *International Classification of Diseases*.[28] In contrast, the classification of diseases *Genera morborum* (1763) by Carl von Linné (Carolus Linnaeus) (1707–78) listed pains as one of the eleven major classifications of disease.[29] The influential classification provided by the French physician François Boissier de Sauvages (1701–67) also listed pains prominently as one of the ten classes of disease.[30] The differences in classification of pain turn on differences in presumptions regarding the reality of diseases. They subtly direct physicians regarding how they should take seriously the pains of their patients. Currently, for example, since pains are not considered diseases in their own right, they tend to be discounted unless they can be shown to have a pathoanatomical or pathophysiological cause. We are led to look for the pathoanatomical or pathophysiological truth value of a complaint before we acknowledge it as being fully bona fide.[31]

The interplay of descriptive, evaluative, explanatory, and social labeling languages in health care thus shapes our appreciation of a medical problem. Though the four languages inseparably intertwine, they can be distinguished. Distinguishing them can allow us to appreciate the roots of different understandings of disease in different cultural contexts. It can also aid us in seeing how hidden value and policy judgments shape the "medical facts" we accept. If the role of such value and policy judgments is not recognized, we are likely to accept uncritically what is offered to us as "the scientific facts." What is presented as a fact, especially as a scientific fact, often has a cachet similar to the deliverances of a divine revelation to a community of believers. It may be considered a value-free timeless reality. This engenders difficulties. If homosexuality is in fact a disease, how could one vote whether it should be recognized as a mental disorder? Should not the determination of its standing be reserved for scientific investigation alone? To answer questions such as these, one will need to examine the languages of medicine in some detail.

## Disease language as evaluative

To see a phenomenon as a disease, deformity, or disability is to see something wrong with it. Diseases, illnesses, and disfigurements are experienced as failures to achieve an expected state, a state held to be proper to the person afflicted. This may be a failure to achieve an expected level of freedom from pain or anxiety. It may involve a failure to achieve an expected realization of human form or grace. Or it may involve a failure to achieve what is an expected span of life. These genres of judgments characterize a circumstance as one of suffering, one of pathology, one of a problem to be solved. Such judgments may be made either by the individuals afflicted or by others regarding those individuals. In being characterized as perverted, diseased, or deformed, an adverse judgment is rendered. This is the case even with a disfigured nose, for which the bearer seeks cosmetic surgery.

THE SEARCH FOR VALUES IN NATURE. How does one encounter medical phenomena as problems? Is it in terms of societally conditioned values? Or are there values ingredient in natural processes that can be disclosed as guidelines for appreciating what should count as biological and psychological norms? Until recently, especially within Western thought, the answer affirmed the latter. The presumption was that nature contained ingredient goals and purposes by which dysfunctions, disfigurements, and disabilities could be judged objectively. One sees this language most fully developed in the language of sexual perversion. Consider the following statutory definition of an unnatural act and perversion.

Every person who is convicted of taking into his or her mouth the sexual organ of any other person or animal, or who shall be convicted of placing his or her sexual organ in the mouth of any other person or animal, or who shall be convicted of committing any other unnatural or perverted sexual practice with any other person or animal, shall be fined not more than one thousand dollars ($1,000.00), or be imprisoned in jail or in the house of correction or in the penitentiary for a period not exceeding ten years, or shall be both fined and imprisoned within the limits above prescribed in the discretion of the court.[32]

How does one know that such acts are unnatural? How does one discover the norm from which the activities deviate? Does one appeal to statistical frequencies regarding what individuals usually or customarily do in a particular society? If so, what moral force would such findings have? How could they disclose a biological or physiological ideal?

The traditional Western answer was given in terms of a view of man and of nature as created by God and therefore designed toward the achievement of the purposes of God. To speak of perverting nature in sexual or other activities thus presupposes a divine standard ingredient in nature from creation. The Western Christian Middle Ages was thus able to synthesize a set of presumptions regarding the Creator God and His designs for nature with an Aristotelian language of essences and final causes. Within the Aristotelian framework, it was presumed that one could discover the essences of things and that an examination of these essences would disclose ingredient purposes. These Aristotelian assumptions, when fortified by Stoic views that one's lot was maximized by following the laws of nature, made a fertile ground for the completion of the Western Christian synthesis in terms of which one could then discover what was natural and unnatural. Such presuppositions supported judgments such as those by Thomas Aquinas that, all things being equal, masturbation is a greater sin than a naturally performed rape, because masturbation violates the very law of nature.[33]

Certain views of a designing Creator God make it plausible to presume that one will be able to discover what are truly and objectively diseases by appeal to the design of nature. One will need only to attend to *the* function of the organs in question in order to decide whether a particular condition should count as a disease. This is plausible as long as one remains within a view that integrates the requirements of morality with a metaphysical theory in order to give a normative account of nature. Things appear quite different within a secular neo-Darwinian perspective. Consider color blindness, which is a disadvantage in a number of environments but which confers an advantage if one needs to recognize camouflage. In environments where spotting camouflage increased reproductive success, color blindness would confer an advantage on the individual with the trait.[34] However, in terms of the creationist view, one could still understand the trait as a defect. It is simply that in a particular deviant environment, a defect may produce an advantage. The same would be the case with respect to homosexuality, which in certain environments might confer an advantage. Those who recognize God as designing human nature, albeit through evolution, still have as a canonical reference point the ideal nature of man adapted for the ideal environment, Eden before the fall.

In terms of presumptions regarding ideal designs, one can make moral, physio-aesthetic, and anatomico-aesthetic judgments regarding proper human form, function, and freedom from pain. However, once one departs from a perspective that acknowledges a design, how can one appeal to a canon of normality that will provide a basis for value judgments? One cannot appeal to a design or to *the* ideal environment. Nor will appealing to what is statistically normal in itself decide what ought to be the case. From the fact that most people may lie or cheat to some extent, it does not follow that such behavior is praiseworthy, proper, or ideal. The same holds for widely distributed, if not nearly universal diseases, such as caries or arteriosclerosis among the elderly. This is not to deny that problems will come to be accepted if they are frequent enough. Individuals may indeed acquiesce in widely distributed diseases. However, when given the opportunity to treat them, such circumstances may be recognized as clinical problems, as illnesses, as diseases. What would be the basis for such a judgment?

Abnormality is recognized as abnormality within a particular context of expectations. For example, if one steps away from moral traditions with strong notions of certain actions being improper, it is difficult to make sense of consensual acts being perverse or unnatural. Consider the example of a brother and sister who are competent, sterile, and unmarried who decide at the age of fifty to have intercourse. Is such an act unnatural? Is it perverse? Is it wrong? If there is consent and no likely harm (e.g., there will be no children who will be harmed), there may be little adverse to say in general secular moral terms. Yet the impropriety of incest is understood within traditional Judaism and Christianity without the metaphysical presuppositions of Roman Catholicism. While acknowledging the all-pervasive fallen character of the world and the role of evolution in biological history, traditional Christianity can recognize acts and inclinations that violate the nature of the moral life as perverse or unnatural. Indeed, all sexual acts outside of the marriage of a man and a woman will be appreciated as perverse and unnatural, with some being worse than others.[35] But such understandings cannot be shared with moral strangers. This whole range of moral and nonmoral wrongness, including the wrongness of sibling incest as just sketched, cannot be appreciated in general secular moral terms or within its vision of human normality and abnormality.

Thus, on the one hand, one again encounters the vacuity of a secular moral account. On the other hand, one must recognize the presence of numerous competing content-full normative visions. Feminist, Roman Catholic, and Orthodox Jewish visions of reality in general, and of medical reality in particular, remind us in their diversity of the contrasting character of different understandings, not just of exploitation and proper action, but of what counts as normal or perverse.

DISEASE AS SPECIES ATYPICALITY, OR THE ATTEMPT TO DISCOVER DESIGN IN THE PRODUCTS OF EVOLUTION. One might, as Christopher Boorse, attempt to discover what should count as a disease by appealing to species-typical levels of species-typical functions, which have been established through evolution. Thus, in his earlier works Boorse attempted to distinguish between a concept of illness, which is value laden, and one of diseases, which is value free. Boorse characterized illnesses as states of affairs in which one has a disease that is serious enough to be incapacitating and that is "(i) undesirable for its bearer; (ii) a title to special treatment; and (iii) a valid excuse for normally criticizable behavior."[36] In contrast, he attempted to fashion a notion of disease that is independent of desires and societal roles. Thus, he framed a concept of disease in these terms:

1. The *reference class* is a natural class of organisms of uniform functional design; specifically, an age group of a sex of a species.
2. A *normal function* of a part or process within members of the reference class is

a statistically typical contribution by it to their individual survival and reproduction. . . .

3. A *disease* is a type of internal state which is either an impairment of normal
   functional ability, i.e. a reduction of one or more functional abilities below
   typical efficiency, or a limitation on functional ability caused by environmental agents.

4. *Health* is the absence of disease.[37]

In this way, Boorse attempts to identify deviations from a norm so as to discover
what ought to count as diseases. Even without creationist presumptions, and
without an appeal to societal values, he hopes to disclose the line between health
and disease.

The difficulties with Boorse's approach are multiple. First, in placing his
accent on individual reproductive fitness, he fails to accent the more generally
acknowledged notion of inclusive fitness. What appears to be important in evolution is not whether a particular individual reproduces, but whether that individual
maximizes the chances of his genes being spread in the gene pool. Thus, if one
does not marry and stays at home as a bachelor uncle or maiden aunt, one may
maximize the reproductive capacities of one's siblings with whom one stays, and
thus in fact maximize the chances of genes such as one's own being passed on.

It is not just that Boorse overlooks the role of inclusive fitness in evolutionary
accounts of "biological design"; he is unsympathetic to the fact that species may
in fact be well adapted because of a balance among various contrasting traits.
There may not be a single design, but rather a number of designs. When such is
the case, one cannot speak straightforwardly of either species design or species
typicality. In contrast, Boorse's approach reflects a somewhat Platonic view that
favors a single typical way to achieve the excellence of humans.[38] A number of
traits undoubtedly exist in balance, because the balance itself maximizes inclusive fitness. Here one might think of the somewhat classic case of sickle cell
disease. If sickle cell disease developed, as it appears, to confer a protection for
pregnant women against falciparum malaria, it is then a successful product of
evolution.[39] What is to count as a species-typical blood type? A particular blood
type, or a balance among types that may include sickle cell? The "human species
typical design" appears to be a balance among a number of different designs or
traits.

It is for this reason that Boorse is so clear that homosexuality should count as a
disease.[40] In the absence of such a notion of typicality, it will not even be clear
how one could determine in general secular terms what should count as homosexuality. Will a single homosexual encounter suffice? It is not clear whether
Boorse has in mind individuals who would rate as Kinsey 5s or 6s on the Kinsey
scale, which ranges from Kinsey zeros, who have never had any homosexual
experience, to Kinsey 5s, whose homosexual experiences dominate their sexual

lives, to Kinsey 6s, who are innocent of any heterosexual activity. What of Kinsey 4s, who although they have predominantly homosexual encounters still have heterosexual experiences, and who may reproduce at the same rate as Kinsey zeros? In short, the more one recognizes how biological and behavioral phenomena often express themselves along a continuum, the more difficult it becomes to speak of species typicality, without explicit appeal to a particular normative viewpoint.

The problem is that it is difficult to decide what is or is not a medical problem, if one does not specify an environment and a set of goals. But appeals to evolution, reproductive fitness, and inclusive fitness do not resolve what should count as a problem to be treated by medicine. One will not be able to decide whether sickle cell disease (i.e., being homozygous for sickle cell trait) is in fact a disease, unless one knows whether one is taking a species-oriented or an individual-oriented perspective. If one is concerned about individual pain and suffering and the circumscription of life expectancy, being homozygous for sickle cell will be a disease. On the other hand, if one is concerned to maximize species survival, one will hope that sickle cell trait remains in the gene pool, in the event that through some worldwide catastrophe falciparum malaria would spread without the ability to control it through drugs (e.g., Jesuit bark). One might thus term it not a disease but an element of an evolutionarily secured advantage.

To decide what is a problem for medicine, one must make reference to a particular environment and a particular set of goals, so that one can understand whether the individual is well adapted. What will be required for the realization of particular goals will differ from environment to environment. If one is a black living in Trondheim without the availability of exogenous vitamin D, then the possession of highly pigmented skin would put one at a disadvantage with regard to survival. One will have a greater risk, for example, of developing rickets. However, if the environment were to include vitamin D–enriched milk, as is the case in modern circumstances, the individual becomes well adapted. So, too, a Norwegian with lightly pigmented skin and without adequate clothing and protection from the sun will run a markedly increased risk of developing carcinoma of the skin if transported to the tropics. The notion of successful adaptation is context specific and determined by what one wishes to achieve in a particular context.

One cannot simply turn to the results of evolution to determine what should count as a disease. From a general secular perspective, we are the product of blind, selective forces, which, if they have been successful, have adapted us to environments in which we may no longer live. Since what is species typical may represent an adaptation to environments in which we no longer live, it may not afford us the same degree of adaptation as that provided by some species-atypical trait. Moreover, evolution is not directly concerned with the comfort and pleasure of humans or with their goals. For all these reasons, one will not be able simply to turn to biological conditions or the outcomes of evolution in order to discover what ought or ought not to be seen as a medical problem. Conditions stand out as problems because they thwart the goals of particular individuals or groups of individuals or because they make difficult the realization of particular understandings of the good or virtuous life.

It might be the case that zoologists would be interested in determining what states of affairs represent species-atypical departures from species-typical levels of function. But one cannot know whether such are good or bad departures until they are seen within the context of particular human goals and values in a particular environment. Since evolution does not aim at the realization of the goals of individuals or of societies, the outcomes of evolution can fail to be in accord with individual and societal goals and values. Indeed, sickle cell anemia offers an example of the lack of coincidence. To speak metaphorically, the individuals who die of sickle cell disease are, from an "evolutionary perspective," sacrificed in the process of maximizing the fitness of heterozygotes. Individuals, however, will be concerned that their physicians treat them, not to maximize the survival potential of their genes or their species, but to achieve the goals of relief of suffering and avoidance of disability, which the patients hold to be proper. They will establish institutions dedicated to relieving pain, avoiding disability, and restoring ability. Such individual or societal perspectives are alien to evolution, which as such has no perspective. Evolution is, after all, a general term for a process in which traits appear through random mutations and are selected by the blind forces of nature. Evolution is a change in gene frequencies from one generation to another.

As a result, one must note yet another difficulty in appealing to the conditions of nature or the results of evolution. Such an appeal makes one's judgments regarding what ought or ought not to count as disease hostage to the past.[41] What one now finds as species-typical levels of species-typical functions are the result of past selective pressures, which may have delivered biological capacities ill adapted to current circumstances. One might think, for instance, of menopause, which is most likely the result of past evolutionary forces in circumstances where few women lived to reach menopause. Consequently, the development of the phenomenon may well have conferred neither an advantage nor a disadvantage. In any event, the species-typical character of calcium metabolism for postmenopausal women is one of negative calcium balance. More calcium is absorbed than deposited, leading to the development of osteoporosis and painful debilities such as collapsing vertebrae and greater exposure to risks of fractures. Such phenomena are as species typical as menopause itself. Yet one would usually want to say that osteoporosis in postmenopausal women is a disease. One must recognize that the blind outcomes of nature are sometimes beneficial, sometimes neutral, and sometimes undermining of our purposes and welfare. As a consequence, a physician will be unable to determine a classification of disease simply by attempting to discover what will count as species-atypical levels of species-typical functions.

In short, a project such as Boorse's must fail. A species-atypical level of a species-atypical function correlated with a decreased reproductive rate will not be a sufficient condition for acknowledging a circumstance as a disease. Even if, for example, one determined that individuals with IQs over 140 tended not to reproduce as effectively as individuals within two standard deviations from the norm, one would likely not wish to characterize high intelligence as a disease. On the other hand, as the example involving menopause suggests, a species-atypical level of a species-atypical function is not a necessary condition for being a disease. One can in fact identify such circumstances as osteoporosis in postmenopausal women as diseases. Having a species-atypical level of a species-atypical function is neither a necessary nor a sufficient condition for having a disease. The point is that appeals to facts of the matter will not sustain an adequate reconstruction or account of the ways in which patients and physicians understand diseases.

How, then, is one to identify the normal and abnormal, the diseased and the healthy? Medicine as a secular science cannot appeal to the design of the Creator. Second, as even Boorse will agree, statistical findings are at best suggestive, but surely not defining, of what should count as diseases for medicine. Third, appeals such as Boorse's to species typicality are of primary interest only to biologists engaged in unapplied scientific research.[42] Here, criticism of approaches such as Boorse's can be put in a qualified positive light. As a zoologist, one may have an interest in determining what levels of function characterize a particular species. One may in addition be interested in discovering the evolutionary processes that led to those circumstances. But such are not the interests of physicians or patients who have nonepistemic goals such as the relief of pain, the preservation of function, the achievement of desirable human form and grace, and the postponement of death. If Christopher Boorse has succeeded at all, he has reconstructed not clinical medicine's concept of disease, but perhaps a notion of disease that would be employed by an unapplied scientist. It is because medicine is applied to the achievement of particular individual and societal goals that Boorse's attempt fails. One must wonder, since he does not consider the notion of inclusive fitness, whether Boorse's account would be in fact adequate for a zoologist. In any event, Boorse has unwittingly done us the very important service of underscoring the special character of medicine's concerns by contrasting them with the concerns of unapplied biological science.[43]

DISEASES AND VALUE JUDGMENTS. Problems stand out as problems for medicine because they are disvalued.[44] They are seen as pathological. They are associated with pathos or suffering, and suffering is judged, all else being equal, to have a disvalue. The very appreciation of a problem as a problem for medicine is tied to its appearing as a failure to achieve a desired state. It may be a failure to achieve a desired or expected level of freedom from pain or anxiety. It may involve a failure to achieve an expected level of function. It may involve a failure to achieve an expected realization of human form or grace. Or it may involve a failure to achieve what is an expected span of life. These genres of judgments depend on a family of values; they characterize circumstances as ones of suffering, of pathology, or as problems to be solved. As we shall see, there is the additional presumption that the problem is of the sort that is beyond immediate willing away and is embedded in a web of causal forces of an anatomical, physiological, or psychological sort open to medical explanation and manipulation. This qualification is needed in order to distinguish these disvalued circumstances that are viewed as causally determined and that are given to medicine vis-à-vis those viewed as due to human choice and given to the charge of law. These negative judgments may be made either by the individuals afflicted or by others regarding those individuals. When a person is characterized as diseased or deformed, an adverse judgment is rendered. This is the case whether one is concerned with tuberculosis or such circumstances as a disfigured nose for which the bearer seeks cosmetic surgery.

One encounters a wide range of problems that lie along a continuum. On one end of the continuum there are circumstances likely to be disvalued in whatever culture an individual lives, and in terms of whatever goals are possessed by individuals or societies. One need not presume transcultural values regarding the proper range of human function or form. One need only recognize that certain circumstances are likely to be impediments to the realization of goals (1) in nearly any foreseeable environment and (2) in terms of any likely cluster of human purposes. Thus, on the one hand, crushing substernal pain radiating down the left arm accompanied by weakness, collapse, and a feeling of impending death is likely to make myocardial infarction a disvalued circumstance across cultures, even if there are appreciable differences in cultural values regarding human function. On the other hand, color blindness, the inability to roll up the sides of one's tongue, or the incapacity to taste phenylthiocarbamide may or may not count as genetic diseases or defects, depending on the environment in which persons live and the goals they and their cultures support.[45] Notions of proper human form and grace are heavily infected by values and cultural expectations.[46]

One can recognize a complex interplay among environment, cultural expectations, individual goals, and the ways in which problems stand out as diseases, while still expecting a considerable amount of cross-cultural agreement regarding what should count as diseases. One will be able to acknowledge that cultures not only influence goals but also shape the environment in which the goals are achieved, while still accounting for the intersubjectivity of disease claims in terms of the many conditions that undermine goals across environments and cultures, whatever the goals might be. Since the treatment of diseases is a societal undertaking, those conditions more generally acknowledged as problems worthy of treatment will be more easily accepted as diseases. Thus, tuberculosis, schizophrenia, myocardial infarction, and osteogenic sarcoma can be straightforwardly acknowledged as diseases and need not be termed ego-dystonic tuberculosis, ego-dystonic schizophrenia, or ego-dystonic myocardial infarction.

There are, however, difficulties when conditions do not generally impede values across cultures and groups. Consider how the categorization of menopause as a disease would meet with greater controversy than a similar categorization of tuberculosis or myocardial infarction. It is not sufficient to note that one may refuse treatment for menopause. The judgment that one has a disease carries a negative valence. The term disease may function adequately for identifying tuberculosis, while being less appropriate for circumstances such as menopause, which only certain persons, in certain circumstances, may regard as clinical problems to be treated. After all, for some, refusing treatment might not be enough. They would also wish to refuse the very categorization of menopause as a disease.

Given these concerns, one might even wish to eliminate or strongly qualify the term *disease* in situations where misunderstandings could arise. One might think of substituting the term *clinical problems* to identify those difficulties that stand out as conditions that ought to be addressed and solved by medicine.[47] Such a term would more accurately indicate the ways in which clusters of value judgments make conditions stand out as problems to be treated. It would also contribute to enlightening the long history of disputes regarding the nature of diseases. One might think here of the disputes between ontologists and physiologists of disease, between those who held diseases to be in some sense things or entities and those who held them to be artificial characterizations of physiological and anatomical phenomena.[48] If what makes a cluster of findings stand out as a disease is that it bothers individuals in a way that medicine can explain or cure, it is more accurate to consider diseases not as enduring entities, but clusters of findings collected together because of their usefulness in giving prognoses and guiding treatment. Clinical, etiological, and pathoanatomical "disease entities" serve as treatment warrants.[49] One draws a line between innocent physiological or psychological findings and pathological findings because of particular human values in a particular circumstance, not because of the discovery of an essential distinction that exists outside of particular human expectations. In determining what should count as a problem warranting therapy, considerations of costs of treatment, quality of outcome, and length of survival may all be incorporated. The more nominalist or instrumentalist views of disease are better justified in that they eschew the ontological quest to discover the essence of disease.

The term *clinical problem* underscores the fact that an attempt to give a neutralist, purely descriptive, account of disease fails. Diseases stand out for us as problems to be solved, all else being equal. Of course, attendant circumstances may make things far from equal. Having the right disease at the right time may provide one with an exemption from military service or a comfortable disability income. However, a disease is a disease because it is disvalued—in a particular way. It is a clinical problem. One may still draw a distinction, somewhat as Boorse drew, between illness and disease in order to discriminate between those physiologically, anatomically, or psychologically rooted circumstances that are in fact currently causing suffering versus those circumstances that will surely or likely lead to suffering for that individual, or those circumstances that usually lead to suffering for humans or for animals of X sort (here one will need to recall the special problem of speaking of the diseases of nonhuman animals). Such does not indicate a contextless disease reality. It acknowledges rather that an individual has a disease, a clinical problem, but is not yet, or is not now, ill. The judgment of illness will then bring with it the special negative evaluations that are associated with current suffering.

The central point is that we encounter diseases, illnesses, disabilities, sufferings through a web of important nonmoral values. The values are not those involved in holding that an individual is evil for violating the rights of others or for failing to be charitable or benevolent. The nonmoral values that structure medicine are also distinguishable from the nonmoral values employed in such judgments as "That is a beautiful sunset," "That is an ugly painting," "That is an attractive person," though they have a similarity in having aesthetic characteristics. They are values invoked in judging human function, form, and grace. They reflect ideals of freedom from pain, of human ability, and of bodily form and movement. They are aesthetic in that deformity and dysfunction are ugly. They have their special sense in depending on ideals of anatomical, physiological, and psychological achievement and realization.

To say that John is diseased, deformed, or disabled is to pass a negative value judgment. The force of such judgments will range from those that are rather mild, such as "Mary has a disfigurement," to those that are rather strong, such as "Herbert is perverted." Often the values lie hidden within the disease term itself, as occurs in "George is a schizophrenic." Schizophrenia is not valued; to be judged schizophrenic is to bear a disvalue. Whether it is athlete's foot, tuberculosis, or a deformed nose, diseases or clinical problems are not good things to have. They are things that are good to prevent, treat, or cure. So, too, concepts of health remind people what ought to be achieved.

Concepts of health function both negatively and positively. On the one hand, concepts of health indicate what states of affairs ought to be avoided. In this sense, concepts of health identify an absence of a particular disease or disorder. To be healthy in this sense is not to be ill. Concepts of health usually work in the very opposite way of that which was invited by the World Health Organization in its 1958 statement, where it argued that "health is a state of complete physical,

mental and social well-being and not merely the absence of disease or infir-
mity.''[50] In this sense, as well as others, there are not only many diseases but
many healths.[51] There are both negative senses of health (health as absence of
particular diseases, deformities, and dysfunctions) as well as positive senses of
health.[52] In their broadest meaning, concepts of health give substantial direction
regarding the significance of well-being and of human flourishing.[53] Because
both concepts of health and disease are shaped by the interplay of numerous
values, it will not be possible to discover a clear line between intervening to
correct abnormalities versus to enhance potentials. For example, would a cure for
menopause correct an abnormality or would it be a mere enhancement of individual well-being? To distinguish between curing a disease and enhancing nature,
one must possess a notion of what is species typical, normative, or natural.
Within the polymorphism of traits within actual species, one must recognize a
guiding design so as to discern what will count as restoring the normal state
versus enhancing function. Outside of a particular understanding of human nature, its purposes, and its values, such distinctions and discernment cannot be
made. We will turn to this issue in greater detail in chapter 9, when we examine
the science-fictional allure of germline genetic engineering. Only by appreciating
the web of nonmoral value judgments that direct our bioethical judgments will
one be able fully to understand the actual social transactions that occur in health
care.[54] One is not simply concerned in health care to maintain one's moral
integrity or to achieve moral virtue. Health care is directed to the realization of a
wide range of nonmoral values regarding bodily and mental function, form, and
freedom from distress.

*Disease language as descriptive*

Diseases do not appear simply through a web of values. They are also appreciated, understood, and seen through a set of descriptive assumptions. Language is
an intersubjective undertaking and therefore requires a standardization of terms
and, as a result, leads to a standardization of concepts as well. The more that
precision is required, the more the standardization becomes formal. One might
think here of the *Systematized Nomenclature of Pathology,* which provides three
alternative ways of describing findings, so that, for instance, Wilson's disease
can be described as ''copper disorder,'' ''ceruloplasmin disorder,'' or ''hepato-
lenticular degeneration.''[55] One can provide descriptive terms that are etiological, anatomical, or clinical, depending on one's context. The choice is not an
innocent one, for it already skews the ways in which one comes to appreciate the
matter at hand. One might think here of the criticism by Alvan Feinstein of *The
Standard Nomenclature of Diseases and Operations and of the International
Classification of Diseases.*[56] He argues that such classifications may press a
clinician to be more specific than the data justify. For this reason Feinstein

defends the clinical category of stroke against the more precise terms *cerebral arteriosclerosis* or *encephalopathy*.[57]

Describing reality is always infected with both evaluative and explanatory expectations. One sees in terms of the interpretations one has in mind. It is for this reason that medicine provides excellent examples of missteps in the psychology of discovery. The fact that one sees reality already in terms of one's expectations has been well explored in science generally.[58] But in medicine it has recurring practical importance, as Henrik Wulff has argued with regard to the impact of diagnostic interpretations. The very description of findings as medical casts them in terms of explanations, often importing unnoticed the influence of values and theories. Such diagnostic data transformations occur when one sees a shadow in a lung as pneumonia. But they also occur when one terms someone's heavy breathing "dyspnea" or "shortness of breath." Even to put matters in medical terms is already to appreciate the findings not as innocent rapid breathing, but as a likely difficulty in need of further diagnostic intervention and possible treatment.[59]

Consider the case of Koplik's spots, which are pathognomonic of measles. Whenever one sees Koplik's spots, one can make the diagnosis of measles with a 100 percent probability of being correct. This is the case because Koplik's spots are by definition an element of the beginning of measles. A diagnostic data transformation takes place, however, when one sees small irregular bright red spots on the buccal and lingual mucosa *as* Koplik's spots. One may see some irregular bright red spots with bluish white specks in the center and yet not be sure that they are Koplik's spots. What one will see will turn in part on one's expectations under the circumstances.

One may attempt to describe medical findings as innocently as possible of values and theories, as has been suggested by Lawrence Weed.[60] But even to see problems as medical problems is to put them in a context rich with expectations and presumptions. Descriptions require standardizations of terms. Such standardizations will be fashioned through quasi-political or societal discussions and against background assumptions about what will be useful in achieving particular goals and purposes. Those assumptions are themselves structured by explanatory views.

### Disease language as explanatory

The language of medicine is structured around its explanatory assumptions. Problems are seen as medical problems because they are presumed to be embedded in a pathophysiological, pathoanatomical, or pathopsychological nexus and because the problems are not experienced as removable at the immediate will of the sufferer. As such, they are not legal problems or religious problems, but problems to be resolved through the manipulation of the elements of a special causal web. How one understands this web has major implications. What one accepts as underlying causal forces will influence one's views of how to frame descriptions and regarding what one should judge to be good or bad prognostic signs. Explanatory models bring coherence, as we have already seen, to the multiplicity of events we encounter in medicine. They give a sense to the stories we tell about illness and disease. As we noted in exploring the clinical accounts offered by Hippocrates, such stories differ in terms of what the storyteller takes to be relevant to a coherent account. Explanatory models structure the very sense of what we see and experience.

Even recognizing and naming a cluster of symptoms and signs is itself a form of explanation. A recent dramatic and painful example has been the evolution of our understanding of AIDS. AIDS as acquired immunodeficiency syndrome began simply as a cluster of findings that slowly became ever more prognostic. Initially, the significance of signs was misgauged. For example, the period of usual infection prior to disease was grossly underestimated. There also was a period of time between identification of a syndrome and the initial understanding of its underlying cause, the human immunodeficiency virus (HIV). Numerous diagnostic data transformations became possible as an underlying understanding of the disease evolved. Moreover, as with all diseases, AIDS was also placed within a particular set of social and moral concerns. For example, it would be impossible to understand the full weight of the diagnosis without also understanding the moral and other values brought to the appreciation of venereal disease and homosexuality. But the concerns that shape the experience of AIDS are not only moral values. They turn also, as with all diseases, on nonepistemic values and particular understandings of what it is to explain correctly.

One must note before proceeding that the very nature of explanation is a puzzle. Here it will be enough to distinguish between the issues raised by the structure of explanation, and the issues raised by its goals. Explanation provides, to use a Hegelian idiom, a structure for reflection. It relates different sorts of elements: appearances and laws, observations and regularities. They are related as the weaving together of being in terms of correlatives. Thus, one comes to understand the fevers, pains, rashes, sweating, diarrhea, and so forth of a patient in terms of underlying laws, intelligible patterns, anatomical understandings, or physiological mechanisms. The laws and regularities acquire their sense through that to which they give regularity and coherence. The hidden pathological forces and disease mechanisms have content in their expressions. The various expressions of disease gain meaning and coherence through the mechanisms they are seen to presuppose and express.

The cardinal example in medicine of this intertwining of findings and understandings is the relation between the data of clinicians and the data of pathoanatomists and pathophysiologists, which is provided by the laws of pathoanatomy and pathophysiology. Two worlds of observations are related. The findings of the clinician are related to the observations of the pathoanatomists and pathophysiologists and take on a new significance through these anatomical and pathological observations. The observations of the pathoanatomist and pathophysiologist take on clinical significance through being related to the world of the clinician. This exchange of meanings is effected through a web of mechanisms, laws, and regularities. Explanation affords a coherence among groups of observations and findings.[61] The development of clinical-pathological and pathological-clinical correlations offers an expansion, as we will see, of the explanatory powers of medicine through allowing two different domains of observation to be correlated and reinterpreted through wide-ranging organizational schemes (e.g., through laws in pathology and anatomy). New explanations of diseases can then be tested in different ways by observations within the domains of both clinicians and basic scientists.

This correlation of observations, one with the other, through mechanisms, laws, and regularities, is undertaken in medicine not just to give insight. It is undertaken primarily in order to manipulate reality, that is, to treat diseases, pains, deformities, disabilities, and so forth, as well as to predict the course of diseases, that is, to provide prognoses. Science is in general concerned to provide explanations and predictions and to allow for the manipulation of nature. However, in health care the concerns with predictions and manipulations have a salient nonepistemic character. One is not predicting primarily in order to know or manipulating primarily in order better to understand. Rather one is framing explanations in order to come to terms with the human pains, anxieties, disabilities, and deformities associated with clinical problems. These goals of explanation, as we will see, direct applied sciences such as medicine to mold the character of explanation in order to facilitate the achievement of these nonepistemic goals. One will highlight those explanations most useful in curing disease, alleviating pain, and giving the kinds of prognostic information with which patients are usually concerned.[62]

Medical findings are seen within prevailing etiological, pathological, and psychopathological theories. The contribution made by theories to the ways in which we experience medical reality can be appreciated if one compares how the description of medical problems changes with explanatory accounts. For instance, the various problems associated with tuberculosis, which were once separated within different taxa of traditional nosologies, can now be gathered together under one rubric, given our current etiological model. We see consumption, King's evil, and Pott's disease as all manifestations of *one* disease. On the other hand, we can now clearly distinguish between typhoid and typhus, which were once seen as one disease. There is a dialectical interplay between the descriptions of diseases and the explanatory models used in accounting for them. As a consequence, if one were to enter the world of a seventeenth- or eighteenth-century clinician, one would not find the same understanding we possess today of the significance of tuberculosis, typhus, gonorrhea, or syphilis. The findings we associate with these diseases today were in the past gathered under different rubrics.

Consider the description given by Thomas Sydenham (1624–89) of venereal diseases. In his description, he mixes in a way we no longer would the signs and symptoms of both syphilis and gonorrhea. They were for him one disease.

This disease proceeds in the following manner. The patient, sooner or later, (according as the woman with whom he has lain was more or less infected, and according as his constitution renders him more or less disposed to receive the infection) is first seized with an uncommon pain in the parts of generation, and a kind of rotation of the testicles; and afterwards, unless the patient be circumcised, a spot, resembling the measles in size and colour, seizes some part of *glans,* soon after which, a fluid like *semen* flows gently from it; which differing every day there from, both in colour and consistency, does at length turn yellow, but not so deep as the yolk of an egg.[63]

We are likely to experience similar changes in classification when we develop better etiological accounts for that cluster of diseases we term cancer. We are likely to discover that what we took to be one particular form of cancer may in fact be caused by more than one cluster of etiological factors, leading us in the future to rearrange our descriptions in accord with our explanatory assumptions. Explanatory assumptions frame how medicine is experienced by both patients and practitioners.

Consider one of the better-known classifications of disease, or nosologies, of the eighteenth century, that of François Boissier de Sauvages (1701–67). Sauvages's final classification was presented in a work entitled *Nosologia methodica sistens morborum classes juxta Sydenhami mentem et botanicorum ordinem.*[64] As the title indicates, it is a systematic classification of diseases that follows the suggestions of Thomas Sydenham and that is placed in a botanical order. Thomas Sydenham was himself highly influenced both by the works of Sir Francis Bacon (1561–1626) and by the successes of botany in the seventeenth century.[65] The influence of Bacon and Sydenham remained strong in medicine throughout the eighteenth century, having not only an impact on Sauvages, but on William Cullen[66] (1710–90), among others. In addition, botany continued to offer a paradigmatic example of a successful classification of reality. One sees the influence of botany on medicine in a number of ways, including the fact that Linnaeus, the well-known naturalist and botanist, also provided a classification of diseases.[67] In addition, Sauvages and Linnaeus maintained a correspondence regarding classifications.[68]

The result was a view of diseases and of the reality of illnesses that is strikingly different from ours. Consider the ten major classes under which Sauvages united 42 orders, some 315 genera, and 2,400 species of diseases (depending on which edition one consults).[69]

| I. | Vitia | Defects, blemishes and symptoms treatable by the mechanisms of surgery (this class includes everything from vitiligo and exophthalmos to fractures and herpes) |
|---|---|---|
| II. | Febres | Fevers |
| III. | Phlegmasiae | Inflammations |
| IV. | Spasmi | Spasms |
| V. | Anhelationes | Difficulties in breathing |
| VI. | Debilitates | Weaknesses |
| VII. | Dolores | Pains |
| VIII. | Vesaniae | Insanities |
| IX. | Fluxus | Fluxes |
| X. | Cachexiae | Constitutional disorders and deformities in volume, symmetry, weight, and color (the class includes such "deprivations" as depigmentation and "deformities" as pregnancy) |

For Sauvages and for others of his time, fevers and pains were diseases in their own right, as the classification shows. Moreover, phenomena were brought together in a way that may appear strange to many of our contemporaries. For instance, under fluxes were included both bloody discharges and diarrhea. The classification was clinical, rather than etiological or anatomical, though Sauvages also provided such classifications.

Sauvages developed his classification for reasons very similar to those that influenced the American Psychiatric Association in the development of its *Diagnostic and Statistical Manual of Mental Disorders* (*DSM-III*), as well as its successors, DSM-III-R and DSM-IV: the provision of a theory-neutral description of diseases. Medicine in general was at the time of Sauvages as ignorant of the causes of diseases, and as overwhelmed by conflicting theories, as psychiatry is today. Sauvages, and those who fashioned similar classifications, pursued as unbiased a description of reality as was possible. In this they followed Sydenham, who with Bacon presumed that (1) the world has a general rational structure that (2) can be disclosed by careful examination, were one only (3) to free oneself from distorting prejudices. Sydenham shared with Bacon a view regarding the intrinsic rationality of reality and the capacity of the human mind to know that structure. Consider, for example, Sydenham's injunction in the preface to the third edition of his 1676 *Observationes medicae:*

In writing, therefore, a history of diseases, every philosophical hypothesis which hath prepossess'd the writer in its favour, ought to be totally laid aside, and then the manifest and natural phenomena of diseases, however minute, must be noted with the utmost accuracy; imitating in this the great exactness of painters, who, in their pictures, copy the smallest spots or moles in the originals. For 'tis difficult to give a detail of the numerous errors that spring from hypotheses, whilst 'writers, misled by false appearances, assign such phenomena for diseases, as never existed, but in their own brains.[70]

Sauvages and the other writers of the eighteenth century who were influenced by Sydenham inherited these presuppositions along with Sydenham's influential commitment to the task of understanding the natural histories of diseases. From Sydenham they inherited as well the assumption that descriptions of the reality of disease would disclose species of disease.

Sydenham, Sauvages, Linnaeus, Cullen, and others were guided by an almost paradoxical distrust in theory combined with faith in empirically inquiring reason. They had no sense that their very attempt to see the world free of theory was itself rich in theoretical assumptions concerning the nature of knowledge and of reality. A sense of this is provided in one of the explanatory footnotes provided with Sydenham's *Observations*.

Hypotheses owe their origin to ostentatious vanity and idle curiosity; whence 'tis easy to conceive how much they must needs obstruct the improvement of physick, which is a science that depends chiefly upon well-conducted experiments and close and faithful observation; whereas hypotheses are always built in great part upon feign'd, precarious, and often very obscure principles.[71]

The endeavors of Sydenham, Sauvages, and Cullen, and the nosologies they produced, which appear to us as highly elaborated products of a theory imposed upon reality, were to their authors attempts to free the mind from the burdensome theorizing that characterized much of medicine in the seventeenth and eighteenth centuries.

Undertakings similar to those of Sydenham and Sauvages remain in areas of medicine where theory has had little success in effectively explaining phenomena. A good example is the nosology developed by the American Psychiatric Association. Robert Spitzer in his introduction to DSM-III observed:

For most of the DSM-III disorders, however, the etiology is unknown. A variety of theories have been advanced, buttressed by evidence—not always convincing—to explain how these disorders come about. The approach taken in DSM-III is atheoretical with regard to etiology or pathophysiological process except for those disorders for which this is well established and therefore included in the definition of the disorder.[72]

Seven years later, in his introduction with Janet Williams to the DSM-III-R, the point remains.[73] Although the claim is that these classifications are "atheoretical" with respect to certain theories, they are surely not innocent of theoretical assumptions, any more than were the classifications of Sauvages and Linnaeus. There is rather an attempt to frame a classification with very little dependence on etiological and pathogenic assumptions.

Through the success of anatomy and physiology in providing etiologic and pathogenetic accounts of medical phenomena, the ways in which diseases were experienced by patients and physicians were refashioned as medicine entered the nineteenth century. Although there were anticipations of the role of pathoanatomical correlations with clinical findings in the *Sepulchretum* (1689) of Theophile Bonet (1620–89)[74] and in the *De sedibus et causis morborum per anatomen indagatis* (1761) of Giovanni Morgagni (1682–1771),[75] it was with the beginning of the nineteenth century that the clinical world was radically restructured in terms of work done in the laboratory and the anatomical dissection room. The world of illness that was open to experience by the patient and the clinician alike became correlated with, and reinterpreted in terms of, the findings of the pathoanatomist and the physiologist. Foucault makes this shift central to his work, *The Birth of the Clinic*.[76] As he documents, the gaze turned inward as a result of the work of Xavier Bichat (1771–1802) and François-Joseph-Victor Broussais (1772–1838), among others. The true disease is no longer that which is experienced by the clinician or the patient; the real disease becomes the lesion. As Broussais put it, "true medical observation is that of the organs and their modifiers, it is in fact an observation of the body itself."[77] In the nineteenth century, diseases become, as Rudolf Virchow (1821–1902) put it, "altered vital state[s] of larger or smaller numbers of cells or cell-territories."[78]

One must appreciate the force of this change. The whole language of disease was altered. Fevers were no longer diseases in their own right, but became merely symptoms. Jaundice was now a symptom of the disease hepatitis. These changes required a major recasting of medical reality and a retreat from taken-for-granted clinical nosologies, such as those of Sauvages. Consider, for example, how this shift was experienced by Bichat.

It is well known into how many errors we have fallen, so long as we had confined ourselves to the simple observation of symptoms. Let us take for example consumption. It has been considered as an *essential malady,* before we had recourse to postmortem examination; since, it has been shown that marasmus was only a consecutive symptomatic malady of the affection of an organ. Jaundice has been for a long time considered by practitioners as an *essential malady;* post-mortem examination has also proved that this affection, though primitive, was in reality only consecutive to diverse alterations of the liver, of which it is always the symptom. The same has happened with respect to dropsies, which although for a long time considered as essential affections, have never been other than the result of some organic disease. It is, then, ignorance of organic affections, resulting from a total neglect of post-mortem examination, which is the cause that has misled the ancient practitioners on most diseases; thus, *Cullen* and *Sauvages* have erred in their classifications.[79]

What had been considered to be diseases became symptoms; the reality of diseases is now to be found in changes in organs. A few remnants of the language of eighteenth-century classifications remained. For instance, the term *essential hypertension* recalls when clusters of symptoms, with an unknown causal basis, were held to be a disease in their own right.

The changes were complex. Because of a loss of confidence in causal and anatomical explanations, Sydenham had turned to a clinical phenomenology. The former explanations were involved in hypotheses poorly secured. The latter phenomenology was directed to a clinical reality manifest to the physician. Sauvages for his part sustained an interest in causal and anatomical classifications. This remained rather marginalized. For example, in the two-volume 1768 edition,[80] of the total 1,562 pages of the body of the work, only 73 pages are devoted to his etiological classifications and a mere 10 pages to his anatomical. At the end of the eighteenth and the beginning of the nineteenth centuries, confidence and energies shifted towards anatomical and then physiological accounts of medical reality. The ontology of the clinician's world as portrayed by Sauvages et al. became discredited and the reality of medicine was reassembled in a novel fashion.

The shift of interest towards anatomical and physiological accounts offered the possibility of explaining under one rubric phenomena that had once been scattered across the nosological frameworks of the eighteenth century. In short, these changes made it possible to unify observations within a new explanatory model. The shift offered insights into the mechanisms of disease that had not previously been available. But most important, it offered a research program through which the bewildering disparate findings and claims of medicine could now be examined, criticized, and organized in terms of emerging understandings of anatomy and physiology. It redirected the energies of medicine in a way that led to major advances in medical understanding during the first part of the nineteenth century and to major advances in therapeutics in the last part of the nineteenth and during the twentieth century.

What one finds in the 1800s is the correlation of two domains of medical description. The first is the traditional domain of clinical findings, which had been the focus of Sydenham, Sauvages, and Cullen. The second is a relatively new domain of descriptions provided by anatomists, physiologists, pathologists, and microbiologists. The two domains were brought together by new accounts of disease that allowed the descriptions to interact. Clinical findings, as well as laboratory findings, could falsify theoretical assumptions. The result was a set of complex opportunities for studying the nature of medical reality. Clinical findings invited the fashioning of theoretical models through which laboratory findings were sought in order to account for those clinical findings, which were then redescribed, now in terms of the emerging basic scientific models. On the other hand, laboratory findings invited clinicians to look for phenomena that could be predicted in terms of the basic scientific models.

A dialectic interaction was established. Clinical findings were redescribed in terms of theoretical models. The redescribed reality could itself then lead to puzzles that would engender further changes in the theoretical models and so on, *ad indefinitum*. The laboratory findings had their real sense as being part of the mechanisms used in explaining the clinical findings. Anatomical findings became lesions because they were the underpinnings for clinical problems. On the other hand, the clinical findings had their sense colored by the theoretical models and the laboratory findings employed in explaining them. There was a dynamic interaction between the explanans and the explanandum, between that which explained and that which was to be explained, each conferring on the other part of its own significance.

Past ways of understanding medicine had come to appear implausible. Consider Broussais's reflections on past medical investigations.

One has filled the nosographical framework with groups of most arbitrarily formed symptoms . . . which do not represent the affections of different organs, that is, the real diseases. These groups of symptoms are derived from entities or abstract beings, which are most completely artificial οντοι; these entities are false, and the resulting treatise is ontological.[81]

However, both Broussais and in fact Foucault failed to appreciate the full significance of these changes. They understood that the world of symptoms had been recast in terms of the presuppositions of a new and powerful research problem. They failed to appreciate that this restructuring carried with it an ideology that discounted the significance of patient complaints. Patient problems came to be understood as bona fide problems only if they had a pathoanatomical or pathophysiological truth value. Absent a lesion or a physiological disturbance to account readily for the complaint, the complaint was likely to be regarded as *male fide*. This requirement was credible because the laboratory sciences had become the basic medical sciences in an important ontological sense. They were seen as disclosing the reality underlying clinical findings. On the other hand, clinical observations, which for Sydenham and Sauvages had been integral to the basic medical science, clinical medicine, now became secondary. Clinical medicine became a manifestation of a deeper reality. This was in a very restricted sense correct with regard to the development of explanatory models. Accounts of disease were now formulated in terms of underlying pathophysiological and pathoanatomical mechanisms. The error lay in failing also to accent the goals and purposes of medicine. As an applied science, medicine remains focused on caring for human suffering. Clinical medicine begins from and returns to the problems of patients. However, the changes in explanatory assumptions, and the development of the basic sciences, led to certain unfortunate changes in the ideology of symptoms.

To appreciate this, one must note that the clinical nosologies accented the problems the patients experienced. Pains constituted, as has been noted, one of the ten classes of disease in the nosology of Sauvages. They were the fourth (dolorosi) of Linnaeus's eleven classes.[82] Consider, for instance, Sauvages's category, "dolores vagi, qui nomen a side fixa non habent" (wandering pains that do not have a name from a fixed site), the first of his five orders of pains.[83] Sauvages's classification allowed him to take patient anxieties and distress as serious problems in their own right. His classification highlighted these symptoms through considering them diseases.

By legitimating such complaints, Sauvages legitimated the social role of those who complained of a wide range of pains and sufferings. By deciding whether a symptom is bona fide or *male fide,* medicine authenticates an individual's claim to particular forms of treatment and a particular social role. Medicine's concern with evaluative, descriptive, and explanatory endeavors is thus also intimately tied to the performative role of language, through which social reality is shaped.

## Disease language as shaping social reality

In addition to describing and evaluating problems as medical and explaining them, physicians and other health care workers place these problems within social practices. Such individuals are gatekeepers of therapy roles, or to use Talcott Parsons's more restrictive term, sick roles.[84] To characterize a patient as sick is not only to say that the patient has a problem that ought to be solved and that the problem can be explained in medical terms. It is also to cast that individual in social roles where certain societal responses are expected. If the individual is placed in a full-fledged sick role, the sick person is usually held not to be responsible for being in that role, is excused from social duties that the illness impairs, and is enjoined to seek treatment from a set of individuals socially recognized as appropriate therapists.[85] A therapeutic imperative is established. In determining that someone is sick one accepts a prima facie claim regarding ways in which the person ought to be treated, in that sickness is a state that, *ceteris paribus,* is not valued, is a state in which people do not want to be. There is thus a defeasible presumption that sick people want to be treated. In addition, a diseased individual may lose particular social rights and prerogatives. Determinations such as insanity will relieve a patient of particular social prerogatives. On the other hand, if the individual is held to be partially or totally disabled, the individual may be able to receive welfare payments.

Medical language thus has a performative character. Just as a sheriff changes legal reality, not simply describes it, when saying to a lawbreaker, "You are under arrest," a physician changes social reality when saying to a patient, "You have cancer"; "You have syphilis"; "You have AIDS"; "You are fifty percent disabled"; or "You have a terminal disease." The patient is placed in a social context with a set of taken-for-granted social expectations. These routinized expectations stabilize the social world through a web of stereotyped roles.[86] This is not to say that without a diagnosis a person will not still die of cancer or AIDS. It is rather that the diagnosis places the various physical and psychological happenings associated with such diseases within a special set of social reactions and expectations. These routine expectations can also direct moral judgments and invite particular responses. It is because medicine focuses primarily on "caused" rather than chosen phenomena that such social roles tend to remove blame for *being* in a state of illness (though blame still may be assigned for becoming ill or remaining ill, insofar as this can be influenced by personal choice, e.g., "You caused your disease through smoking"). It is because states of affairs become clinical problems against the background of health care institutions that offer hope of cure or care that certain individuals (e.g., physicians, dentists) stand out as persons appropriate to address such problems.

The set of expectations that typically defines being sick differs, given different diagnoses. Consider the different ways in which there will be typical, formally or informally established, social responses to a diagnosis of heart disease, cancer, syphilis, AIDS, or acne. There will be different responses on the part of insurance companies, employers, welfare agencies, friends, and lovers. Diagnosis is a complex means of social labeling, as is the process of arresting a criminal. Such labeling shapes social reality toward the achievement of therapeutic goals.

## The social construction of medical reality and the challenge of clinical judgment

Symptoms, signs, pains, deformities, illnesses, diseases, even the body[87] and well-being, appear within a nest of descriptive, evaluative, explanatory, and social expectations. The values presumed in seeing particular circumstances as diseases or clinical problems are conditioned by societies, their views of the good life, and the social roles they support. So, too, common endeavors to describe reality presuppose informal, if not formal, agreements with regard to canonical, descriptive terms. Finally, as the history of medicine has shown, medicine's explanatory goals are pursued by particular groups of scientists with particular understandings of what should count as the proper rules of evidence and inference, which may conflict with lay understandings of disease and treatment or with the understandings of other investigators. To resolve such controversies, those involved will need to make clear what rules of evidence ought to be accepted and why. This question may be confronted by a single scientist when raising the question whether that scientist's explanation should be accepted as *the* explanation, even in the absence of a particular controversy. Explanation is thus always potentially communal, in that one advances knowledge claims with the presupposition that they ought to be accepted by other investigators. Knowledge claims presume their intersubjectivity—that they should be able to be justified generally, even if they are articulated by particular men and women within particular communities and cultures.[88]

There is thus a tension between the universal aspirations of knowers and the particular context in which real individuals actually know and frame explanations. From past experience and on the basis of what one ought to anticipate, given the limitations of human reason, one should expect that not all such controversies will allow of resolution by an appeal to sound arguments alone. One will not always be able decisively to determine what is the correct set of rules of evidence and inference, or the proper set of conclusions. As a result, one will need to appeal even in science to rules of fairness in debate and in the resolution of scientific controversies. One will need to establish procedures, which may often involve committees and votes. A set of nonepistemic considerations will need to be employed in order to bind knowers peaceably in their task of knowing truly.

Science as a social endeavor must mediate the passions, jealousies, and controversies of individual scientists in order to pursue goals that transcend a particular time, culture, and controversy. Much of the mediation is informal. Scientists come to see certain classes of problems as more interesting than others. Common terminologies are fashioned, and incentives such as the approbation of members of the Royal Society direct the inquiries of investigators even in the most abstract of undertakings. The very presence of the Nobel Prize, for instance, motivates scientists across national boundaries and contributes to the cohesiveness of scientific endeavors. The same can be said of funding agencies, which are more likely to support "orthodox" investigations and to shy away from undertakings that appear eccentric.

Such informal constraints are supplemented by formal modes of standardization the more a science is applied. In medicine, this is expressed in the phrase "the usual and customary standards of medical practice." Although these standards may not always have a fully formal articulation, they come to be the object of public discussion and court testimony. In addition, in order for physicians to evaluate the efficacy of different therapies, collective endeavors such as the American Joint Committee on Cancer are organized to fashion rules for the use of descriptive terms in diagnostic categories. In such circumstances the social reality of the applied sciences is settled by votes within committees. The decisions in such circumstances are made not simply in terms of the character of reality as it is taken really to be, but also in terms of which modes of classification will be most useful in organizing treatment and care.

Here one might think in particular of the ways in which cancers are staged.[89] The classification and stagings of cancer are fashioned "to allow the physician to determine treatment for the patient more appropriately, to evaluate results of management more reliably, and to compare statistics reported from various institutions on a local, regional, and national basis more confidently."[90] Such classification and staging is the result of particular social organizations balancing the interests of various groups. One has, for instance, the American Joint Committee for Cancer Staging and End-Results Reporting (organized January 9, 1959) having given the following account of its operation:

Each of the sponsoring organizations designates three members to the Committee. The American College of Surgeons serves as administrative sponsor. Subcommittees, called "task forces," have been appointed to consider malignant neoplasms of selected anatomic sites in order to develop classifications. Each task force is composed of committee members and other professional appointees whose special interests and skills are appropriate to the site under consideration.[91]

As a point of history, there has been a problem in coordinating these classifications of the American Joint Committee on Cancer (AJCC) with the recommendations of the TNM Committee, originally known as the Committee on Clinical Stage Classification and Applied Statistics of the Union Internationale Contre le Cancer. This has involved compromises leading to an observation in 1983: "In a few instances, arbitrary changes have been made to make the recommendations of the AJCC consistent with those of the TNM Committee of the International Union Against Cancer. Consistency at all anatomic sites has not as yet been achieved."[92] The picture is that of the social construction of reality through various formal processes that fashion agreements for common endeavors.

It should be obvious that the ways in which one decides to describe phenomena such as cancer are not of interest to physicians alone. The interests of patients are also involved. The classification of cancer is not like the classification of stars. The choice among different ways of classifying cancers sets the conditions for the ways in which physicians will choose therapeutic interventions. The number of stages selected (why, for instance, use three, four, or five stages for any particular carcinoma?) presupposes cost–benefit calculations and understandings of prudent actions that have direct implications for the ways in which patients are treated. They involve more than purely scientific judgments; they concern as well the proper balancing of benefits and harms in the organization of therapeutic choices around a particular number of stages of cancer. The choice to subdivide stages (e.g., stages IA and B) will reflect the decision that a more complex assessment of therapeutic options is appropriate. There are limitations to the number of subdivisions one can make and still have them remain useful. Human physicians can only remember and easily organize data in terms of a limited number of classifications. Since the treatment of patients and the assessment of the treatment of patients are a collective endeavor, there must be a choice among the competing possibilities for division, subdivision, and classification. There are no unique natural lines in reality to which the classifications correspond. Rather, the categories are as much created as discovered through endowing certain findings with significance.

After one has decided on classifications and systems for staging diseases and clinical problems, one will need to come to terms with the fact that the decisions one will make will at times be wrong. This involves a complex set of moral and prudential concerns that have been gathered under the rubric of clinical judgment and medical decision making, and that can be reconstructed in various artificial intelligence approaches to the problem solving in clinical medicine.[93] In deciding whether an individual has a disease or a clinical problem of a certain sort, one will need to assess the consequences that will follow from being wrong and then take account of that likelihood in establishing the threshold of certainty required to make a diagnosis. One will need, in short, to ask what the costs are of holding a particular diagnosis to be true. For example, if one operates to remove a breast or a prostate on ambiguous data that indicate the presence of a cancer, one may have imposed major costs upon the persons so treated. On the other hand, if one delays the treatment of certain diseases in order to acquire better data, the condition of the patient may worsen. Even the acquisition of diagnostic data is associated with costs. These costs are not only financial but often include risks of morbidity and mortality. Here one might think of the risks of liver biopsy, heart catheterization, and other invasive diagnostic tests. Before one acquires information, one must first judge that the knowledge will likely make a sufficient difference in the treatment of the patient to merit the risks and costs to which the patient will be exposed. In medicine, acquiring knowledge and making knowledge claims have direct implications for the ways in which patients are treated.[94]

Because of the difficulty of deciding what is a proper balance between the risks of over- and undertreating patients, it will often be very difficult to determine whether particular therapeutic interventions are warranted. One will not be able *simply* to discover whether physicians are performing unnecessary hysterectomies or unnecessary tonsillectomies. One will not be able simply to discover, by appeal to factual issues alone, what treatments are indicated, what treatments are appropriate, what treatments are ordinary, or what treatments are extraordinary. Integral to such judgments will be appeals to particular hierarchies of values and to peaceable processes for resolving disputes in these matters. Such judgments will not be purely epistemic. Judgments in such matters depend on deciding how important it is to avoid the problems solved by surgery versus how important it is to avoid the problems that may be caused by surgery (including transfer of funds to surgeons). Because surgical interventions are often predicated on the availability of funds through third-party payers, the definition of necessary versus unnecessary interventions becomes an issue of importance to all who participate in a particular insurance plan (including government welfare policies). Financial considerations, the world of financial reality, will thus play a role in the framing of the world of disease and warranted therapeutic interventions. One needs to find mechanisms for fairly choosing particular criteria. Since a community of individuals is involved, problems of fairness and democratic procedure become salient.

Most of the crucial terms in bioethical debates share in a complexity of this sort. Determinations of death are made against the background of judgments regarding how sure one must be that one can avoid significant numbers of false positive and false negative determinations of death. What will count as a *significant* number is again not a purely factual question. As we will see, what one will mean by a viable fetus in the abortion debate will also not be a purely factual matter. In scientific debates with a heavy ethical and political overlay or in ethical debates with a heavy scientific focus, one will find concerns with values and facts intertwined. By this I do not mean to suggest that the fact–value distinction is not appropriate in many contexts. Rather, the factual and evaluational components, which are distinguishable, occur inseparably bound in everyday debates.

## Seeing a problem as a medical, rather than as a legal, religious, or educational problem

The world of medical findings is only one of a number of finite provinces of meaning controlled by major social institutions. The ability of physicians to create social roles ("You are diseased"; "You are perverted") must be contrasted with the role of bishops to excommunicate or to reconcile, or of judges to declare persons guilty or innocent. As a result, it is not simply a question of how circumstances ought to be construed within medicine, but whether they should be construed within medicine at all, rather than within a collateral and competing institution, such as the law or religion. Each of the major social institutions identifies problems for its care in terms of sets of values that make problem situations stand out as inviting interventions, as failing to meet a standard, as a difficulty to be set aside. The institutions of education, religion, morality, law, and medicine in this fashion variously characterize circumstances as those of ignorance, sinfulness, blameworthiness, criminality, civil liability, or disease. To see a circumstance as one of sinfulness, criminality, or disease is to place it within the province of one of the major social institutions with its peculiar models of explanation and with its own special directing goals.

The facts available within the spheres of religion, law, morality, and medicine are seen as problems of a particular kind in terms of particular webs of values, descriptive conventions, explanatory models, and social roles. Religious accounts of reality involve supernatural causal models dependent on views regarding the final destiny of individuals and the universe. It is in this fashion that religions give ultimate meaning to life, suffering, and death. Legal accounts will incorporate particular systems of evidence and proof, which determine which findings can be assessed in what ways in order to achieve the goals of particular practices of blaming and praising. One might think here of Hart and Honoré's classic account of causation and the law.[95] As they point out, when flowers in a garden wither due to a gardener's failure to tend them, the gardener is held as having caused the flowers to die, though from a more neutral perspective, the failure of a passerby to water the flowers and the absence of sufficient rainfall are equally causes of the flowers dying. It is the social presumptions regarding the duties of gardeners that make these other circumstances assume the role of background conditions and highlight the gardener's failure to water the flowers as *the* cause of their dying. A set of social relevances is employed to establish a particular account of causation, so as to identify certain causes because of their role in a social practice. The result is that a set of social expectations and values frames a context for experience and action.

Medicine similarly accents some causes over others because of the usefulness of this practice. Consider how diseases are characterized as genetic, infectious, or environmental diseases, though the particular disease may be influenced by all three factors. Tuberculosis, for example, is "due" to genetic, infectious, and environmental influences. One usually speaks of it as an infectious disease because of the general usefulness of that designation. Seeing it as an "infectious" disease focuses our attention and directs treatment to the causal factor that is usually most useful to address. Medicine accents those causal factors most amenable to medical intervention.

One must note, even if only in passing, the complexity of the notion of cause.[96] The term *cause* can be used to identify conditions that are sufficient to produce effects, necessary to produce effects, or that contribute to the likelihood of an effect's occurring. In medicine, where the data are often statistical, causal factors are frequently identified in the last sense. Factors are identified that are part of experiencing reality coherently and of explaining how events take place according to rules. In the applied sciences, one is not interested simply in giving a coherent account, but in selecting among the possible coherent accounts those more useful in achieving one's goals and purposes. In most circumstances, it will not be worthwhile to attend to all of the factors involved in giving a complete causal account. One directs one's attention and addresses instead those factors most easily manipulable. Medicine, like the law, tends to underscore those causes that can be eliminated, prevented, or usefully manipulated.[97] Each such major institution underscores certain elements of a neutral, encompassing, scientific account of reality, because of the importance of some elements for the particular social institution, such as assigning sinfulness, determining criminal or civil liability, or directing treatment in a useful manner.

As already indicated, major social institutions such as medicine and the law also differ in the character of the adverse judgments they give in characterizing undesirable circumstances. Consider how antisocial behavior can be understood alternatively as a sin, as a crime, as a moral fault, or as a disease (i.e., as a mental disorder). In seeking to characterize a circumstance as a disease rather than a sin, a moral fault, or a crime, one is not simply attempting to place such behavior in a social institution more able to resolve the problem. One is also choosing among values to be assigned to the phenomenon. Again, terming a circumstance a disease is not a value-free finding. If a circumstance is seen as one of disease, deformity, disability, or dysfunction, it is found to have fallen short of a physiological or psychological norm. So, too, when a circumstance is seen as a crime or a sin. It is disvalued in terms of a special set of value judgments. To decide between regarding a circumstance as a disease, a crime, or a sin is to choose from among competing value frameworks in terms of which to understand a state of affairs and among different social responses by which to respond to a state of affairs.

It is therefore important to decide how a problem will be understood. In deciding where to place a problem, one changes the frame of reference for interventions. In medicalizing a set of problems, one may relieve afflicted individuals of one set of disvaluations and encumber them with another. Consider the shift from holding drug addicts to be immoral to holding them to be diseased. Or consider alcoholism, which can be characterized as a sin, a moral fault, a crime, or a disease. One will need to decide where the accent should fall, in that shifting the accent from one major social institution to another changes the character of the responsibility one expects from individuals alternatively viewed as sinful, sick, diseased, or criminal. However, such choices need not be fully exclusive. Within different social contexts, the same person can consider another as sick, diseased, criminal, or sinful.

Major difficulties have occurred through overmedicalizing problems. One might think here in particular of controversies regarding the use of the insanity plea as a means of determining that an individual's problem is one that justifies treatment, rather than punishment.[98] Or consider the use of psychiatric hospitalization in the former Soviet Union to control political dissidence. Political problems are medicalized, undoubtedly in part, because medicine offers an efficacious way of controlling free expression.[99] Overmedicalization of problems may also represent sincere misuses of the social institution of medicine. It is a matter of considerable importance when to regard behavior not as freely chosen but as causally determined and open to medical cure. Such choices are made regularly when puzzling over disruptive children and adult criminals. They are choices with major moral presuppositions and consequences. They have their past instructive analogues, such as the special diseases assigned to slaves in the American South before the War Between the States, for example, drapetomania and dysaesthesia aethiopis, through which runaway or laggard slaves were seen as diseased.[100]

The problem is not simply to decide on the correct sick role or the correct staging or characterization of a disease, but whether to see a problem as a disease at all. The major social institutions offer competing construals of reality with competing costs and benefits. There are advantages and disadvantages in seeing disruptive behavior as a crime, a sin, a moral fault, or a disease. In some circumstances and from certain perspectives, it is more important, useful, and plausible to see individuals as responsible for their actions and in need of punishment or discipline, not treatment. In others it is more useful and plausible to see behavior as determined and open to technological manipulation. The general moral is to understand that these choices are often not clear-cut. One must make them as best one can in terms of the plausibility of the account and its usefulness.

In many circumstances, anything but a medical account will be highly implausible. Samuel Butler and *Erewhon* notwithstanding, it will be highly implausible to hold individuals responsible for developing appendicitis. In other circumstances, as for instance in drug addiction, the argument may plausibly go more than one way. In some circumstances, it may not make sense to choose between accounts; instead, it will be more plausible and useful to employ two or more accounts. It may make perfect sense to treat alcoholism as a disease, while at the same time regarding it as a moral problem. The proper choice may be one of both . . . and, rather than either . . . or.

In this volume we have explored the possibility of justifying a general secular morality and bioethics. We found that what could be secured was content-less and could gain authoritative content only with the permission of those involved. The same can be said with regard to both applied and unapplied science. Particular scientific communities at particular times embrace particular facts, findings, and rules of evidence and inference that we later find to be idiosyncratic, just as particular moral communities involve the acceptance of particular moral rules and views of the good life. Scientific controversies can occur between individuals united in a general commitment to science as an endeavor of intersubjectively establishing claims regarding the nature of the world, but divided due to different particular understandings of rules of evidence and inference. When the debates involve scientific issues with heavy ethical and political overlays, the conflicts become, as one would expect, complex. The individuals involved in such controversies will be participants in different moral and scientific communities and, as a result, will be in conflict with regard to different understandings of knowing truly and deciding fairly.

Such differences in understandings regarding what it means to know truly and decide fairly are often at the root of conflicts regarding the proper characterization of medical facts, or regarding whether a problem should be understood as a medical, legal, or moral problem. Concerns with evaluation and explanation intertwine in health care in decisions about whether problems are medical problems, and about how medical problems ought to be understood and classified. The choice of how to view a circumstance is not simply an epistemic or knowledge-based determination. It is also a determination based on a set of value considerations. The very characterization of reality can thus become a moral issue.[101] The very naming and characterization of a problem can raise questions of what values ought to be invoked, and of how they ought to be ordered. It will raise as well the question of who should participate in framing the classifications, and whose hierarchies of costs and benefits should have precedence. This issue must be answered in part, as has been indicated, through the practice of free and informed consent. It must also be answered through public acknowledgment of the ways in which problems are classified as medical, legal, religious, and so on. Since medical characterizations of problems depend not just on knowing reality truly, but on deciding in a fair manner among various ways of classifying reality, problems of individual rights, democratic prerogatives, and rights of privacy become salient. If classifications are natural, no one is at fault for describing reality as it is. One may not like the way reality is, but the scientist has not taken away anyone's rights by describing things the way they are. However, if one is fashioning a classification in order to pursue particular goals, the choice of the particular goals is open to negotiation among those involved.

## The democratization of medical reality: some conclusions

Portrayals of reality are cultural products. Although there are constraints placed upon us as knowers by the given character of the objects, objects appear to us through our concepts and in terms of the conditions of our experience. In the case of the unapplied sciences, where one's choice among different construals of reality is dictated by the ideal of a fully intersubjective account free of idiosyncratic values and purposes, there is a commitment to avoid imposing the values and perceptions of one particular group of knowers. Within an unapplied science one attempts to know anonymously and impersonally. But even here portrayals of reality are fashioned through background commitments that involve choices among different epistemic values. The world of unapplied science is a compromise made in the face of controversies.[102] In the applied sciences where the role of nonepistemic values is more salient, the constructed character of reality is easier to recognize. The goals that medicine can apply are manifestly varied and dependent on the visions of particular individuals and communities. We have seen this illustrated by the staging of cancer and by questions regarding medical decision making. Different ways of staging cancer and different balancing between over- and undertreatment depend in part on different understandings of the values involved. There are choices to be made among alternative accounts of medical reality. Since these choices are not simply determined on epistemic grounds, we become accountable for the ways in which we fashion that reality. How should one choose among competing descriptions of reality?

The question is, Who gets to choose? This is not a plea that staging systems for cancer be decided by referendum. But one must recognize that the choice among different understandings of reality within the applied sciences is a matter of communal interest. Communities must begin with a recognition of the constructed character of medical reality. This recognition underscores our choices and indicates our responsibilities as individuals who not only know reality but also know it in order to manipulate it. One must also recognize that these manipulations tend to be communal. The issue of who decides is thus moved from the area of individual free and informed consent to a communal area of negotiations regarding construals of reality. Systematic programs for treatment and for the assessment of treatment, or communal insurance policies, are in principle not the undertakings of isolated individuals. As a result, communities of physicians, insurers, and the various publics will need to negotiate regarding the characterization of medical reality they will employ when they collaborate, including the creation of various notions of futility.[103] Such negotiations may take on either a formal or an informal character; the negotiations can occur through the market or, when that is not possible, by formal democratic procedures. In either case, these represent a democratization of reality. One comes to recognize reality as the outcome of the choices of various communities of individuals.

Because of the principle of permission, individuals have rights to participate freely in such negotiations. The more one recognizes and respects these conditions, the more the medicalization of reality will vary from community to community. A traditional Roman Catholic community is likely to have understandings of health, disease, disorder, deviance, and disability quite different from those of a community of secularized cosmopolitans. Their different constructions of medical reality can then be embedded in alternative health care systems, which carry with them quite different understandings of what should count as a disease to be treated and of what treatment expenses should be sustained by the community.[104] Within different communal systems, there may very well be different notions of the sick role and the role of the physician versus that of the priest.

Since there are numerous understandings of medical reality, those who so wish should be at liberty to act on their own moral and metaphysical visions in the company of consenting collaborators. The limits of secular morality and general state authority leave space for diversity in appreciating and acting on medical reality. These circumstances provide one among the many grounds for not establishing a single all-encompassing health care system. There is no canonical content-full secular vision of medical reality, of illness and disease, of health and proper health care. There are Cuban Communist, Orthodox Jewish, Shiite Moslem, New Age pagan, feminist, male chauvinist, Southern Baptist, and Orthodox Christian visions of medical reality and proper health care. Given the limited secular moral authority of the state, and given the diversity of the moral and metaphysical visions of medical morality, there should be, to paraphrase Mao Tse-tung, space for a thousand views of health care to develop and for a hundred different systems of health care delivery to contend.

## Notes

1. Charles S. Peirce, *Collected Papers of Charles Sanders Peirce,* ed. Charles Hartshorne and Paul Weiss (Cambridge, Mass.: Belknap Press, 1965), 5.316.

    The view I am defending here has, as did Peirce's view, a substantial indebtedness both to Kant and to Hegel. This is a point already acknowledged in chapter 2 but worth repeating and enlarging. First, Kant's arguments are essentially correct (at least when given a Hegelian accent): we know reality only through our concepts. We never know reality uninterpreted by our understandings. To use the Kantian idiom, we do not know things as they are in themselves, as they are totally apart from our categories, but only as they are given to us through our categories of understanding. "What the things-in-themselves may be I do not know, nor do I need to know, since a thing can never come before me except in appearance." Kant, *Immanuel Kant's Critique of Pure Reason,* trans. Norman Kemp Smith (London: Macmillan, 1964), p. 286, A277 = B333. We cannot make out an account of reality apart from our understandings of reality. From Hegel one can derive the suggestion that one might as well cease speaking of an inaccessible reality in itself. Even as a limit on experience, as a direction toward the object, a mere "something = x" (*Critique of Pure Reason,* A250), to which one turns in empirical investigation, the thing-in-itself is itself a product of thought (G. W. F. Hegel, *The Encyclopaedia of the Philosophical Sciences* [1830], sec. 44). If one never encounters the purely other, the object as it is in itself, one can then regard the struggle to know reality as one of overcoming otherness and incompleteness in ever more coherent accounts of reality. The element of otherness directs us to seek accounts that can set that otherness aside.

This undertaking is a cultural endeavor. Consider Hegel's reflections on this task. "By thinking things, we transform them into something universal; things are singularities however, and the lion in general does not exist. We make them into something subjective, produced by us, belonging to us, and of course peculiar to us as men; for the things of nature do not think, and are neither representations nor thought." *Hegel's Philosophy of Nature,* trans. M. J. Petry (London: Allen & Unwin, 1970), p. 198, sec. 246 Zusatz. Our aim is to grasp and comprehend nature, to make it ours, so that it is not something beyond and alien to us. As a result, in our attempt to know nature, we do not simply see nature. We come, as Hegel observes, to see ourselves, "to find in this externality only the mirror of ourselves." Ibid., vol. 3, p. 213, sec. 376 Zusatz.

Hegel recognized, as Kant did not, that categories of knowledge are historical. The ways in which we see nature, the concepts through which appearance is given to us, if those concepts are specified in any detail, will develop through time. Revolutions occur in science when the basic categories change. "All cultural change reduces itself to a difference of categories. All revolutions, whether in the sciences or world history, occur merely because spirit has changed its categories in order to understand and examine what belongs to it, in order to possess and grasp itself in a truer, deeper, more intimate and unified manner." Ibid., vol. 1, p. 202, sec. 246 Zusatz. The quote from Peirce underscores both the direction for investigation, namely, the attempt to find ever more articulated understandings of nature, and the realization that science is a historical process.

For an introduction to the philosophical issues involved in Hegel's notions of knowledge as negation, versus knowledge as an encounter with an object in its otherness, see Werner Flach, *Negation und Andersheit* (Munich: Ernst Reinhardt, 1959). The difficulty is to speak of knowledge when there remain numerous and competing metaphysical and empirical understandings (e.g., feminist and Roman Catholic understandings). One is forced to articulate a science for metaphysical and moral strangers.

2. Ludwik Fleck, *Entstehung und Entwicklung einer wissenschaftlichen Tatsache: Einführung in die Lehre vom Denkstil und Denkkollektiv* (Basel: Benno Schwabe, 1935); English version, *Genesis and Development of a Scientific Fact,* ed. T. J. Trenn and R. K. Merton, trans. F. Bradley and T. J. Trenn (Chicago: University of Chicago Press, 1979).

3. Thomas Kuhn, *The Structure of Scientific Revolutions* (Chicago: University of Chicago Press, 1962; 2d ed., enlarged, 1970).

4. Among the shifts in the historiography of medicine has been the recognition that all accounts of history and of science are from a perspective. Given postmodernity, one has innumerable perspectives from which to choose, ranging from Roman Catholic to feminist. See, for example, Ann Oakley, "Ways of Knowing: Feminism and the Challenge to Knowledge," in *Essays on Women, Medicine and Health* (Edinburgh: Edinburgh University Press, 1993), chap. 16. So, too, like Roman Catholic ethics and epistemology, feminist ethics and epistemology intertwine. See, for example, the essays in Helen Holmes and Laura Purdy (eds.), *Feminist Perspectives in Medical Ethics* (Bloomington: Indiana University Press, 1992).

5. For other discussions of the contextual character of scientific thought, see Peter Achinstein, *Law and Explanation* (Oxford: Oxford University Press, 1971), and *The Nature of Explanation* (New York: Oxford University Press, 1983). Imre Lakatos and Alan Musgrave (eds.), *Criticism and the Growth of Knowledge* (Cambridge: Cambridge University Press, 1970). Larry Laudan, *Progress and Its Problems* (Berkeley: University of California Press, 1977).

6. Isaac Baker Brown, *On the Curability of Certain Forms of Insanity, Epilepsy, Catalepsy, and Hysteria in Females* (London: Robert Hardwicke, 1866).

7. H. Tristram Engelhardt, Jr., "The Disease of Masturbation: Values and the Concept of Disease," *Bulletin of the History of Medicine* 48 (Summer 1974): 234–48.

8. For the reports of death due to masturbation, see, for example, *Report of the Board of Administrators of the Charity Hospital to the General Assembly of Louisiana* (for 1872) (New Orleans: The Republican Office, 1873), p. 30; and *Report of the Board of Administrators of the Charity Hospital to the General Assembly of Louisiana* (for 1887) (New Orleans: A. W. Hyatt, 1888), p. 53.

9. A published autopsy report from Birmingham, England, concerning a dead masturbator showed that masturbation "seems to have acted upon the cord in the same manner as repeated small haemorrhages affect the brain, slowly sapping its energies, until it succumbed soon after the last application of the exhausting influence, probably through the instrumentality of an atrophic process previously induced, as evidenced by the diseased state of the minute vessels." James Russell, "Cases Illustrating the Influence of Exhaustion of the Spinal Cord in Inducing Paraplegia," *Medical Times and Gazette,* London 2 (1863): 456.

10. Baker Brown, *On the Curability of Certain Forms,* p. 11.

11. Ibid., p. 17.

12. Ibid., pp. 51–52.

13. American Psychiatric Association, *Diagnostic and Statistical Manual of Mental Disorders* (Washington, D.C.: American Psychiatric Association, 1952), pp. 38–39, taxon 000-x63. The Manual specifies that, when indicating the diagnosis of "sexual

deviation," "The diagnosis will specify the type of the pathologic behavior, such as homosexuality, transvestism, pedophilia, fetishism and sexual sadism (including rape, sexual assault, mutilation)."

14. American Psychiatric Association, *Diagnostic and Statistical Manual of Mental Disorders,* 2d ed. (Washington, D.C.: American Psychiatric Association, 1968), p. 44, taxon 302.0.

15. American Psychiatric Association, *Diagnostic and Statistical Manual of Mental Disorders,* 3d ed. (Washington, D.C.: American Psychiatric Association, 1980), p. 281, taxon 302.00.

16. *Diagnostic and Statistical Manual of Mental Disorders,* 3d ed. rev. (Washington, D.C.: American Psychiatric Association, 1987), p. 296, taxon 302.90.

17. *Diagnostic and Statistical Manual of Mental Disorders,* 4th ed. (Washington, D.C.: American Psychiatric Association, 1994), p. 538, taxon 302.9.

18. DSM-III-R, pp. 367–74. These politically and otherwise contested diagnostic categories appear under the general taxon "Proposed Diagnostic Categories Needing Further Study." In DSM-IV one finds Premenstrual Dysphoric Disorder (pp. 715–18), although the other taxa do not find a canonical representation.

19. For an overview of some of the debates focused on the fashioning of psychiatric classifications, see Bernard Gert, "A Sex Caused Inconsistency in DSM-III-R: The Definition of Mental Disorder and the Definition of Paraphilias," *Journal of Medicine and Philosophy* 17 (Apr. 1992): 155–71; and Sue V. Rosser, "Is There Androcentric Bias in Psychiatric Diagnosis," *Journal of Medicine and Philosophy* 17 (Apr. 1992): 215–31. For a discussion of some of the philosophical issues in DSM-IV, see David B. Allison and Mark S. Roberts, "On Constructing the Disorder of Hysteria," 239–59; David DeGrazia, "Autonomous Action and Autonomy—Subverting Psychiatric Conditions," 279–97; Allen Frances, Avram Mack, Micheal First, et al., "DSM-IV Meets Philosophy," 207–18; John Sadler, Yosaf Hulgus, and George Agich, "On Values in Recent American Psychiatric Classification," 261–77; and Mark J. Sedler, "Foundations of the New Nosology," 219–38, *Journal of Medicine and Philosophy* 19 (June 1994).

20. T. Gaillard Thomas, *A Practical Treatise on the Diseases of Women* (Philadelphia: Henry C. Lea's Son, 1880), p. 778.

21. For example, François Boissier de Sauvages places his some 2,400 diseases under four classes, the first of which is fevers. He characterizes fevers as "syndromes frigoris, successivique caloris cum artuum debilitate & pulsus vi adaucta, saepe quoad frequentiam." Sauvages, *Nosologia methodica sistens morborum classes* (Amsterdam: Fratrum de Tournes, 1768), vol. 1, p. 243. William Cullen in his *Nosology* groups diseases under four classes, the first of which is "Pyrexie," which is divided into five orders, the first one "Febres" or fevers. He gives the following definition of fever: "Praegressis languore, lassitudine, et aliis debilitatis signis, pyrexia, sine morbo locali primario." William Cullen, *Nosologia methodica,* 3d ed., (Edinburgh: J. Carfrae, 1820), p. 21.

22. Hippocrates, *Epidemics* 3, case 16, in *Hippocrates,* trans. W. H. S. Jones (Cambridge, Mass.: Harvard University Press, 1962), vol. 1, pp. 285, 287.

23. Hippocrates, *Epidemics* 1.1, vol. 1, pp. 147, 149.

24. Ivan Illich, *Medical Nemesis* (New York: Pantheon Books, 1976).

25. Lee B. Lusted, *Introduction to Medical Decision Making* (Springfield, Ill.: Thomas, 1968), pp. 98–140.

26. Ronald Bayer, *Homosexuality and American Psychiatry* (New York: Basic Books, 1981).

27. American Joint Committee on Cancer, *Manual for Staging of Cancer,* 2d ed. (Philadelphia: Lippincott, 1983). This social construction of the reality of oncology maintains its character in subsequent editions. See Oliver Beahrs, Donald Henson, Robert Hutter, and B. J. Kennedy (eds.), *Manual for Staging of Cancer,* 4th ed. (Philadelphia: Lippincott, 1992).

28. U.S. Department of Health, Education, and Welfare, *Eighth Revision International Classification of Diseases,* 2 vols. (Washington, D.C.: U.S. Government Printing Office, 1968).

29. Carolus Linnaeus, *Genera morborum, in auditorum usum* (Upsalae: Steinert, 1763).

30. François Boissier de Sauvages de la Croix, *Nosologia methodica sistens morborum classes juxta Sydenhami mentem et botanicorum ordinem,* 5 vols. (Amsterdam: Fratrum de Tournes, 1763); 2d ed., 2 vols. (Amsterdam: Fratrum de Tournes, 1768), vol. 2, pp. 1–149.

31. Horacio Fabrega, Jr., "Disease Viewed as a Symbolic Category," in H. T. Engelhardt, Jr., and S. F. Spicker (eds.), *Mental Health: Philosophical Perspectives* (Dordrecht: Reidel, 1977), pp. 79–106.

32. Maryland Annotated Code (1979 Cumulative Supplement), art. 27, sec. 554. One might note that the punishment for unnatural acts was once more severe in America. Consider Benjamin Goad, who was hung and his mare executed in his sight after he had been discovered in 1673 committing the "unnatural & horrid act of Bestillitie on a mare in the highway or field." *Records of the Court of Assistants of the Colony of the Massachusetts Bay 1630–1682* (1901), vol. 1, pp. 10–11.

33. Thomas Aquinas, *Summa Theologica* 2–2, 153–54. Matters are quite different within traditional Christian beliefs which understand the immorality of acts without having to embed them in a particular metaphysical account. Within this viewpoint masturbation evokes a far less serious response than fornication or adultery. See, for example, the canons of St. John the Faster (d. 595), Sts. Nicodemus and Agapius, *The Rudder of the Orthodox Catholic Church,* trans. D. Cummings (1957; reprt. New York: Luna Printing Society, 1983), pp. 936, 939, 940, 942, Canons 8, 11, 13, and 18.

34. Richard H. Post, "Population Differences in Red and Green Color Vision Deficiency: A Review, and a Query on Selection Relaxation," *Eugenics Quarterly* (Mar. 1962): 131–46.

35. The traditional Christian understanding is that those who do not close or harden their hearts to God will find His laws written on their hearts. Unlike the view of Thomas Aquinas, one recognizes these laws not simply through reason, but by grace, by the energies of God. The relation is not merely epistemic, but indeed personal. For an account of this view, see Archimandrite Hierotheos Vlachos, *A Night in the Desert of the Holy Mountain,* trans. Effie Mavromichali (Levadia: Birth of Theotokos Monastery, 1991); Archimandrite Sophrony, *The Monk of Mount Athos,* trans. Rosemary

Edmonds (Crestwood, N.Y.: St. Vladimir's Seminary Press, 1989); Archimandrite
Sophrony, *Wisdom from Mount Athos,* trans. Rosemary Edmonds (Crestwood, N.Y.:
St. Vladimir's Seminary Press, 1975); Archimandrite Vasileios, *Hymn of Entry,*
trans. Elizabeth Briere (Crestwood, N.Y.: St. Vladimir's Seminary Press, 1984).
36. Christopher Boorse, "On the Distinction between Disease and Illness," *Philosophy
and Public Affairs* 5 (Fall 1975): 61.
37. Christopher Boorse, "Health as a Theoretical Concept," *Philosophy of Science* 44
(1977): 562, 567.
38. Robert Trivers, "Parent–Offspring Conflict," *American Zoologist* 14 (1974): 259–
64.
39. F. B. Livingstone, "The Distributions of the Abnormal Hemoglobin Genes and Their
Significance for Human Evolution," *Evolution* 18 (1964): 685. Christopher Boorse
acknowledges the existence of polymorphic traits and intraspecific variations. He
does not come to terms with the way various balances among traits maximize fitness,
often at the price of individual suffering. Boorse, "Health as a Theoretical Concept,"
542–71 especially pp. 546–47, 558, and 563.
40. Boorse, "On the Distinction between Disease and Illness," 63.
41. William K. Goosens, "Values, Health, and Medicine," *Philosophy of Science* 47
(Mar. 1980): 100–15.
42. A helpful distinction among the different senses of normality and a discussion of the
difference between a biologist's taxonomic interest in normality and that of a physician are provided by Marjorie Grene, "Individuals and Their Kind: Aristotelian
Foundations of Biology," in Stuart Spicker (ed.), *Organism, Medicine, and Metaphysics* (Dordrecht: Reidel, 1978), pp. 121–36.
43. For a neo-Aristotelian attempt to discover the boundaries between health and disease,
see Georg Henrik von Wright, *The Varieties of Goodness* (New York: Humanities
Press, 1963).
44. There is a considerable literature supporting what could be termed a weak normativist
account of disease, that is, a view that concepts of disease, though in part based on
empirical determinations, have an essential evaluative component. These views contrast with the neutralist views of individuals such as Christopher Boorse who hold that
concepts of disease are descriptive and explanatory, but not evaluative. For a classic
article supporting the weak normativist view, see Lester King, "What is Disease?"
*Philosophy of Science* 21 (July 1954): 193–203. One should note that the normativist
view suggests that concepts of diseases for animals and plants depend on human
understandings of the purposes of animals and plants. Therefore, the paradigm examples of diseases in animals and plants are those that afflict pets, or animals and plants
grown for food, and so on. It is difficult to speak of feral animals and plants as being
diseased (or at least diseased in a clinical sense) except by analogy. One would also
be able to develop a Boorsian, neutralist notion of the diseases of wild animals and
plants in terms of species-atypical levels of species-typical functions. But such would
not focus on the sufferings experienced by animals. The concept of disease held by
veterinarians or agricultural scientists is, in contrast, dependent on what humans hold
to be the proper functions, levels of pain, and characters of grace and form for
particular groups of living entities. "Diseases" universal to a particular species of

animals and plants could be recognized as diseases only if the animal or plant is being raised as a pet or for profit, and the "disease" impedes such goals. See, for example, Peter Sedgwick, "Illness—Mental and Otherwise," *Hastings Center Studies* 1 (1973): 19–40, and H. T. Engelhardt, Jr., "Is There a Philosophy of Medicine?" in F. Suppe and P. D. Asquith (eds.), *PSA 1976*, vol. 2 (East Lansing, Mich.: Philosophy of Science Association, 1977), pp. 94–108.

45. For a development of this point, see Joseph Margolis, "The Concept of Disease," *Journal of Medicine and Philosophy* 1 (Sept. 1976): 238–55; H. T. Engelhardt, Jr., "Ideology and Etiology," *Journal of Medicine and Philosophy* 1 (Sept. 1976): 256–68.

46. For an appreciation of the variety of vision of human form and ability, one might compare the disparate appreciations offered by the diversity of feminist and nonfeminist understandings of bodily form and disability. See, for example, Barbara Stafford, John La Puma, and David Schiedermayer, "One Face of Beauty, One Picture of Health," *Journal of Medicine and Philosophy* 14 (Apr. 1989): 213–30; Susan Wendell, "Toward a Feminist Theory of Disability," *Hypatia* 4 (Summer 1989): 63–81; Iris Marion Young, "Breasted Experience: The Look and the Feeling," in Drew Leder (ed.), *The Body in Medical Thought and Practice* (Dordrecht: Kluwer, 1992), pp. 215–30.

47. One should note that attempts such as those by Clouser, Culver, and Gert to introduce a term such as malady will not provide what is needed here. K. Danner Clouser, Charles M. Culver, and Bernard Gert, "Malady: A New Treatment of Disease," *Hastings Center Report* 11 (June 1981): 29–37. They offer the following definition of malady: "A person has a malady if and only if he or she has a condition, other than a rational belief or desire, such that he or she is suffering, or at increased risk of suffering, an evil (death, pain, disability, loss of freedom or opportunity, or loss of pleasure) in the absence of a distinct sustaining cause" (p. 36). See also Bernard Gert, *Morality* (New York: Oxford University Press, 1988), pp. 60–61. Medicine, however, treats a number of "maladies" with distinct sustaining causes as, for instance, infertility by providing artificial insemination from a donor. Such a "malady" is not a malady under the rubrics of Clouser et al., since there is a distinct sustaining cause, that of the husband's low sperm count. Hence, a more general term is required. I have proposed the term *clinical problem*. H. T. Engelhardt, Jr., "Clinical Problems and the Concept of Disease," in L. Nordenfelt and B. I. B. Lindahl (eds.), *Health, Disease, and Causal Explanations in Medicine* (Dordrecht: Reidel, 1984), pp. 27–41. See, also, L. Nordenfelt, *On the Nature of Health: An Action-Theoretic Approach* (Dordrecht: Kluwer, 1987).

48. For a review of the conflicts between so-called ontological accounts of disease (those that portray diseases as entities, as in some sense things) and physiological or functional accounts of disease (those that articulate nominalists in their views of the reality of diseases and portray disease taxa as artificial designations), see A. L. Caplan, H. T. Engelhardt, Jr., and J. J. McCartney (eds.), *Concepts of Health and Disease* (Reading, Mass.: Addison-Wesley, 1981), especially pp. 143–263.

49. John L. Gedye, "Simulating Clinical Judgment," in H. T. Engelhardt, Jr.,

S. F. Spicker, and B. Towers (eds.), *Clinical Judgment: A Critical Appraisal* (Dordrecht: Reidel, 1979), pp. 93–113.

50. Constitution of the World Health Organization (preamble), *The First Ten Years of the World Health Organization* (Geneva: World Health Organization, 1958).

51. Chester R. Burns, "Diseases Versus Healths: Some Legacies in the Philosophies of Modern Medical Sciences," in H. T. Engelhardt, Jr., and S. F. Spicker, (eds.), *Evaluation and Explanation in the Biomedical Sciences* (Dordrecht: Reidel, 1975), pp. 29–47.

52. Christopher Boorse, for example, has not only distinguished between negative and positive concepts of health but among positive notions of health understood in terms of whether they accent enhancement of individual potential, species potential, or have global concerns of increasing human ability. "Health as a Theoretical Concept", 542–73. For a general study of issues associated with concepts of health, see Nordenfelt, *On the Nature of Health.*

53. It is within particular communities that particular notions of well-being are nurtured and flourish along with particular content-full moralities. It is within particular communities that one not only learns about virtue, character, and right action; one learns as well about what inclinations and actions are appropriate and desirable, perverse and unnatural. Particular communities bring with them understandings of age-, gender-, and role-specific notions of well-being, health, and flourishing. See, for example, K. P. Wesche, "Man and Woman in Orthodox Tradition: The Mystery of Gender," *St. Vladimir's Theological Quarterly* 37 (1993): 213–51.

54. For a study of some of the ambiguities of the concept of a "health science," see R. John Bench, "Health Science, Natural Science, and Clinical Knowledge," *Journal of Medicine and Philosophy* 14 (1989): 147–64.

55. Committee on Nomenclature and Classification of Disease, *Systematized Nomenclature of Pathology* (Chicago: College of American Pathologists, 1969), p. xvii.

56. *The ICD-10 Classification of Mental and Behavioural Disorders: Clinical Descriptions and Diagnostic Guidelines* (Geneva: World Health Organization, 1992); *International Statistical Classification of Diseases and Related Health Problems* (Geneva: World Health Organization, 1992).

57. Alvan R. Feinstein, *Clinical Judgment* (Huntington, N.Y.: Kreiger, 1974), p. 968.

58. Norwood R. Hanson, *Patterns of Discovery* (Cambridge: Cambridge University Press, 1961); *Perception and Discovery* (San Francisco: Freeman, Cooper, 1969). For a thoroughgoing study of the character of discovery and explanation in medicine and the biological sciences, see Kenneth F. Schaffner, *Discovery and Explanation in Biology and Medicine* (Chicago: University of Chicago Press, 1993).

59. Henrik Wulff, *Rational Diagnosis and Treatment,* 2d ed. (London: Blackwell Scientific, 1981), pp. 30–41.

60. One might think here of Lawrence Weed's problem-oriented medical record, which includes an injunction to describe patient problems at least in part in terms of how they are experienced by the patient. See *Medical Records, Medical Education, and Patient Care* (Chicago: Year Book Medical Publications, 1970).

61. These points are explored by Hegel in the second book of *The Logic,* "Wesen" (Essence), and in the second section of the first part of the *Encyclopedia,* "Die Lehre

vom Wesen" (The Doctrine of Essence). These points are developed as well in Hegel's *Phenomenology of Mind,* his *Phaenomenologie des Geistes,* in his study of sense certainty, perception, and force and understanding. Hegel provides a detailed analysis of the ways in which the meaning of appearance and the laws that are held to lie behind appearance presuppose each other in the very structure of explanation.

62. For an introduction to some of the issues raised by the roles of prediction and manipulation in the fashioning of scientific explanations, see R. G. Collingwood, *The Idea of Nature* (New York: Oxford University Press, 1960). See also Stephen Toulmin, *Foresight and Understanding* (New York: Harper & Row, 1961), and *The Philosophy of Science* (New York: Harper & Row, 1953).

63. Thomas Sydenham, "Answer to Henry Paman, M.D. Fellow of St. John's College in Cambridge, publick Orator of that University; and Professor of Physic in Grethan College; containing the History and Treatment of the Venereal Disease," in *The Entire Works of Dr. Thomas Sydenham,* ed. and trans. John Swan, 3d ed. (London: E. Cave, 1753), p. 339.

64. Sauvages, *Nosologia methodica.*

65. The history of the development of scientific medicine in the sixteenth and seventeenth centuries is complex and tied to numerous reassessments of science, medicine, and the role of observer bias. Much of previous medical practice was being reconsidered. One might think of the sport made of necromancers and water-casters: Thomas Brian, *The Pisse-Prophet or Certaine Pissepot Lectures* (London: R. Thrale, 1637). There is also the influence on Sydenham, the English Hippocrates, of his fellow physician and practice partner John Locke: Patrick Romanell, *John Locke and Medicine* (Buffalo, N.Y.: Prometheus Books, 1984). Lester King provides two important studies of the eighteenth century and the beginning of the period of medical nosology: Lester King, *The Medical World of the Eighteenth Century* (Chicago: University of Chicago Press, 1958), and *The Philosophy of Medicine* (Cambridge, Mass.: Harvard University Press, 1978).

66. William Cullen, *Synopsis nosologiae methodicae* (Edinburgh: William Creech, 1769). For a study of this work, see Robert Kendell, "William Cullen's Synopsis Nosologiae Methodicae," in A. Doig, J. P. S. Ferguson, I. A. Milne, and R. Passmore (eds.), *William Cullen and the Eighteenth Century Medical World* (Edinburgh: Edinburgh University Press, 1993), pp. 216–33.

67. Carolus Linnaeus, *Genera morborum, in auditorum usum.*

68. Fredrik Berg, "Linné et Sauvages: Les rapports entre leurs systèmes nosologiques," *Lynchonos* (1956): 36.

69. Sauvages, *Nosologia Methodica* (1768), vol. 1. pp. 92–95.
    The reader must note that it is difficult to convey to contemporary readers the significance of the major classes in Sauvages's clinically oriented nosology. The classification brings diseases and problems together in unaccustomed ways. For example, underclass X, *cachexiae: coloris, figurae, molis in corporis habitu depravatio* (constitutional disorders: distortion of the body's condition in color, figure, and shape) [vol. 1, p. 95] is the order *tumores, corporis generalis intumescentia, seu adauctum volumen* (swellings: general tumescence of the body or increase of volume), which includes the *genus graviditas,* or pregnancy. It might appear peculiar to

list pregnancy within a classification of diseases. That peculiarity is in part dispelled
if one recognizes that the classification is one of clinical problems and that pregnancy
can occasion clinical difficulties, including swelling of the feet, etc. The difficulty
lies in seeing pregnancy under the classification of swellings and then regarding
swelling as a form of constitutional disorder. The sense of inappropriateness is tied to
our contemporary accepted views of how one should classify clinical phenomena. It
is tied as well to the difficulty of giving *cachexiae* (wastings, consumptions, and bad
conditions of the body) sufficient breadth of meaning.

In addition to his clinically oriented classification of diseases, Sauvages provided
some eighty-plus pages devoted to an etiological classification (*Classes morborum
aetiologicae*) and an anatomical classification (*Methodus anatomica morborum*). In
short, Sauvages developed three alternative classifications from which one could
select, depending on the circumstances.

For an overview of the accomplishments of Sauvages, see Lester S. King, ''Boissier de Sauvages and 18th Century Nosology,'' *Bulletin of the History of Medicine* 60
(Spring 1966): 43–51.

70. Sydenham, in *The Entire Works,* sec. 9, pp. iv–v.
71. Ibid., p. v.
72. *DSM-III,* pp. 6-7.
73. *DSM-III-R,* p. xxiii.
74. Theophile Bonet, *Sepulchretum sive anatomica practica ex cadaveribus morbo
    denatis* (Geneva: L. Chouet, 1679).
75. Giovanni Morgagni, *De sedibus et causis morborum per anatomen indagatis* (Venice:
    Ex Typographis Remondiniana, 1761).
76. Michel Foucault, *Naissance de la clinique* (Paris: Presses Universitaires de France,
    1963). *The Birth of the Clinic: An Archaeology of Medical Perception,* trans.
    A. M. Sheridan Smith (New York: Random House, 1973).
77. F.-J.-V. Broussais, *On Irritation and Insanity,* trans. Thomas Cooper (Columbia,
    S.C.: S. J. McMorris, 1831), p. ix. *De L'irritation et de la Folie* (Paris: Delaunay,
    1828).
78. Rudolf Virchow, ''One Hundred Years of General Pathology (1895),'' in *Disease,
    Life, and Man,* trans. L. J. Rather (Stanford, Calif.: Stanford University Press, 1958),
    p. 214.
79. Xavier Bichat, ''Preliminary Discourse,'' in Bichat, *Pathological Anatomy* (Phila-
    delphia: John Grigg, 1827); reprinted in Caplan et al., *Concepts of Health and
    Disease,* pp. 167–68.
80. Sauvages, *Nosologia methodica sistens morborum classes juxta Sydenhami mentem et
    botanicorum ordinem,* 2d ed., 2 vols. (Amsterdam: Fratrum de Tournes, 1768).
81. F.-J.-V. Broussais, *Examen des Doctrines Medicales et des Systems de Nosologie*
    (Paris: Meguignon-Marvis, 1821), vol. 2, p. 646. Of special interest is Broussais's
    use of the term *ontology* (*ontologie*) to describe medical accounts referring to disease
    entities. I am in debt to Prof. Yoshio Kawakita for his suggestions regarding
    Broussais's usage of the term and his Greek neologism οντοι. See also Thomas J.
    Bole, ''The Neologism οντοι in Broussais's Condemnation of Medical On-
    tology,'' *Journal of Medicine and Philosophy* 20 (Oct. 1995).

82. Carolus Linnaeus, *Genera morborum in auditorum usum* (Hamburg: Buchenroeder & Ritter, 1773 [?]), pp. 16–17.

83. Sauvages, *Nosologia methodica* (1768), vol. 2, pp. 1–42f.

84. Talcott Parsons developed this point in a number of works. See, in particular, *The Social System* (New York: Free Press, 1951); and "Definitions of Health and Illness in the Light of American Values and Social Structure," in E. G. Jaco (ed.), *Patients, Physicians and Illness* (Glencoe, Ill.: Free Press, 1958), pp. 165–87.

85. M. Siegler and H. Osmond, "The 'Sick Role' Revisited," *Hastings Center Studies* 1 (1973): 41–58.

86. Alfred Schutz and Thomas Luckmann, *The Structures of the Life-World*, trans. R. N. Zaner and H. T. Engelhardt, Jr. (Evanston, Ill.: Northwestern University Press, 1973).

87. For an exploration of the body in medical experience, see Drew Leder (ed.), *The Body in Medical Thought and Practice* (Dordrecht: Kluwer, 1992).

88. For a discussion of the social construction of medical reality, see P. Wright and A. Treacher (eds.), *The Problem of Medical Knowledge* (Edinburgh: Edinburgh University Press, 1982).

89. Consider as an example the following staging scheme for lymphoma quoted in a pocket handbook for clinicians. The classification presents a taken-for-granted social construction of clinical reality.

Stage    I     Limited to one area
Stage    II    Involvement of two or more areas on the same side of the diaphragm
Stage    III   Involvement of two or more areas on both sides of the diaphragm
         $III_1$  Upper abdomen, spleen, splenic & hilar nodes
         $III_2$  Lower abdominal nodes
Stage    IV    Disseminated extralymphatic disease

Leonard Gomella, *Clinician's Pocket Reference*, 7th ed. (Norwalk, Conn.: Appleton & Lange, 1993), pp. 272–73.

90. American Joint Committee on Cancer, *Manual for Staging of Cancer*, p. vii.

91. Ibid., p. viii.

92. Ibid., p. xi. For a similar set of reflections in the fourth edition, see pp. ix–x.

93. See A. S. Elstein, L. S. Shulman, and S. A. Sprafka (eds.), *Medical Problem Solving* (Cambridge, Mass.: Harvard University Press, 1978); Feinstein, *Clinical Judgment;* Edmond A. Murphy, *The Logic of Medicine* (Baltimore: Johns Hopkins University Press, 1976); Wulff, *Rational Diagnosis and Treatment;* and Steven Schwartz and Timothy Griffin, *Medical Thinking* (New York: Springer-Verlag, 1986).

94. For a exploration of some of these issues, see José Luis Peset and Diego Gracia (eds.), *The Ethics of Diagnosis* (Dordrecht: Kluwer, 1992). See, in particular, Edmund Pellegrino, "Value Desiderata in the Logical Structuring of Computer Diagnosis," pp. 173–195.

95. H. L. A. Hart and A. M. Honoré, *Causation in the Law* (Oxford: Clarendon Press, 1959); see especially pp. 35–36.

96. For some studies of the concepts of causality employed in medicine, see José Luis Peset, "On the History of Medical Causality," pp. 57–74; Dietrich von Engelhardt, "Causality and Conditionality in Medicine around 1900," pp. 75–104; Anne Fagot-

Largeault, "On Medicine's Scientificity," pp. 105–26; Eric Juengst, "Causation and the Conceptual Scheme of Medical Knowledge," pp. 127–52; and Anne Marie Moulin, "The Dilemma of Medical Causality and the Issue of Biological Individuality," pp. 153–62, in Corinna Delkeskamp-Hayes and Mary Ann Cutter (eds.), *Science, Technology, and the Art of Medicine* (Dordrecht: Kluwer, 1993). See, also, Paul Humphreys, *The Chances of Explanation* (Princeton: Princeton University Press, 1989) and Kenneth F. Schaffner, *Discovery and Explanation in Biology and Medicine* (Chicago: University of Chicago Press, 1993).

97.  For an exploration of the notions of causality and causation in medicine, see Kenneth F. Schaffner, "Causation and Responsibility: Medicine, Science and the Law," pp. 95–122, and H. T. Engelhardt, Jr., "Relevant Causes: Their Designation in Medicine and Law," pp. 123–27, in S. F. Spicker et al. (eds.), *The Law–Medicine Relation: A Philosophical Exploration* (Dordrecht: Reidel, 1981).

98.  B. Brody and H. T. Engelhardt, Jr. (eds.), *Mental Illness: Law and Public Policy* (Dordrecht: Reidel, 1980).

99.  A. Koryagin, "Unwilling Patients," *Lancet* 1 (1981): 821; Harold Mersky, "Variable Meanings for the Definition of Disease," *Journal of Medicine and Philosophy* 11 (Aug. 1986): 215–32.

100.  S. A. Cartwright, "Report on the Diseases and Physical Peculiarities of the Negro Race," *New Orleans Medical and Surgical Journal* 7 (May 1851): 691–715. It is unclear whether Cartwright was captured by the expectations of the times or had advanced his views in order to protect slaves.

101.  Indeed, the experience of illness and disease is structured by evaluative, explanatory, and social expectations. For a recent study, see S. Kay Toombs, *The Meaning of Illness* (Dordrecht: Kluwer, 1992).

102.  For a comparison of the role of epistemic and nonepistemic values in shaping the unapplied and applied sciences, see H. T. Engelhardt, Jr., and A. L. Caplan, *Scientific Controversies* (New York: Cambridge University Press, 1987).

103.  One must note the heterogeneity of futility concepts as well as the necessity of authorizing rather than discovering which should apply and where. Loretta M. Kopelman, "Conceptual and Moral Disputes about Futile and Useful Treatments," *Journal of Medicine and Philosophy* 20 (April 1995): 109–21; Baruch A. Brody and Amir Halevy, "Is Futility a Futile Concept?" *Journal of Medicine and Philosophy* 20 (April 1995): 123–44.

104.  Within particular health care systems fashioned around a particular moral vision, it will be possible to recognize certain states of affairs as perverted or unnatural, because such health care systems can carry with them content-full moral and other value commitments so as to allow a much richer appreciation of medical reality than is possible in terms of a general secular account of disease, illness, disorder, and disability.

# 6

## The Endings and Beginnings of Persons: Death, Abortion, and Infanticide

Persons are central to morality. As chapter 4 recounted, only persons have moral problems and moral obligations. The very world of morality is sustained by persons. The problem is that not all humans are persons in terms of general secular morality. To be a person for secular morality, one must be able to give morally authoritative permission. Or, to put matters somewhat differently, only those entities who can give permission, who can convey moral authority concerning themselves and their possessions will be termed persons. Person in the strict sense will be used to identify those entities who can establish by their agreements a web of moral authority for their collaboration, or who can refuse to be involved with others. Persons in the strict sense are the active participants in the morality that can bind moral strangers, for only persons can negotiate their areas of joint labor and by their refusals set limits to the intrusions of others. As such, persons in the strict sense are moral agents who may be held responsible for their actions.

Not all humans are persons in this strict sense, in the sense of being moral agents. As we saw in chapter 4, infants are not persons in this sense. The severely senile and the very severely or profoundly mentally retarded are not persons in this very important and central way. Nor are those who are severely brain damaged. Again, it is because general secular morality derives its authority and scope from the permission of persons that persons as moral agents, as permission givers, are central.

Other understandings of persons and humans, however true, cannot be acknowledged or given standing within the sparse fabric of general secular morality. The believer should recognize this account of secular morality as disclosing how dreadfully little moral substance can be secured in general secular terms and how what is secured seems distorted and partial.[1] Nothing of the intrinsic worth or significance of humans can be acknowledged. All that one can recognize is the moral authority that can come from persons. Yet, at least this is secured, despite other failures to ground a general secular morality.

Medicine is concerned with persons in the strict sense of moral agents, which includes patients who discuss their problems with their physicians and come to agreements about treatment. Medicine is concerned as well with humans to whom a portion of the rights and prerogatives of persons, in general secular terms, is imputed. Infants and the senile are regarded in many ways as if they were persons. *Person* in ordinary practice is used to refer to both competent adults and the profoundly mentally retarded. This potential ambiguity is significant because definitions of death may appear to focus on the death of persons in the strict sense, while in fact their focus is on the death of persons in other senses as well. So, too, at the beginning of life, one might think that most arguments regarding abortion and infanticide focus on the point at which persons in the strict sense come into being.[2] But, of course, this cannot be the case, since humans do not become persons in the strict sense of moral agents until years after their birth. There are significant tensions between what individuals know in faith or take as assumptions from their received culture and what can be sustained in general secular terms.

These philosophical issues have already been explored in chapter 4. Here we turn to their further elaboration and application. Physicians, after all, must apply abstract concepts of being alive or being dead to actual situations. Physicians declare individuals dead. As the preceding chapter has shown, such determinations are not merely factual, if for no other reason than that such findings can usually not be made without taking into account the costs of the possible false positive and false negative determinations. Deciding on which side one ought to err requires a balancing of costs and benefits. The question is how ought one to approach the world, once it is clear that the entities to whom we have the strongest secular moral obligations, persons in the strict sense, come into being only some time, likely years, after birth, and likely cease to exist sometime before the death of the organism. One must recall here the distinction in chapter 4 between human biological and human personal life. Mere human biological life precedes the emergence of the life of persons in the strict sense, and it usually continues for a while after their death. Because of this circumstance, because of the concerns that persons have to raise children, and because of the interests that persons have to nurture sentiments of sympathy and care, even in secular morality a social sense of person is often imputed to nonpersonal, human biological life. Thus, in general secular morality, infants are treated as if they were persons. So, too, the severely senile are regarded as persons, though they are not such in the strict sense.

## The definition of death

The controversies concerning definitions of death spring in great part from un-clarities regarding the kind of life that is being declared at an end. One can have a sense of this from the different wordings in American statutes defining death. The first two statutes in the United States, that of Kansas, which was enacted in 1970,[3] and that of Maryland, enacted in 1972,[4] speak to the determination of the death of a person.

It is one thing to be interested in the point in time at which human biological life ceases and another to be interested in when persons cease to exist. To speak of the death of a human body suggests an organismic focus on human biological life. The development from a whole-body-oriented definition of death to a whole-brain-oriented definition of death can be interpreted as a move away from a definition focused on human biological life to one focused on the life of a person. Indeed, the history of the debates concerning the definition of death can be seen to hinge on this point, as well as on two others. First, what is the kind of life, the death of which one is to determine? Here the controversy focuses on the contrast between human biological and personal life and can come to involve the various senses of person discussed in chapter 4. Second, how and where is that life embodied? The issue at stake is whether the brain or some other part of the brain is the unique locus, embodiment, or sponsor of the kind of life whose death one seeks to determine. Third, how many false positive and false negative determinations of death ought one to tolerate or find acceptable?

### Bodies, minds, and persons

The first issue concerns the development of a distinction between the life of a human organism and the life of a person. Those two concepts were tied more closely together when the human body was seen in Western philosophical accounts as enlivened by a rational soul. The soul was understood not only to be the source of moral agency, but also to include animal and vegetative functions, which enlivened the body. Thus, Aquinas argued that all of the soul was in every part of the body: "tota in toto" and "tota in qualibet parte." One must recall that Aquinas distinguished among nutritive, sensitive, and intellectual souls,[5] though the intellectual soul included the reality of the other souls in its embodied life. This led to the soul being seen as a kind of catalyst for organic processes. Such views gave special significance to the work of Friedrich Woehler (1800–82), who in 1828 first synthesized urea in vitro. Such was considered impossible by many vitalists, who held that organic compounds required life for their synthesis.

The development of the life sciences has contributed to our knowledge of the ways in which biological functions can be understood without an appeal to a vital principle. It has contributed as well to our mastery of the ways in which those processes can be produced artificially. Life as a biological process has ceased to be a mystery requiring special soul-like catalysts. The systematic integration of the body can be understood without invoking the presence of either the soul or a moral agent. On the other hand, moral agency requires the presence of self-consciousness. Self-consciousness has a sense and meaning that contrast with mechanical, chemical, and biological structures. The life of minds, if it is to be understood adequately, must be captured, at least in part, in introspective psychological terms.[6]

It is for this reason that the principles of biological life contrast with the principles of mental life, and here in particular, the life of persons.[7] The biology that has been marked by successes such as Woehler's helps us to come to terms with various biological functions, including the systematic integration of the body, though it does not suffice for understanding the lived experiences of minds. This is the case, even if one might imagine the artificial synthesis of organisms that would have a mental life and perhaps even be persons, as was HAL in the novel and movie *2001*.[8] To make a judgment about the moral standing of entities, one will need to decide about their capacities for consciousness and self-consciousness, as well as their abilities to conceive of moral goods and to have a rational plan of life. One must know if they are self-conscious, able to choose on the basis of reason and able to make moral claims, and thus be held morally accountable. However, entities that fall short of this status but that can suffer and have pleasure will still be worthy of our moral attention. As chapter 4 has shown, one must distinguish between entities that have mental lives but are not persons, and those that are persons. In general secular moral terms, as expressed in the principle of beneficence, we ought to have regard for entities with a mental life because they suffer and have pleasure. We ought to show respect for those entities which are persons because they (and that respect) sustain the practice of morality. We may not use them without their permission.

This should be plain when one considers the contrast between a human body in which all of the brain except for the lower brain stem has been destroyed, and an adult human body with a fully functioning brain. To understand the first, one need only appeal to the principles of biological life. To understand the second, one will need to appeal to the principles of mental entities, including here that of persons. It is not mere biological life that is of central moral interest. A human body that can only function biologically, without an inward mental life, does not sustain a moral agent. The death of a mere animal marks the passing of a mental life that can suffer and have pleasure. The death of a person marks the passing of an entity that can make promises and fashion strong moral claims. To underscore this point with regard to definitions of death: a body with whole-brain death, or with death of the whole brain except for the brain stem, does not support a mental life, much less the life of a person.

To look at things in this way requires a momentous conceptual step. It requires recognizing that mere human biological life is of little moral value in and of itself. It requires acknowledging that it is the life of human persons in the strict sense that is central to moral concerns. It also means confronting a whole set of new puzzles. One must decide how to regard those levels of human mental life that are not yet the life of a person. In particular, one must decide how to regard the standing of young children, the severely demented, and those who are brain injured. The focus shifts to determining when a particular level of human mental life has ceased.

*Embodiments*

When the determination of the death of a human person involves ascertaining whether human mental life has ceased, problems of the embodiment of human life have taken on their modern character. If one asks simply about the embodiment of human life, one can come to an answer somewhat similar to Aquinas's: human life is in all of the parts of the human body. One might think here of the classic definition of death given in the fourth edition of *Black's Law Dictionary* as "the cessation of life; the ceasing to exist; defined by physicians as a total stoppage of the circulation of the blood, and a cessation of the animal and vital functions consequent thereon, such as respiration, pulsation, etc."[9] Once one's interest is not in the preservation of mere biological life, but in the continuance of a mental life, the focus is on the brain as the sponsor of sentience and consciousness. It is the brain that sustains mental life. The body, in contrast, comes to be seen as a complex, integrated mechanism that sustains the life of the brain, which sponsors the life of a person. One can replace various parts of the body with transplanted organs or prostheses and the person remains the same person. But if one successfully transplanted a brain, one would successfully transplant a person from an old body to a new body. As Roland Puccetti has phrased it, where the brain goes, there goes the person.[10]

This leads to distinguishing among the various embodiments of various mental functions. One may recall the historical antecedents of this debate in the nineteenth-century disputes regarding these issues. Much of our modern ways of understanding cerebral localization are deeply indebted to the phrenologists Franz Josef Gall (1758–1828)[11] and Johann Spurzheim (1776–1832),[12] who argued for the strict localization of mental functions. The phrenologists were attacked by such latter-day Cartesians as M. J. P. Flourens (1794–1867), who in 1845 dedicated one of his books to Descartes in defense of a view that the mind acted as a unity upon the cerebral hemispheres.[13] Gall and Spurzheim in a complex and important fashion influenced the development of the notion that mental functions can, however nonstrictly, be mapped upon various parts of the brain.[14] They also influenced, although indirectly, the work of John Hughlings Jackson (1835–1911), who created the modern idiom of neurology and of cerebral localization.[15] It is from this debate and through this idiom that we come to distinguish among various levels of mental life with different embodiments.

*Living and dying with less than absolute certainty*

Understanding the criteria for being a person as criteria for being a participant in the morality of permission-giving that binds moral strangers, and determining what parts of the brain sponsor the life of persons as participants in this general secular practice of morality will not suffice for fashioning acceptable tests for death. Even after one has achieved sufficient conceptual clarification regarding what it means to be alive as a mind or as a person, and a sufficient understanding of the embodiment presupposed by that life, one will still need to find ways to test safely for when that life's embodiment has gone. Even if one is clear conceptually regarding what it means to be alive in this world, one will still need to fashion reliable operational tests to determine when that life has ceased.

As the President's Commission report on defining death (1981) shows, there have been periods of obsessive fear about avoiding false positive tests even with whole-body-oriented definitions of death. For example, affluent individuals in the eighteenth and nineteenth centuries were occasionally interred with complex mechanisms to allow them to signal others if they revived in their coffins.[16] Such coffins were supplied as well with special provisions for ventilation. So, too, whole-brain definitions of death have raised the issue of what tests are reliable indicators that the brain has died. One might think here of contemporary discussions regarding how often one need repeat tests for reflexes or for EKG activity, or under what circumstances one should test for the capacity of spontaneous respiration in order to declare an individual dead. However, one may not need to be as concerned with false positives as one might think, when one considers that possible survivors with severe brain damage may not have wanted to be treated under such circumstances. On the other hand, one may be properly concerned with false negative tests. If one falsely finds an individual to be alive who is really dead, one may see oneself committed to discharging costly moral obligations of care and treatment.

Such concerns are only indirectly focused on what it means to be alive or on the embodiment presupposed by such life. They are rather primarily focused on ways of determining the end of that life or the destruction of that embodiment with as few false positives as possible. This may lead to an important ambiguity. One may select a whole-body- or whole-brain-oriented test for death, not because one holds that the life of persons is sponsored by the body or the brain as a whole, but because one fears false positive determinations of death that may result from employing a neocortical definition. Or to take a more colorful example, just because one does not wish to be declared dead until one is odoriferous in the Texas summer sun does not necessarily imply that one believes one will be alive up until that very point—the point employed for determining death.

To avoid some of these potential ambiguities, I will use the term *concept of death*, and such variants as *whole-brain-oriented concept of death* and *neocortically oriented concept of death*, to identify conceptual understandings regarding the significance of mental life or of the life of a person and/or the embodiment of that life, such as would lead one to hold that persons are embodied in the brain as a whole or in the neocortex. In contrast, I will use the term *test for* or *determination of death* to identify particular operations used to ascertain whether death according to a particular concept of death has occurred. I will use the term *definition of death* to encompass both concepts of death and tests for death.

## The development of a whole-brain definition of death

To a great extent, all of the conceptual distinctions for a whole-brain-oriented, if not a higher-brain-centers-oriented definition of death were well in hand at the end of the nineteenth century. It was clear that the brain was the sponsor of consciousness and that in fact the cerebrum was the necessary condition for consciousness.[17] The major problems were operational, not conceptual. The difficulty would have been in establishing a whole-brain- or a neocortically oriented test for death that would not have involved an unacceptable number of false positive determinations. The twentieth century contributed not simply more information, but a practical need to develop whole-brain-oriented, if not neocortically oriented, tests for death.

This need sprang from the development in the 1950s of intensive care units and of respirators able to sustain brain-dead but otherwise alive human bodies for a number of hours if not days. This technological advance engendered new financial and psychological costs, due to the false negative determinations delivered by whole-body-oriented definitions of death under contexts of high technology. In the 1950s the development of kidney transplant techniques and in 1967 of heart transplantation further underscored the need to develop a whole-brain definition. If one waited for the individual to be dead on the basis of whole-body tests, one ran the risk of severe damage to the kidneys and profound damage to the heart, which one hoped to transplant. Technological advances, rising costs, and an interest in transplantation pressed the question of whether one could not hold brain-dead but otherwise living human bodies to no longer be the bodies of living persons.

The first hesitant step toward a whole-brain-oriented definition of death was taken in 1968 by the Ad Hoc Committee of the Harvard Medical School, chaired by Henry Beecher. It is important to note that the committee did not forward a definition of death *in sensu stricto,* but rather concluded that individuals with irreversible coma could be declared dead. The committee did not clearly equate destruction of the entire brain with death of the person.[18] Despite these limitations, this proposal had immediate and substantial impact on the understanding of what was to be meant by death. Shortly after the committee's publication of its criteria, the Twenty-Second Congress of the World Medical Association in its "Declaration of Sydney" acknowledged the possible usefulness of encephalographic determinations in declaring death.[19] In the next year, 1969, the Ad Hoc Committee of the American Electroencephalographic Society on EEG Criteria for Determination of Cerebral Death published criteria that equated death with brain death. Though the title suggests a cerebrally oriented definition of death, the committee in fact supported only a whole-brain-oriented definition.[20] It is important to note that the so-called whole-brain definition of death has been widely accepted and employed, though there has been evidence for a considerable time that the whole brain is in fact not dead, that some tissue remains alive.[21] This policy success can only be explained by presuming that it incorporates an implicit *de minimis* criterion.

These developments led to changes in the law by statute, beginning in 1970. Whole-brain-oriented definitions of death became well established over the next decade. The initial and potentially pernicious confusion between when a person is dead and when one is no longer obliged to sustain a person's life began to be clarified. It was generally acknowledged that when the whole brain was destroyed, it was not simply that one was no longer obliged to sustain that individual, but rather that that individual was dead, no longer existing in this world. This was a painful and difficult step. Brain-dead but otherwise alive human bodies are warm to the touch and are respiring, albeit with mechanical assistance. They appear to be alive because they are in fact alive. It is because human biological life continues unabated that transplant surgeons are interested in such bodies as an ideal source for harvesting organs. There is no reason why a brain-dead but otherwise alive male could not function as a sperm donor. In addition, neocortically dead but otherwise alive pregnant women have been sustained until parturition.[22] Such bodies meet one of the significant criteria for biological liveliness, namely, reproductive capacity.

It is because brain-dead but otherwise alive human bodies are biologically alive that it was so difficult for the general public to accept whole-brain-oriented definitions of the death of persons. An example of this difficulty is provided by a 1952 Kentucky case, *Grey et al. v. Sawyer et al.,* in which it was important for purposes of inheritance to determine which of two individuals died first. One individual, who was decapitated in an accident, had continued to spurt blood from her carotids after her companion no longer demonstrated a pulse. As the court record indicates, she was found "decapitated, her head lying about ten feet from her body, which was actively bleeding 'from near her neck and blood was gushing from her body in spurts . . .'" However, physicians testified to the court that "a body is not dead so long as there is a heartbeat and that may be evidenced by the gushing of blood in spurts."[23] For us, the determination of the court is ludicrous, in that we accept a whole-brain-oriented standard. When we read this case, we understand that the head of the decapitated woman began to suffer from anoxia at least at the same time as the brain of her companion. We have gone through a major paradigm shift in our understanding of what it means to be alive and embodied in this world.

*Being there*

These philosophical reflections concerning the life of persons and the meaning of embodiment can be put in terms of a rather straightforward fantasy. Imagine that one consults one's neurologist and is diagnosed as suffering from a serious neurological disease. The bad news is that it will destroy one's whole brain. The good news is that due to the advances in medicine a normal life expectancy can still be assured. If one's reaction to this information is not simply that such a life would be of no use to oneself, but that one would *not be there* for the life to be either useful or useless, one has embraced a whole-brain-oriented concept of death.

The step toward a neocortically oriented (or more precisely, a higher-brain-centers-oriented) definition of death is taken when the physician returns the next day, stating that the bad news is not that bad. Though the patient will lose the entire cerebrum, the lower brain stem, pons, and cerebellum will be able to be preserved. The patient will be able to continue normal breathing unsustained by a respirator. However, there will be no sentience, no experience of the world; the patient will be permanently comatose. If one still concludes that one would not be there, not just that such life would be useless, one has taken the further step toward a higher-brain-centers-oriented concept of death. One has concluded that whatever it means to be in the world as a person requires at a minimum some level of sentience and consciousness. The mere persistence of biological functions is not sufficient. One recognizes the higher brain centers as a necessary condition for the life of persons because they are required for even a minimum of conscious awareness. When there is no cerebrum, there is no person. One also recognizes that the mere existence of a brain stem, pons, and cerebellum is insufficient for the life of a person (or even the life of a mind). A functioning and intact brain stem, pons, and cerebellum do not of themselves secure the existence of a person, because they are not sufficient for consciousness. In short, if the cerebrum is dead, the person is dead.

One may still wish not to employ higher-brain-centers-oriented tests for determining death, even though one accepts as an intellectual point a higher-brain-center-oriented concept of death, because of a concern that there will be an inordinate number of false positive determinations of death. Such a concern could lead one to decide that avoiding such risks is worth the costs of false negative determinations of death. There is also the problem of the emotional and social costs of disposing of a body whose higher brain centers are dead, but that is still spontaneously breathing. As a result, one may judge that individuals such as Karen Quinlan, at least in general secular moral terms, were dead years before they were pronounced dead, though one may not wish to establish a policy of declaring such individuals dead because of possible adverse consequences.

Despite these hesitations, we appear to be moving to higher-brain-centers-oriented definitions in much the same way we moved toward whole-brain-oriented definitions of death.[24] Although the law does not allow such individuals to be declared dead, it is becoming acceptable to stop all treatment for such individuals if their relatives agree. The tone of a number of reflections goes beyond regarding only (1) the wishes of the patients and the next-of-kin or (2) the burdens and costs that might make such treatment disproportionate, and (3) in addition recognizing that no further life is being lived, at least in general secular terms. The President's Commission for the Study of Ethical Problems in Medicine and Biomedical and Behavioral Research made the following recommendation in its March 21, 1983, report:

The decisions of patients' families should determine what sort of medical care permanently unconscious patients receive. Other than requiring appropriate decisionmaking procedures for these patients, the law does not and should not require any particular therapies to be applied or continued, with the exception of basic nursing care that is needed to ensure dignified and respectful treatment of the patient.[25]

There is a recognition that there is nothing more one can do for the permanently unconscious. Indeed, permanently unconscious individuals currently can be seen as falling into a limbo between those individuals recognized to be persons alive and in the world, and those unambiguously recognized as dead. That it is licit in general secular moral terms to stop all treatment, including intravenous hydration and nutrition,[26] seems only reasonable. There is no one to suffer from dehydration and starvation or to derive pleasure from hydration and nutrition. On the other hand, would it be justifiable for patients or their families to demand treatment under such circumstances? Should one convict an individual of murder who killed such a body? The arguments to this point suggest an answer in the negative on all these points, at least in general secular terms. Such bodies, since they are no longer the embodiment of persons or even of a mind, would count, at least in general secular terms, as biologically living corpses. Indeed, the Ethics Committee of the Society of Critical Care Medicine recommends that patients "in a persistent vegetative or permanently unconscious state . . . should be excluded from the ICU."[27] If some wish to sustain such a corpse, that should be their prerogative, if they use their private funds. Also, an individual who killed such a body may very well be guilty of a secularly cognizable moral offense, as is the desecrator of a corpse but the offense would not be that of murder. There would be no one there in the body to kill. Particular moral communities could require special laws that recognized acts against such bodies as acts of murder if committed on their property or facilities. Malpractice awards should not generally be made to sustain the lives of such entities.[28]

The problem is where to draw the line. One may not be clear how much consciousness is required for there to be the life of a person. Again, it is for such reasons that one may err on the conservative side. Thus, in applying a whole-brain-oriented concept of death, one may require the lack of all electroencephalographic activity, in the absence of hypothermia or central nervous system depressants, to declare death, even though the presence of some EEG activity will surely be insufficient to establish the presence of a person. Such an approach may be acceptable because it is clear that the capacity for EEG activity is a necessary condition for the embodiment of human persons, although it is far from clear how much EEG activity, and of what kind, is *sufficient* for the life of a person. One may be willing to accept the absence of all sentience and consciousness as a criterion for the death of a person, though the presence of minimal sentience and consciousness will not be sufficient for the presence of a person, at least in general secular terms. Even a higher-brain-centers-oriented definition of death, which required destruction of the *entire* neocortex, would be conservative.

An illustration of the problem of such borderline cases is provided by *In re Claire C. Conroy,* which involved a petition to discontinue nasogastric feeding on an eighty-four-year-old woman, who suffered from organic brain syndrome. She was still able to move her hands voluntarily and smile when her hair was combed, although she was unable to communicate and was severely demented. One's view of cases such as Conroy's will depend on (1) how much of a mental life one judges to be sufficient for the life of a person, and (2) the protection one holds is due to entities that are the successors of persons. The facts of the Conroy case appear to make the claim implausible that she was still a moral agent. However, there may still be generally justifiable secular moral claims (in addition to rather significant religiously based moral claims) to be made on behalf of entities that succeed on persons and which still have some sentience, not to mention those whose lives are still dimly lit by reason.

This is an ontological problem: how ought we to regard the imperfectly unified mental life of the severely senile? It is too easy, even in general secular moral terms, simply to say that they should be regarded only on a par with other animals that possess similar levels of mental life. The senile surely possess at least the secular moral rights (i.e., beneficence-based rights) of such animals. The senile were also once persons in the strict sense. One knows who they were. Such entities have a moral status quite different from that of children and the profoundly mentally retarded, who are not yet, or who will never become, persons in the strict sense. Here one may have moral obligations out of prior agreements to those former persons with respect to their bodies as one has obligations to honor the testamentary wishes of the dead. Indeed, in such borderline cases one will have duties to such entities (1) because of commitments to the persons they were, (2) because of the actual persons to whom they belong (i.e., their family), (3) because of unclarity regarding the extent to which such former persons live on in a successor entity (i.e., a mental life that is no longer that of a moral agent), as well as (4) because of secular moral obligations of beneficence to these entities, and (5) because of concerns regarding the values associated with the moral persons they were.

The first and second points by themselves could justify obligations beyond those that support respectful treatment of the body as one now treats corpses. Such considerations could surely justify basic nursing care, at least as long as the body of a former person is alive. Though the person is dead, a human is alive regarding which one can have substantial secular moral obligations because of past agreements or because of agreements to current guardians. These considerations have the greatest force. One must discharge obligations one has assumed. Much of this perhaps cannot be sorted out, except through establishing different forms of long-term nursing care embedded in particular clusters of moral commitments. From the outside, these alternative approaches would appear simply as special contractual arrangements. From the inside, they may be sustained by content-full moral visions, as, for instance, those that shape Orthodox Jewish or Roman Catholic nursing facilities. By making permanent loss of consciousness the point at which humans are declared dead, one would be able to establish a practice that would provide uniformity in general secular moral contexts for the declaration of death for infants, the retarded, adults, and the senile. Particular communities with their own understandings of death might exempt themselves. Still, one would have resolved in a conservative fashion, at least from the perspective of general secular morality, the issue of the treatment of entities with a mental life that may succeed the life of a human person. This approach would not support imputing a social sense of person to anencephalic infants or other infants born with similar profound neurological defects. Individuals such as Claire Conroy would be treated as alive and individuals such as Karen Quinlan declared dead. This, however, would not exclude special practices in these regards from being established for particular moral communities.

## Toward a higher-brain-centers definition of death

We have been brought to the conclusion that a whole-brain-oriented concept of death is insufficient for the concerns of secular morality. Whatever we mean by persons as permission givers, as the cardinal sources of general secular moral authority, requires at least the presence of that sentience that is lost forever to the permanently comatose. Whole-brain-oriented definitions of death focus on structures that are insufficient for the embodiment of persons, moral agents who could participate in the morality binding moral strangers. Even with an appropriate conservatism that treated all sentient individuals as if they remained persons, the focus of whole-brain definitions of death is misplaced. This error, implicit in whole-brain definitions generally, was made even worse by the Uniform Determination of Death Act proposed by the President's Commission for the Study of Ethical Problems in Medicine and Biomedical and Behavioral Research in its July 9, 1981, report, *Defining Death*. That act retreated from proposals that clearly accented the brain as the embodiment of the life of persons. Consider here the sparse clarity of the American Bar Association's 1975 model statute: "For all legal purposes, a human body with irreversible cessation of total brain function, according to usual and customary standards of medical practice, shall be considered dead."[29] In contrast, the President's Commission underscored the importance of brain stem function for the life of individuals. It also explicitly incorporated a circulatory and respiratory test for death.

An individual who has sustained either (1) irreversible cessation of circulatory and respiratory functions, or (2) irreversible cessation of all functions of the entire brain, including the brain stem, is dead. A determination of death must be made in accordance with accepted medical standards.[30]

The definition supports a view of the body that cannot be made out if it is persons who are central to secular moral standing. It may be important for traditional religious concerns, yet this is not clearly stated.

First, there is no need explicitly to incorporate a circulatory and respiratory test for death. If circulatory and respiratory functions fail for only a short period of time, the brain will die. Failure of circulatory and respiratory function can be used in most circumstances as a test for brain death in accord with "the usual and customary standards of medical practice." One need only explicitly focus on a determination of brain function when circulatory and respiratory function continues after possible brain death. Second, and even more difficult, is the commission's attempt to construe the importance of the brain, not as the sponsor of consciousness, but rather as either the primary organ for integrating the functions of the major organ systems, or as a hallmark for bodily integration.[31] The commission's report represents an endeavor to reconstrue the whole-brain definition of death in organismic and vitalistic terms, rather than to acknowledge its implications for an understanding of the special significance of the brain for the embodiment of persons. To put it somewhat bluntly, the commission has attempted to turn the whole-brain definition of death into a special test for whole-body death. For the commission, the death of the brain was seen to be important in signaling the death of the body as an integrated whole.

Given the circumstance that human bodies whose higher brain centers are dead have no mental life (and are therefore not moral subjects, much less persons), the only general, secular grounds for hesitation with respect to the adoption of higher-brain-centers-oriented definitions of death (in the absence of special, e.g., religious considerations) will be consequence-oriented (issues in part recognized by the commission). First, one may be concerned whether higher-brain-centers-oriented tests for death will not involve the risk of a significant number of false positive determinations. Such is a technological problem that is likely superable. The enduring moral issues will turn on the psychological costs involved in discontinuing treatment as a matter of course on permanently comatose individuals. For example, the commission finds it difficult to declare cerebrally dead but otherwise alive bodies to be no longer the embodiments of persons.[32] Will generally allowing such individuals to die of dehydration and starvation have an adverse impact on important moral virtues and practices? Would active steps to effect death have significant adverse effects? The reflections of the President's Commission appear to be in the negative on the first point (the Commission presumably would be positive on the second point). Societies would need to investigate carefully the costs of the second.

Certain communities because of their beliefs will not be able to accept a higher-brain-centers-oriented definition, as many currently cannot accept a whole-brain-oriented definition of death. One might think here of the Orthodox Jewish position that an individual is dead only when the last breath is drawn.[33] Indeed, as one moves to a neocortical definition of death, others in addition to Orthodox Jews may wish to employ a different standard. Different definitions of death could be established for different communities. Having community-specific rules as to when estates should devolve upon heirs should pose the least difficulty. One would need only to register as a member of a particular community whose definition of death is publicly known. Concerns with costs could be met insofar as communities requiring further treatment because of a definition that postpones the determination of death then paid for the additional care involved. In some cases this might require those communities to create special treatment units or hospitals. In the absence of payment, the general secular standard could apply. With regard to homicide, one of at least two approaches might be taken. First, the general neocortical definition of death could be established as a defense against homicide, but not against aggravated abuse of a corpse. Second, individuals could be prosecuted for murder when they end the human biological life of individuals understood and recognized as still alive within communities that hold such persons not to be dead until a nonneocortical definition of death is applied. Given the possibility of many and diverse religions that may not even accept the usual whole-brain definition of death, the first approach may be more feasible and still sufficiently meet the claims of members of particular moral communities, at least when the events occur in areas open to all. Still, particular religious communities should be able to establish their own health care facilities where special tort and criminal law could apply.[34]

## Abortion, harm to fetuses, and infanticide

The previous section of this chapter focused on the endings of human life. Because the deaths of persons are not always coincident with the cessation of the biological lives of their bodies, we faced a number of puzzles. In the absence of any canonical content-full moral guidance, the puzzles were explored in terms of when persons cease to be conveyors of permission, persons in the strict sense. This unavoidable approach led to some troubling discoveries regarding the vacuity of secular morality. Among these was, for example, the reevaluation of the senile.

Matters with regard to the beginning of human life are even more disturbing and collide even more substantially with moral concerns regarding the impropriety of abortion and infanticide. Secular morality is blind to the intrinsic immorality of either. In significant measure, this stems from the circumstance that the start of human biological life is not the beginning of the life of a person as a moral agent. Rather, in human ontogeny months of biological life transpire before there is good evidence of the life of a mind, and years go by before there is evidence of the life of a person as a moral agent. As a result, the moral status of zygotes, embryos, fetuses, and even infants is problematic in general secular morality. As we saw in chapter 4, it is not plausible to hold that fetuses are persons in the strict sense of being moral agents. In fact, there is not even evidence to hold that infants are persons in the strict sense. Whatever sort of mental life might exist for fetuses and infants, it is not that of self-conscious moral agents, so that the moral standing of adult mammals, *ceteris paribus,* would be higher than that of human fetuses or infants.

Despite this state of affairs, established secular moral practices in Western culture discourage the killing of human fetuses and newborns, more so than killing adult great apes. From the vantage point of arguments sustainable in general secular terms, these practices can at best be understood as imputing, because of its usefulness, certain rights of persons to these forms of human biological life. As argued in chapter 4, these practices involve treating instances of human biological life within a social sense of person. These practices have similarities with the ways in which we treat the very senile and severely demented adults. There is a difference in that one does not yet know the persons that the fetuses or newborns may with luck become, as one knows who the very senile once were.

In the case of death, we saw the recognized secular moral line between personhood and nonpersonhood move from whole-body-oriented concepts of death to whole-brain death to a proposal to employ higher-brain-centers-oriented concepts of death. This movement constitutes a retreat from imputing the status of persons to a set of individuals who are not persons strictly, but who were once treated as persons in the social sense. A superficial symmetry had existed between the use of whole-body definitions of death and life as the lines of demarcation for the imputing of personhood. One withdrew the status of being a person when the last breath was drawn; one gave the status of personhood when the first breath was drawn. With the introduction of a whole-brain definition of death one might in error seek a new symmetry in secular morality. Unfortunately, it cannot be found. This search might falsely suggest that the criterion of the absence of EEG activity, which had been adopted as a test for death, might in reverse serve as a test for the beginning of the life of a person. One would then in error decide that when EEG activity begins, at least insofar as the concept of person can be justified in general secular moral terms, a person begins, at least insofar as the concept of person can be justified in general secular moral terms. In the declaration of death the presence of EEG activity is used as a test for a necessary, not a sufficient, condition for the presence of a person. The presence of EEG activity does not show the presence of a person. There is no evidence at all that fetuses are moral agents.

The symmetry, lost when one moved to a whole-brain definition of death, will not be regained with a higher-brain-centers definition. At the end of life one is trying to mark when consciousness ceases. When, with the partial death of the higher brain centers, consciousness becomes greatly obtunded, it may still not be certain that the life of the person has ended. On the other hand, when only the first most meager indications of consciousness begin, one can be sure that there is not yet a person in the strict sense of a moral agent. The presence of some neocortical activity is not sufficient for the presence of a moral agent. This asymmetry stems from the fact that with dying persons one knows who is dying and one may have special duties to them to protect their interests, even in a twilight zone of nonpersonal mental life. In the case of fetuses and newborns, one does not yet know who they will be. There are no special secular moral duties to persons who are not yet extant. It is only persons in the strict sense who can give permission and whose use without permission violates the core of secular morality. Secular moral authority to use entities that are not persons depends on those who already are persons. The secular moral standing of entities that are not yet persons in the strict sense is derived from those who already are. In contrast, one can have made special promises to dead persons regarding the care of their corpses. Also, in the case of death, one has a concern to avoid practices that may expose oneself to the risks of false positive or premature determinations of death. In the case of fetuses and newborn children, there is no such risk that can be understood in general secular moral terms. One will never be a child. In secular morality, one at most has a duty not malevolently to injure the future persons the fetuses may become.

## The status of zygotes, embryos, and fetuses

To understand the moral status of the beginning of human biological life, one will need to examine how that life is important for persons as moral agents. Since that life is not the life of a person strictly, the persons involved will not be embodied in that life. If a human fetus has more than the moral status of an animal with a similar level of development, in general secular terms it will be because of the significance of that life for the woman who has conceived it, for others around her who may be interested in it, and for the future person it may become. As incongruous as this comparison of animals and human fetuses will appropriately appear to those who with religious faith understand the evil of abortion, it is a comparison affirmed in secular criminal codes that allow women to abort their fetuses, but not torture their pets.

For this reason, in general secular morality one turns to those to whom fetuses belong in order to determine their worth. The fetus of a woman who wants a child takes on considerable significance. It gains value from her interests and love, and that of others around her. The would-be mother, father, grandmothers, grandfathers, uncles, and aunts can vest a wanted embryo or fetus with great value. The opposite can obtain as well. Because of the circumstances of the conception, the probable circumstances of the birth, or because the fetus is defective or deformed, a negative worth may be given. Such fetuses may be regarded by many as threatening or harmful.

Those who produced a fetus, at least within general secular morality, have the first claim on effectively determining its use. This is usually unambiguously the father and mother who conceived it, especially the mother since she bears it. They produced it, they made it, it is theirs. The fetus can be regarded as a special form of very dear property: the biological lineage of a family, a couple's attempt to fashion another person on whom to bestow their love and give their care and concern. Others may become involved with the gamete producers through special agreements, so that the terms "father" and "mother" become ambiguous. One might think of surrogate motherhood where the gestational mother has an embryo unrelated to her inserted in her womb. The gamete producers may have contracted with a couple (either directly or indirectly) to produce an embryo that will be carried by a gestational mother for the couple. Or the couple may contractually transfer its rights, as would happen if an embryo is donated. But the point remains the same. In general secular morality, it is persons who endow zygotes, embryos, or fetuses with value. Those who made or procreated the zygote, embryo, or fetus have first claim on making the definitive determination of its value. Privately produced embryos and fetuses are private property. They would be societally owned only if societal groups or cooperatives produced them.

Although society may offer incentives for reproductive actions or omissions of various sorts, the limited secular moral authority of the state and the status of the fetus as private property make it improper in general secular morality to use unconsented-to force to determine the abortion choices of women. Unless the procreators have transferred their rights to others (e.g., by donating the embryo to another woman or couple), they have a secular moral right to abort the fetus, even if others would gladly adopt the child it could become. The parents, and especially the woman, have produced the fetus. Next to one's own body, the sperm, ova, zygotes, and fetuses one produces are, in secular moral terms, primordially one's own. They are extensions of and the fruit of one's own body. They are one's own to dispose of until they take possession of themselves as conscious entities, until one gives them a special standing in a community, until one transfers one's rights in them to another, or until they become persons. The sense of right here draws attention to the lack of others' authority to impose their will on such private choices. In a secular morality grounded on the authority of permission, large moral spaces open to do what others will recognize as evil.

One might imagine courts being invited to resolve conflicts between prospective fathers and mothers with respect to conflicting wishes regarding whether to procure an abortion. Here we will imagine that the individuals are rootless yuppies. Since it will be quite difficult to determine who promised whom what, and out of respect for the privacy of the family as a social unit, it would appear prudent to follow the example of the U.S. Supreme Court in not intervening with general secular state force to resolve such issues.[35] Since the woman is investing the major energies in developing the fetus, and in that it would be her body that would be the subject of control, it would be appropriate to allow her the legally protected choice, absent special agreements. However, protection against costs of child care imposed by a secular state should be available to men who renounce all interests in having a child as a part of a prenuptial or similar agreement. Also, state force may with moral probity be used to prevent a surrogate mother from aborting a fetus she has contracted to bring to term.

The foregoing account of the moral status of zygotes, embryos, fetuses, and infants can be nothing but shocking from the perspective of received traditional Western culture, not to mention that which one understands properly in traditional Christian faith. This shock is in part a recognition of the distance between what can be secured through general secular morality and what one knows in faith. In general philosophical terms, this shock or disappointment should be regarded as an invitation to realize the impossibility of reconstructing Judeo-Christian moral sensibilities through general secular moral reasoning. As has already been noted, this struggle to achieve the impossible distinguished the Enlightenment and characterizes the disappointments of postmodernity. In this respect, Kant as a figure marking both the high point and the close of the Enlightenment is an excellent illustration. One might think of his attempt to prove by reason alone that masturbation is an immoral act worse than suicide.[36] Kant was attempting to justify in reason his particular Protestant understanding of sexuality. From our perspective this attempt is a hilarious failure. But similarly the attempt in general secular terms to show the evil involved with abortion and infanticide fails as well. No matter how truly one knows the evil of abortion and infanticide, this cannot be established in general secular moral terms.[37] The contrast between general secular morality and content-full moral commitments is stark and disappointing.

The implications of this contrast are adverse to the general secular authority of the state to impose or require only one criminal law in such matters. Consent of the governed cannot be adequately achieved for the imposition of a particular content-full morality. The visions of proper reproduction are multiple, divergent, and incompatible. Sufficient permission will not be forthcoming for a uniform approach in these matters. If governments derive their moral authority from the permission of those who participate, and if such permission is limited, as has been seen in chapter 4, there remain moral spaces within the general umbrella of geographically located secular states for communities to derive authority to establish particular criminal laws and welfare rights that apply only to their own members. The development of special communal civil and welfare laws would recognize the moral limits of the authority of geographically based states. Within such moral spaces individuals could with ease give expression to the sentiment: "If the government does not like my particular moral commitments, it can leave me alone to realize them peaceably by myself and with consenting others." Such community-specific law would recognize the limits of secular moral authority, while acknowledging the importance of the content-full commitments of particular moral communities.

The law, following the example of New Jersey in allowing communally specific definitions of death, should also allow particular communities to establish and live by their own appreciations of the status of zygotes, embryos, fetuses, and infants, as long as this does not involve the direct, unconsented-to use of persons. Individuals who are members of particular communities should be able to realize their moral commitments in these areas by binding themselves to laws forbidding the killing of their own zygotes, embryos, fetuses, and children, even though such laws would not apply to those outside their own communities. Those who recognize the importance of respecting the special status of human life before general secular law allows it to be treated as human personal life, could then both affirm their moral sentiments for themselves and witness to their importance for others. In whatever way, within the constraints set by the principle of permission, the law comes to terms with those outside particular communities killing individuals held secularly to be dead, but who are members of particular communities that still consider them to be alive, the same could be applied to similar acts against zygotes, embryos, fetuses, and infants. In a world of moral diversity,

THE FOUNDATIONS OF BIOETHICS

limited general secular moral content, and increasing sophistication in storing and transferring data internationally, individuals should be able to carry with them their special criminal and welfare rights and obligations.

### Wrongful life

There is an important limitation in general secular morality with respect to what one may do with fetuses. If one decides not to abort a fetus, if one decides not to kill it, one must take care not to injure the future person it may become. Injuring the fetus, unlike killing it, sets into motion a causal chain that may injure the future person the fetus will become. The moral obligation to refrain from actions that will injure a fetus likely in the future to become a person has been explored in the law under the rubric of tort for wrongful life. Tort-for-wrongful-life suits contrast with tort-for-wrongful-conception and tort-for-wrongful-birth suits, in which individuals have sued because they have been harmed by the failure of contraception or of sterilization and must now care for a child or indeed a handicapped child.[38] In tort-for-wrongful-life suits, the child itself sues for being born under circumstances connected with injury or harm.

In such suits the plaintiff complains of a harm that could have been avoided only by not having conceived the individual or by having aborted that individual. The history of these suits has been somewhat colorful. They have included an action by an illegitimate son against his father, arguing that to be born a bastard in Illinois was a harm (perhaps, unlike some other states, where such antecedents appear to be a qualification for political office), for which the child should be able to collect financial damages.[39] That suit was unsuccessful, as were others such as one brought by a baby girl conceived when her mother was raped by a fellow mental-hospital inmate in the state of New York.[40]

New ground was broken by a California appellate court in *Curlender v. Bio-Science Laboratories*.[41] The court not only awarded damages to the couple but to the child of the couple, who had been misinformed that they were not carriers of Tay-Sachs disease. The court also added in a dictum that, had the information been properly transmitted by the laboratory and by the physician, the parents could have been sued by their child. The court argued that there is a parental duty to children to avoid their birth as defective even if this means avoiding their birth. Knowing procreation of a defective child was held to be a negligent act, actionable under tort law. This holding was subsequently set aside. As a secular moral issue, this view appears implausible if the future life of the child is such that harms do not outweigh benefits. One will on balance not have harmed *that* future person by bringing it into existence. If it is reasonable for the parents to assume that there will be a favorable balance of goods over harms to the child, procreation would appear morally justified as long as the child did not constitute an unagreed-upon burden to others.

Because malevolent actions are forbidden, there remains the problem of distinguishing between foreseen and intended harms. Parents may not intend harm. But it appears permissible to foresee but not intend harm to one's child.[42] One can imagine a king in a constitutional monarchy who must reproduce to pass on his line and where in the absence of an heir a repressive government would be established, but where the heir would inherit a very painful disease. The issue is whether procreating a person under circumstances in which the conception is unavoidably tied to future harms should count as an unconsented-to injury to that future person. If existence is tied to the injury itself, and the injury is not intended but only foreseen, has one violated another's autonomy in the sense of using that person against his wishes? Or has one been morally protected by a variety of double effect?

This question must be answered in part by understanding what it means to produce a child. One need not produce a child for that child's sake. A great number of the children born are neither directly intended nor explicitly planned. They are rather the result of habit, accident, and passion. Even those planned may not be procreated for their sake alone. In fact, such is likely rarely the case. People conceive children because of the need for agricultural laborers as well as for support in old age. They also do so because of a deep human desire to have children, to have the companionship and love of others, not simply to do good to those others by giving them existence. Children may also be produced through an understanding in faith of the meaning of marriage. There are as well traditional goals such as the continuation of families and traditions that require engendering another generation. Such can make procreation a fairly selfless and dedicated act, even if it is not directed primarily to the child. In any event, children are produced for goals that are not theirs, but that may become theirs, and to which they have not consented.

The gift of life is given along with burdens. Children are set at risk when their parents choose dangerous areas to live, work, or vacation. The choice to live in an inner-city rather than a small town frequently entails risks not only to the parents, but to their children. Individuals in the last century who migrated to the American West often made a choice that exposed themselves and their children to danger. So, too, individuals who maintain certain traditional ways of life, such as the BaMbuti discussed in chapter 2, may expose their children to a higher infant mortality than would be the case were they to live otherwise. Parents usually embrace such choices to secure a favorable balance of benefits for the family. Such choices are made because of the availability of jobs or social support, because of the virtues of a traditional way of life, or because the promises of a new frontier make the risks worthwhile. They are usually understood as proper choices in terms of a particular understanding of the good life to which the parents subscribe. Parents also expose their children to risks as a part of their lifestyle, and without a justification in terms of their vision of the good parent. Parents often smoke, drink, or ski, not because they believe such actions will benefit their children, but simply because they enjoy them. Are such actions to be stopped by state force? Are such actions wrong in secular terms?

Given the opacity of the future, which includes our ignorance of the wishes of future individuals, and because future persons by definition do not yet exist as persons strictly, if one acts in a nonmalevolent way toward those future individuals, one has not violated the very notion of a peaceable community. This is so even if in the future those individuals who are conceived do not celebrate the circumstances of their existence. First, there will not be specific duties of beneficence to future individuals. Such cannot, without agreement, be established even to already existing individuals. One will not be required (in general secular terms) to provide children with any special legacy of goods (though providing a legacy could be praiseworthy). Without appealing to a particular moral community and its vision of the good life, perhaps the most that can be required is to attempt to provide a state of life where there would plausibly be more benefits than harms in terms of the moral vision of the procreators. Any action by procreators will to some extent impose a particular vision of the good life on their children. Such impositions on future persons are unavoidable and not improper, since such persons do not exist, not to mention not yet possessing a particular understanding of the good life.

Choosing for them does not violate the principle of permission, unless it is clear that their permission would not be given (i.e., as in the case of the bomb that will explode in twenty years and kill future persons). The notion of the peaceable community will preclude certain acts against future persons. If the bomb setter mentioned in chapter 4 sets a bomb to explode years in the future so as to kill future individuals, it seems plausible that the bomb setter has not only acted in a nonbeneficent, indeed malevolent fashion, but has violated the autonomy rights of those future individuals. The bomb setter would have acted in a way that can reasonably be presumed to be against the wishes of those future persons. In addition, he acts malevolently, thus justifying the use of defensive force. But where the wishes of future persons are far from certain, the most one can say with surety is that one should not directly act to affect those persons in ways that are very likely to be against their wishes. This consideration cuts against the mad bomber who might hold that the children in the future would be better off dead.

One is allowed a great deal of leeway in acting on one's own view of the good life when it comes to possible future persons, because of the difficulty in showing that one is acting against the general notion of a peaceable and beneficent community of persons. To live in the future is to be at the mercy of past visions of the good life, including past visions of benefits and banes. Current persons cannot ask permission from future persons. Still, the foregoing arguments establish certain constraints. In increasing the order of stringency, one can secure some guidance from the principles of beneficence and permission. First, one may not, according to one's own moral vision, act against future persons in ways that are likely to cause more harms than benefits. Violations of the principle of beneficence in general will not warrant coercive restraints. However, malevolent actions can warrant such intrusions. More strictly, using future persons in ways that seem to be against what they will wish violates the principle of permission. So, too, does using future persons contrary to the wishes of those who produce them.

These constraints apply in general to the relationship between current and future persons. They are least severe in the case of parents who can argue (1) "take it or leave it, we would not have produced you except in circumstances marked by harms to you"; or (2) "take it or leave it, we would not have produced you unless we could raise you in circumstances marked by harms to you." As long as (1) there is no malevolent intent, and (2) there is no expectation that the child will likely not wish to live under such circumstances, then there is no violation of either the principle of beneficence or that of permission. The second condition underscores as best one can with regard to children the obligation of parents consequent upon the principle of permission not to do injury to their children without their permission.[43] The principle is especially attenuated because parents can argue that they would not consider reproducing if they had to forgo smoking with their children, hang-gliding with their children, or trekking through the Amazon rainforest with their children. This applies as well to the view that one would not reproduce if this required prenatal testing and abortion. The child is at least receiving a nonmalevolent gift of life that is not clearly against the future child's wishes. With respect to the moral issues raised by tortfor-wrongful-life suits, we can then conclude that, within certain constraints, it is not morally forbidden to conceive a child and allow it to go to term, knowing that it carries with it genetic or other congenital harms. Within particular moral communities there may be special moral principles, including special principles of beneficence, to forbid such reproduction. We will return to this issue in the next chapter in exploring the circumstances in which children may be taken from parents. However, a special application of these reflections still remains to be made.

*State interventions on behalf of the fetus, cesarean sections,*
*fetal surgery, and civil commitment*

These reflections apply not only to decisions to reproduce, knowing that the child will carry a genetic defect. They apply as well to the putative right of the state to force a woman to submit to surgical and medical interventions to prevent damage to her fetus or to cure fetal diseases or defects. This issue has been joined in a number of cases in which women have been compelled to submit to cesarean sections to preserve the life and/or health of the fetus. One of these, *Jessie Mae Jefferson v. Griffin Spalding County Hospital Authority,* was decided by the

Supreme Court of Georgia, which ordered a cesarean delivery.[44] The case concerned a woman with a placenta previa in her thirty-ninth week of pregnancy. As a member of the Shiloh Sanctified Holiness Baptist Church of Butts County, Georgia, her religious scruples brought her to refuse a cesarean section. A vaginal delivery would have led to profuse bleeding avoidable only by a cesarean section. The court was given evidence that the fetus stood a 99 percent chance of dying and the woman a 50 percent chance of dying if a cesarean were not approved. Given this information, Justice Hill observed, "We weighed the right of the mother to practice her religion and to refuse surgery on herself, against her unborn child's right to live. We found in favor of her child's right to live."[45] The woman delivered vaginally without malevent.

This court ruling raised a number of puzzles. Why should it be wrong in general secular moral terms for a woman to refuse lifesaving treatment for herself and for her fetus? Again, an answer will depend on the extent to which a foreseeable but nonintended risk to a future child is compatible with the notion of the peaceable, beneficent community. If it were to violate the notion of the peaceable community, a community functioning with generally justifiable secular moral authority, it would be forbidden under the principle of permission. If it were to violate the notion of the beneficent community (i.e., by being malevolent), it would be forbidden under the principle of beneficence. My proposal in chapter 3 was that malevolent actions against unconsenting persons can legitimate others coming to their defense. But what of those who await a miracle (e.g., movement of a placenta previa)? What about irresponsible actions? What of those individuals who recognize that their actions are not beneficent, but who deny that the actions are malevolent? Consider the case of a woman who smokes or drinks, recognizing that this may pose a hazard to her fetus. She does not smoke or drink in order to injure her fetus; in fact, she wishes the fetus well. She is simply of the opinion that the claims of the fetus on her are not strong enough to force her to change such habits. She may claim that the future person who that fetus may become should be happy that it has the gift of life and that it should not protest about possible detriments due to her habits. If the child is not satisfied with the gift it receives, she adds, then it is surely free in general secular terms to liberate itself through suicide.

If one willfully harms a fetus, believing that it is likely that the future person will not find its life worth living, providing the option of suicide will not be sufficient to defend against the charge of having acted contrary to the principles of permission and beneficence. At the very least, the person produced may recognize the moral obligation not to commit suicide and therefore be condemned to suffer. One will have also acted to produce a future person, believing that the individual will have to live with an unfavorable balance of benefits to harms. Under such circumstances one may presume that the individual will not consent to those harms. When it appears that banes will outweigh benefits in terms of one's own vision of the good, one must presume that one will injure an unconsenting future person.

Given the reflections in the previous section, we are brought to conclude that state force may be used to compel cesarean sections, fetal surgery, or other invasions of a woman's body or to constrain her freedom so as to protect the future health of a child then in utero, if and only if the woman's harmful omissions or commissions are (1) malevolent or (2) such that the anticipated state of the future possible person is so disadvantageous as to make it very plausible that the child would not wish to live under such circumstances. A violation of either of these two conditions will justify force to protect an innocent future person. The case of true malevolence will allow intervention as was argued in chapter 3. The case of a harm so great as to make life unacceptable will justify intervention on behalf of a nonconsenting innocent. The liberty to intervene is limited in recognition of the woman's prima facie secular moral right to be left alone in pursuing her own vision of the good. The pregnant woman's liberty in these matters does not extend to third parties acting to cause such harms or to women who have ceded some of their liberties in these matters by specific contract, as with surrogate mothers.

This limitation of state authority on the basis of general secular morality does not limit (1) condemnation of the woman's actions from the perspective of a particular moral vision nor (2) interventions that have been agreed to as a part of being a member of a particular moral community, most plausibly a non-geographically located community. Although these reflections have focused on women, as it becomes clearer how various circumstances impact on the gametes of both men and women to the detriment of their future children, these reflections will have even wider significance.

These reflections concerning secular morality do not leave us with novel conclusions. Until recently, there was no serious threat of women being forced to forgo the use of major tranquilizers to control their psychoses and to being committed instead to a mental hospital in order to avoid possible risks to their fetuses, or to submit to cesareans against their will.[46] The arguments in this section would secure matters more or less as they have traditionally been: women would not need to fear being forced to submit to cesarean sections or fetal surgery without their consent, except in circumstances in which they act malevolently or willfully under the assumption that the child would under the circumstances prefer nonexistence to life.

## Letting defective newborns die

Although one may recognize robust limits to the secular moral authority of the state to impose treatment on women for the benefit of their fetuses, it might seem easier to justify protecting the lives and well-being of infants and children. One might attempt to justify requiring their treatment and forbidding intended killings (i.e., infanticide), even though young children and infants are not persons in the strict sense of moral agents, on the basis of the good consequences of such rules on the beneficent rearing of children. Even if such a practice could be justified because of its consequences, exceptional circumstances would override the rule (1) when the consequences of not breaking the rule are more costly than adhering to the rule, and (2) when the reasonableness of such exceptions is sufficiently apparent as not to undermine the rule itself. The more the exceptions are incorporated into the operative understanding of the protecting rule, the more this will seem acceptable.

For a while this appeared to be how American law and public policy would develop regarding decisions to discontinue treatment for severely defective newborns. A 1973 review of cases suggested that treatment be stopped when there are serious questions regarding the quality of life of the child and substantial costs likely to be borne by the family or society if the child were treated.[47] Another review in 1973 showed that of 299 deaths in a special-care nursery, 43 (14 percent) were related to a choice to withhold treatment. Of this group 15 newborns had multiple abnormalities; 8, trisomies (i.e., as occurs in Down's syndrome, when there are three of one chromosome, rather than a pair); 8, cardiopulmonary disease; 7, meningemyelocele (a herniation of part of the spinal cord and its covering through a defect in the vertebral column); 3, other central nervous system disorders; and 2, short bowel syndrome (insufficient small intestine).[48]

This approach endorsed the general rule of protecting and caring for newborns; it allowed exceptions when the quality of outcome was low and costs associated with treatment were high. It is under such circumstances that we have generally acknowledged that duties of beneficence are defeated. The greater the difficulties in discharging a duty in beneficence, the easier it is to show that the duty has been defeated. The lower the likelihood of success, the weaker the duty in beneficence to perform it. Although I may generally have a duty to come to the aid of a friend dying of thirst, that duty can be defeated if the friend is at the top of a high mountain, accessible only at great risk. In addition, the less likely it is that the friend would find the quality of life acceptable if saved, the weaker the duty: the friend would likely forward a less strong claim. Also, if the friend is injured and is likely to die soon even if saved, the duty weakens as the amount of life to be secured decreases. Put simply, a duty justified in terms of achieving a good weakens as the good is on balance diminished. The actual strength of the duty and the character of the balance among the competing considerations will depend on the content of the particular moral vision invoked in making the calculations.

In general secular morality there is a further complication. In the case of the infant, it is not yet a person to make a claim directly. It is not a person in the strict sense. Some may wish to avoid persons in the strict sense coming into existence with severe handicaps, who could make burdensome claims upon duties of beneficence. In addition, others may wish to expend significant resources in order to bring persons into existence, only if their lives will be of sufficient quality and quantity. The concept of quality of outcome is itself complex, for it must include both quality of life as it is likely to be judged by those associated with that life and quality of life as it is likely to be perceived by the individual living it. The principle of beneficence can encompass both interpretations. We derive both benefits and harms from our perceptions of the quality of the lives of others. In summary, in almost all moral understandings there will be circumstances when it will be proper to let an infant die, and for the couple to attempt again to produce a child who will grow to be a person without serious handicaps.

Although quality of life considerations may constitute flagrant, illegal discrimination under the Americans with Disabilities Act, such is not proscribable (no matter how opprobrious it may appear within particular moral visions) with general, secular moral authority.[49] Such coercive interdiction of discrimination on the basis of one particular vision of justice, fairness, or beneficence (unfortunately or fortunately) cannot be justified without appeal to a particular moral vision or ideology. However one might wish to the contrary, Nozick seems on this point to be correct. "Any private owner can regulate his premises as he chooses."[50] Private hospitals and private health care systems should always be free to make choices based on quality-of-life considerations. In illustration, one might consider one of the ways in which the Americans with Disabilities Act has been invoked to compel treatment in the instance of the Baby K case, in which it was argued that a baby with anencephaly should be treated as would a normal baby.[51] After all, when one is anencephalic, one is blind, deaf, and dumb—a truly severe constellation of disabilities.

These considerations, with certain qualifications, can lead one to articulating the following algorithm regarding how one can appreciate secular duties of beneficence with respect to providing health care:

$$\frac{\text{Strength of the duty}}{\text{of beneficence}} = \frac{\text{Chance of} \times \text{Quality} \times \text{Length}}{\text{success} \quad \text{of life} \quad \text{of life}}$$
$$\text{Costs}$$

The duty to preserve the life of a newborn is generally defeated as the chance for success diminishes, as the quality or quantity of life for the newborn decreases, and as the costs of securing that quality of life increase. Appealing to such an algorithm to justify selective nontreatment pays tribute to a general commitment to save lives, while recognizing how exceptions become plausible.

This approach was generally that of American case law until recently. Parents were at liberty to choose any course of treatment or nontreatment endorsed by a body of accepted medical opinion. If a physician, representing a view within the range of accepted medical opinions, judged that treatment was not indicated, parents could follow that recommendation. Concepts of indicated and nonindicated treatment incorporated considerations of likelihood of success, quality of outcome, likely length of survival, and costs. This approach left treatment choices in the hands of parents unless their decisions were egregious.

This approach in American public policy was undermined through the controversies precipitated by the birth on April 9, 1982, of a child with Down's syndrome complicated by esophageal atresia (i.e., no passage from the mouth to the stomach) and tracheal esophageal fistula (i.e., an anomalous connection between the windpipe and the gullet). The case of Infant Doe of Bloomington came to an informal hearing before the Indiana Supreme Court, which upheld the parents' right to refuse treatment.[52] The foregoing analyses of general secular morality support the court, in that significant costs in raising a child with physical and mental handicaps can defeat the usual duties of beneficence to an entity not yet a person in the strict sense, indeed, even those who are already moral agents.

In response to this case, the American federal government first imposed and then, after a judicial reversal, proposed regulations on March 7 and July 5, 1983.[53] These were contested on a number of procedural and other grounds.[54] On January 12, 1984, the government imposed the following rules on all hospitals receiving federal funds:

(i) Withholding of medical beneficial surgery to correct an intestinal obstruction in an infant with Down's Syndrome when the withholding is based upon the anticipated future mental retardation of the infant and there are no medical contraindications to the surgery that would otherwise justify withholding the surgery would constitute a discriminatory act, violative of section 504.

(ii) Withholding of treatment for medically correctable physical anomalies in children born with spina bifida when such denial is based on anticipated mental impairment, paralysis or incontinence of the infant, rather than on reasonable medical judgments that treatment would be futile, too unlikely to succeed given complications in the particular case, or otherwise not of medical benefit to the infant, would constitute a discriminatory act, violative of section 504.

(iii) Withholding of medical treatment for an infant born with anencephaly, who will inevitably die within a short period of time, would not constitute a discriminatory act because the treatment would be futile and do no more than temporarily prolong the act of dying.

(iv) Withholding of certain potential treatments from a severely premature and low birth weight infant on the grounds of reasonable medical judgments concerning the improbability of success or risks of potential harm to the infant would not violate section 504.[55]

The government was joined in this view by the American Academy of Pediatrics, which stated that:

When medical care is clearly beneficial, it should always be provided. When appropriate medical care is not available, arrangements should be made to transfer the infant to an appropriate medical facility. Considerations such as anticipated or actual limited potential of an individual and present or future lack of available community resources are irrelevant and must not determine the decisions concerning medical care. The individual's medical condition should be the sole focus of the decision. These are very strict standards.[56]

These rules and this viewpoint clearly reject reliance on quality-of-life considerations in decisions to withhold lifesaving treatment.

In late 1984 the rules by the Department of Health and Human Services regarding nondiscrimination on the basis of handicaps continued to be the focus of considerable controversy. One of the judicial challenges sprang from the case of Baby Jane Doe, whose parents initially attempted to choose a conservative over a surgical approach for the treatment of their child born with multiple birth defects, including spina bifida manifesta (exposure of the spinal cord and membrane).[57] Because of the questions raised in the courts regarding the authority to implement such regulations on the basis of section 504 of the Rehabilitation Act of 1973, the American Congress passed amendments to the Child Abuse Prevention and Treatment Act requiring that states accepting funds under the statute adopt such regulations.[58] This has led to yet further proposed rules[59] and to final regulations.[60] The 1984 law provided that withholding medically indicated treatment will constitute child abuse when it involves

the failure to respond to the infant's life-threatening conditions by providing treatment (including appropriate nutrition, hydration, and medication) which, in the treating physician's or physicians' reasonable medical judgments, will be most likely to be effective in ameliorating or correcting all such conditions, except that the term does not include the failure to provide treatment (other than appropriate nutrition, hydration, or medication) to an infant when, in the treating physician's or physicians' reasonable medical judgment, (A) the infant is chronically and irreversibly comatose; (B) the provision of such treatment would (i) merely prolong dying, (ii) not be effective in ameliorating or correcting all of the infant's life-threatening conditions, or (iii) otherwise be futile in terms of the survival of the infant; or (C) the provision of such treatment would be virtually futile in terms of the survival of the infant and the treatment itself under such circumstances would be inhumane.[61]

No provision is made for quality-of-life judgments; in fact, such judgments are forbidden, save with respect to chronically and irreversibly comatose existence. It should be clear, given our analyses of the principles of permission and beneficence, that both the federal government and the American Academy of Pediatrics are mistaken, if their goal was to justify their position in general secular terms. The circumstance that the child, which is not yet a person in the strict sense, falls within the authority of the parents as their possession sets limits to the authority of the state to intervene. In addition, the use of force to impose a particular federal understanding on unwilling parents should oblige the government, at the very least, to sustain the costs incurred in the child's care.

The American Medical Association at the same time accepted "quality of life

[as] a factor to be considered in determining what is best for the individual.''[62] Moreover, it endorsed the role of parents in making such quality-of-life decisions.

In desperate situations involving newborns, the advice and judgment of the physician should be readily available, but the decision whether to exert maximal efforts to sustain life should be the choice of the parents. The parents should be told the options, expected benefits, risks and limits of any proposed care; how the potential for human relationships is affected by the infant's condition; and relevant information and answers to their questions. The presumption is that the love which parents usually have for their children will be dominant in the decisions which they make in determining what is in the best interest of their children. It is to be expected the parents will act unselfishly, particularly where life itself is at stake. Unless there is convincing evidence to the contrary, parental authority should be respected.[63]

Although the AMA did not characterize the burden to the family or society involved in treating severely defective newborns as a primary consideration, the AMA did not exclude it.[64] Since these debates in the mid-1980s, decisions to limit treatment to severely disabled newborns have been further complicated by the Americans with Disabilities Act, which has raised the specter of mandating equal treatment for anencephalics. After all, an anencephalic child brings with it almost every imaginable disability, among them being blind, deaf, dumb, and paralyzed.[65]

Western societies have generally allowed infants to die when the costs of treatment have been significant and the likelihood of success restricted.[66] Given nonsecular moral grounds against directly intending the death of the child, such omissions have not been described as infanticide, though death was often a foreseen consequence of discontinuing treatment. One is generally excused from providing treatment if that treatment constitutes a serious burden on oneself or on society. As Pope Pius XII declared,

normally one is held to use only ordinary means—according to the circumstances of persons, places, times, and culture—that is to say, means that do not involve any grave burden [*aucune charge extraordinaire*] for oneself or another. A more strict obligation would be too burdensome [*trop lourde*] for most men and would render the attainment of the higher, more important good too difficult.[67]

Within such understandings it is also proper to consider the likelihood of success. In this fashion, one can identify a class of newborn infants for whom treatment would be so costly and so unlikely to succeed that one is excused in most moral visions from providing or accepting treatment. However, one would not be forbidden to provide treatment as an act of supererogation. In acts of supererogation one may discriminate. Out of the class of children one is not obliged to treat, one may decide to treat those likely to survive without serious mental or physical handicaps. Traditional Roman Catholic doctrine of extraordinary treatment provides a moral framework for discriminating against newborns who will likely be encumbered by serious physical or mental handicaps.

Once one loses religious insight as to why directly intending death is evil, matters change significantly. In general secular moral terms there are no grounds for holding that it is wrong to intend the death of those infants whom one is at liberty no longer to preserve with life-sustaining treatment. Indeed, since one may intend death, it will not be possible in general secular moral terms to show that one may not actively expedite death. In general secular moral terms where permission is cardinal, it is not possible to make out the evil in murder, *ceteris paribus,* other than that of taking a person's life without permission or with malevolence. Since infants are not persons strictly whose autonomy can be violated or entities who can suffer by having their goals thwarted, a painless death through active euthanasia may appear to cause less harm than withdrawing treatment while foreseeing but not intending death. Indeed, general secular morality, which draws its authority and substance from the permission or concurrence of moral agents, cannot give standing to the wrongness of any intentions save those of direct malevolence. The result is that distinctions between intending death versus foreseeing but not intending death, as well as between active versus passive euthanasia, can in general secular moral terms be understood, if at all, only with reference to past agreements or likely future consequences.[68] This would appear in general to support tolerating frank infanticide.

## Infanticide

An examination of infanticide must begin with the observation that it has been widely practiced throughout the world as a means not only of disposing of deformed newborns, but of controlling population growth. It is difficult to argue that there is a close connection between the practice of infanticide and the general civility of a population. In the Western Middle Ages, when infanticide was officially condemned, there was persecution of heretics and Jews alike. Twentieth-century Germany, which forbade infanticide, produced the tyranny of Hitler. The same may be observed with respect to the vast slaughter of the innocents perpetrated by the Soviet Union, which was also officially free of infanticide. Though one might associate infanticide with primitive cultures or non-European traditions, it has deep roots in Western cultural foundations. There was a wide acceptance of infanticide in the Greco-Roman world. Plato endorsed the practice of infanticide (*Republic* 5.460c). Infanticide was also recommended by Aristotle in his *Politics:* "Let there be a law that no *deformed* child shall live."[69] One should note that infanticide among the Athenians goes back at least to the lawgiver Solon, one of the seven wise men of Greece. Sextus Empiricus states that Solon legalized infanticide, though in fact he seems only to have tolerated infanticide through exposure, a practice generally accepted by the Greeks: "Solon gave the Athenians the law 'concerning things immune,' by which he allowed each man to slay his own child."[70] Rome in the Twelve Tables acknowledged parental rights to commit infanticide. There even appears to have been a duty to kill deformed children. Cicero remarks in his *De Legibus*, "A dreadfully deformed child ought to be killed quickly, as the Twelve Tables ordain" (*De Legibus* 3.8.19).

These views were reflected in medical practice. In the oldest extant textbook of gynecology, Soranus (A.D. 98–138) included a section on how to determine whether a newborn child is worth rearing. As Soranus put it, the midwife

should also consider whether it is worth rearing or not. And the infant which is suited by nature for rearing will be distinguished by the fact that its mother has spent the period of pregnancy in good health, for conditions which require medical care, especially those of the body, also harm the fetus and enfeeble the foundations of its life. Second, by the fact that it has been born at the due time, best at the end of nine months, and if it so happens, later; but also after only seven months. Furthermore by the fact that when put on the earth it immediately cries with proper vigor; for one that lives for some length of time without crying, or cries but weakly, is suspected of behaving so on account of some unfavorable condition. Also by the fact that it is perfect in all its parts, members and senses; that its ducts, namely of the ears, nose, pharynx, urethra, anus are free from obstruction; that the natural functions of every [member] are neither sluggish nor weak; that the joints bend and stretch; that it has due size and shape and is properly sensitive in every respect. This we may recognize from pressing the fingers against the surface of the body, for it is natural to suffer pain from everything that pricks or squeezes. And by conditions contrary to those mentioned, the infant not worth rearing is recognized.[71]

This passage may give a sense of what it meant to act upon Cicero's injunction to follow the Fourth Table. It provides a sketch by a physician close to that period regarding how one should take into account factors that are predictive of futility, cost of treatment, and quality of life. Soranus's recommendation need not be interpreted as supporting active infanticide, only nontreatment.[72]

The inability to disclose the evil of infanticide collides with the remnants of the Judeo-Christian ethic still shaping many particular secular moral understandings. As with abortion, strong condemnations of infanticide were made by Christians from the very beginning. The Didache states, "Thou shalt do no murder; thou shalt not commit adultery; thou shalt not commit sodomy; thou shalt not commit fornication; thou shalt not steal; thou shalt not use magic; thou shalt not use philtres; thou shalt not procure abortion, nor commit infanticide."[73] Though murder and infanticide (as well as abortion) are condemned separately, both condemnations are strong. Moreover, there is in another passage a condemnation of "murderers of children" (5.2). In addition, "The Epistle to Diognetus" specifically describes Christians as people who "do not expose their offspring" (5.6). Many secular cosmopolitans, not to mention observant Jews and Christians, feel justified disquiet as their society is returned to the practices of a pluralistic pagan past.

The secular moral status of infanticide is by default. It results from the inability of secular morality to justify a general canonical content-full account of the moral status of either fetuses or young children. This failure limits the secular moral authority of the state to intervene. A legal proscription would require a particular canonical ordering of harms and benefits. Such can be justified only within a particular moral vision. The conclusion is very unpleasant. The equivalent of the Athenian and Roman noninterference with infanticide is unavoidable, given the limited secular moral authority of the state. To prohibit infanticide legally on the basis of considerations of beneficence (e.g., in order to realize a particular view of good parenting) would require establishing governmental authority for overriding parental autonomy when no person in the strict sense will be harmed. The difficulty is in showing secular moral authority to impose a particular view of how to protect the morality of either individuals or communities. Those who defend infanticide will see the virtue of their practice outweighing the goods that accrue from its prohibition. Because of the centrality of the principle of permission, the burden of proof lies on the shoulders of the interveners to demonstrate that parental actions may be forbidden, rather than on the parents to show that they have liberty to act.

## Fetal experimentation and in vitro fertilization

A general moral understanding within a secular pluralist society of the significance of fetal experimentation and in vitro fertilization must be secured in terms of the status of the fetus, since secular morality cannot provide a content-full understanding of reproduction. Fetuses do not have the standing of persons for general secular morality. They are the biological products of persons. They become persons in the strict sense only some time after birth. They may become persons in the social sense if a community ascribes to them some of the fundamental rights to protection usually accorded to persons in the strict sense, as moral agents. Early-gestation fetuses appear to have minimal, if any, mental life. They do not appear to have sufficient mental capacity to suffer as can normal adult mammals. It is for these reasons that this volume has already concluded that their secular moral status must be understood primarily in terms of their being the special possessions of persons and in terms of our concerns for the persons they may become. The first of these considerations reminds us why we must gain the consent of those who produce an embryo or fetus, or their assignees, before experimenting on or otherwise using an embryo or fetus. The second of these considerations reminds us why we must be concerned about injuring fetuses. If those fetuses are allowed to go to term, so that the harms finally settle on the persons those fetuses become, one will have injured persons in the strict sense.

As a consequence, there will be no sustainable secular moral arguments in principle against nontherapeutic experimentation with fetuses, or against in vitro fertilization. There may be somewhat persuasive arguments that will establish rules of decorum for such endeavors. One may be able to indicate where certain practices may erode the very fabric of respect toward fetuses, infants, or the helpless. However, such arguments are unlikely to be clearly decisive or open to unambiguous articulation. They will depend on various hunches or suppositions regarding the effect of possible future practices on the anticipated activities of humans.

Consider the case of nontherapeutic fetal experimentation done with the permission of the immediate progenitors of the fetus and with reasonable certainty that the fetus will be destroyed if injured, rather than allowed to go to term. The more useful the research, the easier it will be to regard this undertaking, in general secular terms, as a beneficent and warranted act despite the adverse judgments it will evoke from many. A better understanding of fetal development will produce knowledge not only interesting in its own right but also useful toward the end of preventing congenital abnormalities and thus harms to future persons. If fetuses are not persons in the strict sense, it will be difficult to understand why in general secular moral terms women may seek abortions for any reason but researchers may not engage in fetal experimentation with the altruistic goal of producing knowledge and well-being.

These secular moral reflections are not hostile to restrictive rules on the use of governmental funds in fetal experimentation.[74] It is one thing to determine what persons have a right to do with their own resources, and another thing to decide to what extent common funds may be employed to support projects disapproved of by those who contribute those funds. These reflections do lead to justifying a very permissive policy with regard to fetal experimentation in deep conflict with Judeo-Christian understandings. Current state laws that categorically forbid fetal experimentation are without secular moral justification.[75] Fetal experimentation may be categorically forbidden when it is done with malevolent intent, or without reasonable provision for the destruction of the fetus if it is harmed to such an extent so as to make nonexistence preferable to existence. But otherwise, the restrictions set by the moral considerations raised by tort-for-wrongful-life are insufficient to set significant secular moral barriers.

There are further unpleasant conclusions. Since people are at liberty to act with themselves and consenting others, and since fetuses are not persons strictly, it will not be possible in general secular moral terms to forbid engendering fetuses as sources of organs or particular tissues.[76] Nor will it be possible to do so when these fetuses are engendered for pay or aborted for financial profit, much less when they are produced in order to secure fetal tissue likely to be of use in treating relatives. Again, any constraints would depend on a particular content-full moral vision, and no such vision is available in general secular terms.

Given this understanding of fetal experimentation, it becomes very difficult to place restrictions on in vitro fertilization (IVF) and embryo transfer (ET) done with the goal of producing a healthy child for parents who would otherwise be incapable of reproducing. There have been objections to in vitro fertilization on traditional moral grounds of its being unnatural in presupposing the acquisition of sperm through masturbation or because of the fashioning of human life under direct technological control. The first contention is difficult to sustain in terms of arguments generally accessible in a secular pluralist context. One would need special premises to show that masturbation, rather than being a morally neutral act that can be engaged in either for recreation or for special procreative goals, violates the laws of nature or is otherwise immoral.[77] As to the second objection, it likely trades on a sense of the sacred that cannot be made out in general secular morality. For secular morality, human reproduction is no more or less the proper focus of objectification and technological manipulation than cardiac physiology. To see reproduction as special would require a content-full moral vision or account of reproduction. Again, for secular morality, permission will be central, leading to carefully crafted consent forms that will make clear to the parties involved what is at stake in third-party-assisted reproduction.

From the perspective of many moral communities with content-full understandings about the meaning and significance of reproduction, permission or agreement will not be seen to be sufficient to set aside certain evils and improprieties. Surrogacy as well as artificial insemination by a donor has been recognized as illegitimately introducing a third party into the act of reproduction.[78] As has already been noted, the evil of such intrusions has been understood within traditional Christianity. There have been attempts, however unsuccessful, to appreciate this evil in general secular terms. The Warnock Report presents an argument against surrogacy, which it also recognizes in its consideration of artificial insemination from a donor. "The objections turn essentially on the view that to introduce a third party into the process of procreation which should be confined to the loving partnership between two people, is an attack on the value of the marital relationship."[79] Similar arguments have been made with regard to in vitro fertilization and embryo transfer in general. The idea is that all third-party-assisted reproduction improperly inserts an individual or individuals who have no place in the reproductive act. Without a content-full understanding of proper reproduction, it will not be possible to show that introducing a third person in the case of either a gamete donor or technological assistants makes reproduction take on a quasi-adulterous character, or whether enlisting such persons should be regarded positively as an affirmation of a good realized through the free collaboration of persons.

Another charge against in vitro fertilization, that it involves an improper objectification of human reproduction, has been voiced by a number of thinkers, primarily theologians. The concern has been that the use of technological artifice in the very heart of human reproduction distorts its sense and meaning.[80] A classic statement of opposition is provided by Paul Ramsey:

To put radically asunder what God joined together in parenthood when He made love procreative, to procreate from beyond the sphere of love (AID, for example, or making human life in a test-tube), or to posit acts of sexual love beyond the sphere of responsible procreation (by definition marriage), means a refusal of the image of God's creation in our own.[81]

Similarly, the Roman Catholic declaration *Donum Vitae* states:

The moral relevance of the link between the meanings of the conjugal act and between the goods of marriage, as well as the unity of the human being and the dignity of his origin, demand that the procreation of a human person be brought about as the fruit of the conjugal act specific to the love between spouses. . . . But even in a situation in which every precaution were taken to avoid the death of human embryos, homologous IVF and ET dissociates from the conjugal act the actions which are directed to human fertilization. For this reason the very nature of homologous IVF and ET also must be taken into account, even abstracting from the link with procured abortion.[82]

This view is incomprehensible without the provision of special theological premises.

As the theologian Joseph Fletcher indicated, rationally planned reproduction is natural to rational beings.[83] Human reproduction becomes the object of the intervention of persons because human biology imposes factual constraints while persons plan and aspire to goals and purposes that may be realizable only in part through the biological means at hand. There is a recurring tension between humans as persons, as planning, aspiring entities, and humans as bodies, as individuals possessing what they may regard as the idiosyncratic deliverances of a particular biological past. Self-conscious, rational reflection can thus engender an instructive dualism of object and subject. The human body is experienced as an object that only imperfectly embodies the goals of persons. Persons become pregnant at the wrong time, with the wrong person, or not pregnant at the right time, with the right person. These failures of aspiration can be set aside in part through the interventions of human technology. Outside of a vision of the fallen character of human nature and of a canonical content-full understanding of how this is to be set aside, the use of technology in the fashioning of children will be regarded as integral to the goal of rendering the world congenial to persons. Such interventions can be seen as in principle improper only by appeal to special theological or ideological premises.

Finally, it will not be possible in general secular moral terms to condemn in vitro fertilization because it may involve the wastage of fertilized embryos. If early abortion can be chosen without let or hindrance because fetuses are not persons, it follows a fortiori that there is no injury to a person in disposing of excess embryos produced in the process of in vitro fertilization. The fact that one can (1) minimize pain and discomfort to the woman by harvesting a number of ova at one time, (2) avoid the risk associated with the gestation and birth of triplets and quadruplets, by fertilizing all of them but implanting only one or two at a time, and still (3) freeze the extra embryos in the event that further implantations are required to secure a successful pregnancy or a second pregnancy does not render the intervention immoral because defective or unused embryos may be discarded. Embryos are not persons as moral agents.

The substantial secular moral issues in in vitro fertilization are those that involve promises, trust, and commitments. The relations of persons bound together in the production of a child may be complex. In an extreme case, a man $A$ and a woman $B$ may donate an ovum and sperm for in vitro fertilization and implantation in a woman $C$, who will be the host mother and deliver the child for adoption to a man $D$ and a woman $E$ who are both infertile, the woman without ovaries and a uterus, and for whom the woman $C$ is willing to serve as the host to gestate a child. There will need to be understandings with regard to the qualities of care and attention that will be provided by the in vitro fertilization clinic. There will need to be a web of promises defining the obligations of the host mother $C$ to avoid teratogenic agents or other circumstances that might injure the fetus. One will need to make clear who will accept responsibility for the child if it is born with serious congenital deformities.[84] The limits of the obligations of $A$ and $B$ will also need to be defined, as well as those of all the parties involved.[85] These are important issues, but they are not unique to in vitro fertilization. They are, rather, a part of the web of mutual obligations that generally binds persons together and that is sustained through moral concerns for mutual respect and beneficence.

Most of these issues are not new ones. They have already been raised by practices such as the artificial insemination of the wives of infertile husbands, as well as the artificial insemination of a woman to bear a child for a couple when the wife is infertile. One does not need a complex technology such as in vitro fertilization in order to outline the central moral issues of trust and confidence that such interventions raise. Given the arguments in this volume, a secular moral evil is not involved if all the parties are freely consenting and there is likely to be a positive balance of benefits over harms. Certain religious groups will understand the evils that remain. Roman Catholics, for instance, will recognize that such activities involve not only the moral evil of masturbation but that of adultery as well.[86] Such views require a very particular appreciation of the nature of marriage and of proper reproduction, one that cannot be sustained in general secular terms.[87] The general secular moral focus is instead on a consensual and beneficent involvement of individuals in the important goal of reproduction.

The contrast between a general secular moral understanding and traditional Judeo-Christian understandings of reproduction is perhaps made more salient by considering the case of commercial surrogacy. If women are persons, moral agents, they should be able to contract as they wish to use their bodies as they want. Without a particular canonical moral perspective, it will not be possible to see why it is any more or less demeaning or exploitative to hire a woman as a surrogate mother than to hire her as a ballet dancer or opera singer. In each case one is hiring her to use certain capacities of her body for the enjoyment or goals of others. For those who see some special argument against commercial surrogacy through a comparison with prostitution, they will confront the need to make out in general secular terms why it is more demeaning for a woman to work as a prostitute than as a ditchdigger. Nor will appeals to exploitation help, for one will not be able to understand who is the exploiter and who is the exploited without a particular canonical content-full moral vision. Is the woman exploited who is hired by an affluent couple to function as a surrogate mother, or is the woman exploited by those with special moral intuitions who use the law to stop her from hiring herself out as a surrogate mother and thus restrict the range of her choices? To understand what counts as exploitation, one has to have a canonical content-full moral understanding of appropriate choices and contracts.

## The patient as person: the secular moral vision

Medicine, as opposed to veterinary medicine, is the medicine of persons. It is not aimed at the mere prolongation of biological life. It is undertaken in order to postpone death, to prevent and alleviate illness and deformity, to cure diseases, to amplify biological and psychological capacities, and to care for the sufferings of persons. Medicine is the agent of persons. It is engaged on their behalf. It is restrained by obligations to respect the wishes of persons and directed by the goal of doing good to persons. It is therefore crucial to recognize when persons begin and when they end in order to know to whom medicine, and health care in general, has its obligations. Physicians, nurses, and allied health workers must know when they are faced with a person whose wishes must be respected and who may set bounds to the desires of physicians and others to realize particular understandings of the good life. It is for this reason that this chapter explored the issues of brain death and abortion.

This examination reveals an in part unanticipated moral landscape. Besides showing the implications and character of a morality that can bind moral strangers, a general secular morality, this chapter discloses its differences from and contrasts with traditional Judeo-Christian understandings of moral probity. By laying out the implications of what can be shared by moral strangers, it is meant both to show the implications of such a morality as well as to account for many of the changes in our mores as we enter a post-Christian, neopagan era. The West since the Renaissance has in various ways been reconsidering, rethinking, and recapturing its pagan past. This process is far from over and its implications for bioethics are still only dimly perceived.

At present, the tensions between general secular morality and traditional moralities are less severe with respect to the definition of death. These tensions are likely to increase as one is able reliably to identify individuals who are no longer moral agents but still maintain a certain level of consciousness without self-consciousness. In general secular morality they will not count as moral agents. Other, less conceptually driven definitions of death may already pose more difficulties, but of a less conceptual nature. One might think here of proposals to apply cardiac-oriented definitions of death in order to harvest organs from individuals who do not wish to be resuscitated. Under such proposals, organs might be taken from individuals who have not suffered higher-brain-centers damage (e.g., individuals with amyotrophic lateral sclerosis) who do not wish to be resuscitated and who have suffered a two-minute asystole. If one holds that the importance of definitions of death lies in their indicating when the possibility for sentience and action in the world has been destroyed, then such individuals may not truly be dead in this conceptual sense; they may from a higher-brain-centers-oriented definition of death be regarded as having volunteered to be organ donors while they are dying.[88]

When one examines the contrast between traditional Judeo-Christian understandings of the status of embryos, fetuses, infants, and reproduction, the difference between what can be established in general secular morality and in traditional Judeo-Christian appreciations is most stark. It is impossible to make out the evil not only of abortion but of infanticide. Further traditional notions of appropriate reproduction can radically be set aside in a technology that allows Bubba Jones and Betty-Lou Smith to make extra money selling their gametes, which may then be purchased by F. Fitzhugh Yuppie and Q. Alessandra (Buffy) Cosmopolitan, in order to have zygotes produced at the Holistic Fertility Clinic to be carried to term for them by Henrietta Mercenarius. The traditional Judeo-Christian appreciation of reproduction as a sacred act and union of the couple[89] cannot be appreciated within a secular context. A secular context lacks either the values to supply such content or the openness to the grace of God to disclose such values. Anything content-full, anything substantial about the meaning of sexuality or the purpose of reproduction can only be appreciated within a particular, content-full moral context. Outside of such a context, no one can even understand why it is important to have children. Indeed, outside of such a context it will not be possible to make out in general secular terms (aside from financial and similar concerns, including tax consequences) why one should even bother to be married.

## Notes

1. Traditionally, the Christian appreciation of the profound moral evil of abortion does not depend on a philosophical argument, but rather on tradition and worship. See, for example, *Didache* 2, 2; Tertullian, *Apology* 9, 8. See, also, the feasts of the Conception of the Theotokos, December 9, and of the conception of St. John the Baptist, September 23.
2. It must be underscored that it is not the goal of secular morality to endorse infanticide,

abortion, and the like. Rather, what one discovers is that the morality available to bind moral strangers, that morality which we find available without grace, cannot appreciate most substantive issues of morality. On the one hand, this discloses the full intellectual force of the failure of the modern philosophical project to ground substantive morality in reason. On the other hand, this discloses the moral impoverishment of the moral life without grace.

3.  Kan. Stat. Ann., §77–202 (Cum. Supp. 1979) [enacted 1970].
4.  Md. Ann. Code, art. 43, §54F (1980) (effective July 1, 1972).
5.  St. Thomas Aquinas, *Summa Theologica,* 1, Q. 118, art. 2, reply to objection 2.
6.  For an exploration of the contrast between the experienced significance of mental life and the presented significance of physical objects, see H. T. Engelhardt, Jr., *Mind–Body: A Categorial Relation* (The Hague: Martinus Nijhoff, 1973).
7.  I use the term *principle* here to indicate essential or characteristic constituents. The principles of mental life require as a part of their explication an account of the interiority of that life.
8.  Arthur C. Clarke, *2001: A Space Odyssey* (New York: New American Library, 1968).
9.  *Black's Law Dictionary,* 4th ed. rev. (St. Paul, Minn.: West, 1968).
10. Roland Puccetti, "Brain Transplantation and Personal Identity," *Analysis* 29 (1969): 65.
11. François Joseph [Franz Josef] Gall, *On the Functions of the Brain and of Each of Its Parts: with Observations on the Possibilities of Determining the Instincts, Propensities, and Talents, or the Moral and Intellectual Dispositions of Men and Animals, by the Configuration of the Brain and Head,* trans. Winslow Lewis (Boston: Marsh, Capen and Lyon, 1835).
12. J. G. Spurzheim, *Phrenology or the Doctrine of the Mental Phenomena,* 2 vols. (Boston: Marsh, Capen and Lyon, 1833).
13. M. J. P. Flourens, *Examen de la Phrenologie,* 2d ed. (Paris: Paulin, 1845).
14. For a treatment of this point, see Robert M. Young, *Mind, Brain, and Adaptation in the Nineteenth Century* (Oxford: Clarendon Press, 1970).
15. See H. T. Engelhardt, Jr., "John Hughlings Jackson and the Mind–Body Relation," *Bulletin of the History of Medicine* 49 (Summer 1975): 137–51.
16. President's Commission for the Study of Ethical Problems in Medicine and Biomedical and Behavioral Research, *Defining Death* (Washington, D.C.: U.S. Government Printing Office, 1981), pp. 13–15.
17. John Hughlings Jackson, "Remarks on Evolution and Dissolution of the Nervous System," in *Selected Writings of John Hughlings Jackson,* ed. James Taylor (New York: Basic Books, 1958), vol. 2, pp. 76–91.
18. Ad Hoc Committee of the Harvard Medical School to Examine the Definition of Brain Death, "A Definition of Irreversible Coma," *Journal of the American Medical Association* 205 (Aug. 5, 1968): 337–43.
19. World Medical Association, "Declaration of Sydney," *Medical Journal of Australia Supplement* 58 (1973): 2.
20. Ad Hoc Committee of the American Electroencephalographic Society on EEG Criteria for Determination of Cerebral Death, "Cerebral Death and the Encephalogram," *Journal of the American Medical Association* 209 (Sept. 8, 1969): 1505–10.

21. Amir Halevy and Baruch Brody, "Brain Death: Reconciling Definitions, Criteria, and Tests," *Annals of Internal Medicine* 119 (Sept. 15, 1993): 519–25.

22. There have been reports in the press of brain-dead women who have been brought to term. Some may not have been fully brain dead in terms of rigorous whole-brain criteria. Still, one should note that there would be nothing paradoxical in such an event. The living body of a dead woman would have sustained her fetus until birth. For a discussion of some recent cases, see Ernst Reichelt, "Hirntod und Schwang-erschaft," 4–9, Inge Wolf, "Gynäkologische Überlegungen zu Hirntod und Schwangerschaft, 13–20, Hans-Martin Sass, "Hirntod und Schwangerschaft. Eth-ische Aspekte," 21–31, *Medizinethische Materialien* 88 (January 1994).

23. Gray et al. v. Sawyer et al., Gray et al. v. Clay et al., 247 S. W. 2d 496, 497 (Ky. App. 1 952).

24. For a recent exploration of higher-brain-centers-oriented definitions of death, see Richard Zaner (ed.), *Death: Beyond Whole-Brain Criteria* (Dordrecht: Kluwer, 1988). Interest in reassessing the whole-brain-oriented definition of death has in part been spurred by concern to harvest organs from anencephalic babies. See Fritz Beller and Julia Reeve, "Brain Life and Brain Death—The Anencephalic as an Explanatory Example," *Journal of Medicine and Philosophy* 14 (Feb. 1989): 5–23; and James Walters and Stephen Ashwal, "Anencephalic Infants as Organ Donors and the Brain Death Standard," *Journal of Medicine and Philosophy* 14 (Feb. 1989): 79–87. See also American Academy of Pediatrics Committee on Bioethics, "Infants with Anen-cephaly as Organ Sources: Ethical Considerations," *Pediatrics* 89 (June 1992): 1116–19; Donald Medearis and Lewis Holmes, "On the Use of Anencephalic Infants as Organ Donors," *New England Journal of Medicine* 321 (Aug. 10, 1989): 391–93; Joyce Peabody, Jane Emery, and Stephen Ashwal, "Experience with Anencephalic Infants as Prospective Organ Donors," *New England Journal of Medicine* 321 (Aug. 10, 1989): 344–50; and Robert Truog and John Fletcher, "Anencephalic Newborns: Can Organs be Transplanted before Brain Death?" *New England Journal of Medicine* 321 (Aug. 10, 1989): 388–90.

25. President's Commission for the Study of Ethical Problems in Medicine and Biomedi-cal and Behavioral Research, *Deciding to Forego Life-Sustaining Treatment* (Wash-ington, D.C.: U.S. Government Printing Office, 1983), p. 6.

26. Roland Puccetti, "The Life of a Person," in W. B. Bondeson et al. (eds.), *Abortion and the Status of the Fetus* (Dordrecht: Reidel, 1983), pp. 169–82. It should be noted that there is considerable dispute in some areas whether it is morally obligatory to provide artificial hydration and nutrition to permanently comatose individuals. Some Roman Catholics, for example, have held that it is obligatory. Office of the Vicar General, Archdiocese of New York, "Principles in Regard to Withholding or Withdrawing Artificially Assisted Nutrition/Hydration," *Issues in Law and Medicine* 6 (1990): 89–93. In contrast, Roman Catholic bishops in Texas have held that the provision of artificial hydration and nutrition can quite plausibly involve an extraordi-nary burden. Texas Bishops, "On Withdrawing Artificial Nutrition and Hydration," *Origins* 20 (June 7, 1990): 53–55.

27. Society of Critical Care Medicine Ethics Committee, "Consensus Statement on the

Triage of Critically Ill Patients," *Journal of the American Medical Association* 271 (Apr. 20, 1994): 1202.

28. There could be an exception where individuals belong to a religion that would require that such bodies be maintained until whole–brain or whole-body death occurs. Physicians and hospitals should be free to charge such patients higher fees.

29. American Bar Association, *Annual Report* 231–32 (1978) (Feb. 1975 midyear meeting).

30. President's Commission for the Study of Ethical Problems in Medicine and Biomedical and Behavioral Research, *Defining Death*, p. 3.

31. Ibid., pp. 31–34, 37–38.

32. Ibid., p. 40.

33. Immanuel Jakobovits, *Jewish Medical Ethics* (New York: Block, 1959), p. 277; also *Tzitz Eliezer*, 9:46 and 10:25:4, and *Babylonian Talmud*, Yoma 85a, Soncino ed.

34. For a study of the New Jersey law allowing a religious option to use only a whole-body definition of death, see Robert S. Olick, "Brain Death, Religious Freedom, and Public Policy: New Jersey's Landmark Legislative Initiative," *Kennedy Institute of Ethics Journal* 1 (1991): 275–88. This religious exemption is likely to be of importance not only for Orthodox Jews, but also some Japanese and American Indians. If higher-brain-centers-oriented definitions of death were adopted, it might be requisite in terms of traditional Christian understanding for Christians to make use of such exemptions as well.

35. Planned Parenthood of Central Missouri v. Danforth, 428 U.S. 52 (1976).

36. Immanuel Kant, *Metaphysik der Sitten*, AK VI 425.

37. This volume's exploration of the general secular moral significance of such acts as abortion and infanticide should be interpreted not as a defense of those acts, but as a disclosure of the impotence of secular morality and the tensions and disappointments of postmodernity.

38. For a review of the issues raised by tort-for-wrongful-life cases, see Angela R. Holder, "Is Existence Ever an Injury?: The Wrongful Life Cases," in S. F. Spicker et al. (eds.), *The Law-Medicine Relation: A Philosophical Exploration* (Dordrecht: Reidel, 1981), pp. 225–39. Also, G. M. Lehr and H. L. Hirsh, "Wrongful Conception, Birth and Life," *Medicine and Law* 2 (1983): 199–208; and E. Haavi Morreim, "Conception and the Concept of Harm," *Journal of Medicine and Philosophy* 8 (1983): 137–57. See, also, Derek Parfit, *Reasons and Persons* (Oxford: Clarendon Press, 1984), especially pp. 371–77.

39. Zepeda v. Zepeda, 41 Ill. App. 2d 240, 1963.

40. Williams v. New York, 223 N.E. 2d 849, 1963.

41. Curlender v. Bio-Science Laboratories and Automated Laboratory Sciences, 165 Cal. Rptr. 477 (Ct. App. 2d Dist. Div. 1, 1980). This holding of the court in Curlender has been superseded on appeal and by statute. In a second case involving tort for wrongful life, California courts held that the parents would not be liable. Turpin v. Sortini, 31 Cal. 3d 220, 643, P.2d 954, 182 Cal. Rptr. 337 (1982). In addition, California precluded by statute suit by children against their parents on such grounds. Cal. Civ. Code, Sec. 43.6 (1982), enacted in 1981. For another tort-for-wrongful-life case that also did not involve recognizing an avenue of recovery against parents, see Harbeson

v. Parke-Davis, Inc., 98 Wash. 2d 460, 656 P.2d 483 (1983). For two further discussions of some of these issues, see Jeffrey Botkin, "The Legal Concept of Wrongful Life," *Journal of American Medical Association* 259 (Mar. 11, 1988): 1541–45; Deborah Mathieu, *Preventing Prenatal Harm* (Dordrecht: Kluwer, 1991).

42. The reader will notice here a distinction drawn from the traditions of Roman Catholic moral theology between foresight and intention. This distinction is central to the concept of double effect. Individuals may act foreseeing consequences they do not intend, but that, had they intended, would render the act immoral. Thus, a good Roman Catholic may not directly intend to kill himself. However, if he is engaged in a just war, he may throw himself on a grenade that lands in his foxhole to save his comrades. This is permissible as long as he does not intend to kill himself but only to absorb the shrapnel with his body, although he can surely foresee that this will lead to death. One effect is intended (the absorbing of the shrapnel); the second effect (his death) is foreseen but not intended.

Traditionally, there are four points to the doctrine of double effect: (1) the evil outcome is not intended, (2) the good outcome does not follow from the evil outcome, (3) the action engaged in is not intrinsically immoral, and (4) the good consequences outweigh the bad. In secular moral circumstances these considerations can be employed to distinguish between those circumstances in which one may foresee a harm one is not obliged to avoid, but where it would be immoral (malevolent) to intend that harm. For a discussion of these issues, see Thomas J. Bole III, "The Theoretical Tenability of the Doctrine of Double Effect," *Journal of Medicine and Philosophy* 16 (Oct. 1991): 467–73; Joseph Boyle, "Who Is Entitled to Double Effect?" *Journal of Medicine and Philosophy* 16 (Oct. 1991): 475–94; Alan Donagan, "Moral Absolutism and the Double-Effect Exception," *Journal of Medicine and Philosophy* 16 (Oct. 1991): 495–509; Frances Kamm, "The Doctrine of Double Effect: Reflections on Theoretical and Practical Issues," *Journal of Medicine and Philosophy* 16 (Oct. 1991): 571–85; Donald Marquis, "Four Versions of Double Effect," *Journal of Medicine and Philosophy* 16 (Oct. 1991): 515–44; and Warren Quinn, "Actions, Intentions, and Consequences: The Doctrine of Double Effect," *Philosophy and Public Affairs* 18 (1989): 334–51. The role of double effect will be further explored in chapter 7.

43. The issue of when children may consent to harms will in part be explored with the emancipation of children in chapter 8. Here it is enough to note that one will need to decide when children are indeed competent. One will need to come to a judgment as to when they understand and appreciate the significance of their choices, such that they must be respected, at least through noncoercion. There are limitations on the extent to which parents must comply even under circumstances of competent decision making on the part of their children. As was argued in chapter 4, children are in certain respects examples of indentured servants who have special duties to their masters.

44. Jessie Mae Jefferson v. Griffin Spalding County Hospital Authority, 247 Ga. 86, 274 S.E. 2d 457 (1981). *Mirabile factu,* Jessie Mae Jefferson delivered her child vaginally and without difficulty. Depending on one's religious convictions or one's views of false positive diagnoses of placenta previa, one may come to the conclusion that

prayer does indeed work miracles. For an account of this case, see George Annas, "Forced Cesareans: The Most Unkindest Cut," *Hastings Center Report* 12 (June 1982): 16–17, 45.

45. Jefferson v. Griffin Spalding, at 460.

46. P. H. Soloff, S. Jewell, and L. Roth, "Civil Commitment and the Rights of the Unborn," *American Journal of Psychiatry* 136 (1979): 114–15. For a review of some court actions and of circumstances that could lead to court actions to force women to accept cesarean sections, see, for example, Watson A. Bowes, Jr., and Brad Selgestad, "Fetal Versus Maternal Rights: Medical and Legal Perspectives," *Obstetrics and Gynecology* 58 (Aug. 1981): 209–14; J. R. Lieberman, M. Mazor, W. Chaim, and A. Cohen, "The Fetal Right to Live," *Obstetrics and Gynecology* 53 (Apr. 1979): 515–17; Thomas L. Shriner, Jr., "Maternal Versus Fetal Rights—A Clinical Dilemma," *Obstetrics & Gynecology* 53 (Apr. 1979): 518–19; Ronna Jurow and Richard H. Paul, "Cesarean Delivery for Fetal Distress without Maternal Consent," *Obstetrics and Gynecology* 63 (Apr. 1984): 596–99. See also Veronika Kolder, Janet Gallagher, Michael Parsons, "Court-Ordered Obstetrical Interventions," *New England Journal of Medicine* 316 (May 7, 1987): 1192–96; Mathieu, *Preventing Prenatal Harm*; Laurence McCullough and Frank Chervenak, *Ethics in Obstetrics and Gynecology* (New York: Oxford University Press, 1994); and Lawrence Nelson and Nancy Milliken, "Compelled Medical Treatment of Pregnant Women," *Journal of American Medical Association* 259 (Feb. 19, 1988), 1060–66. There have as well been statements that recognize at last some limited autonomy for women in these circumstances. See American College of Obstetrics and Gynecologists, "Patient Choice: Maternal-Fetal Conflict," *ACOG Committee Opinion* 55 (Oct. 1987); and Board of Trustees, "Legal Interventions during Pregnancy," *Journal of American Medical Association* 264 (Nov. 28, 1990): 2663–70.

47. Anthony Shaw, "Dilemmas of 'Informed Consent' in Children," *New England Journal of Medicine* 289 (Oct. 25, 1973): 885–90.

48. Raymond S. Duff and A. G. M. Campbell, "Moral and Ethical Dilemmas in the Special-Care Nursery," *New England Journal of Medicine* 289 (Oct. 25, 1973): 890–94. A review of these issues in terms of contemporary law and public policy is provided in R. C. McMillan et al. (eds.), *Euthanasia and the Newborn* (Dordrecht: Reidel, 1987).

49. Americans with Disabilities Act of 1990, 42 U.S.C.A. §§ 12101 et seq. (West 1993).

50. Robert Nozick, *Anarchy, State, and Utopia* (New York: Basic Books, 1974), p. 323.

51. In the Matter of Baby "K," 1994 WL 38674 (4th Cir. Va).

52. Robert F. Weir, "Sounding Board: The Government and Selective Nontreatment of Handicapped Infants," *New England Journal of Medicine* 309 (Sept. 15, 1983): 661–63; and *Selective Nontreatment of Handicapped Newborns* (New York: Oxford University Press, 1986).

53. *Federal Register* 48 (Mar. 7, 1983): 9630–32; *Federal Register* 48 (July 5, 1983): 30846–52; final regulations were issued in *Federal Register* 49 (Jan. 12, 1984): 1622–54.

54. American Academy of Pediatrics v. Heckler, 561 F. Supp. 395 (D.D.C. 1983).

55. *Federal Register* 49 (Jan. 12, 1984): 1654. These regulations, as well as the proposed

regulations that have followed, outline and suggest the use of infant care review committees. This has led to a growing interest in developing institutional ethics committees. The extent to which such committees will be useful will depend on the extent to which they provide access to special expertise and a chance for the arbitration of disputes or for the diffusion of responsibility. They will not have authority morally to substitute for the agreements of physicians and patients without the consent of those parties. This will be true not only in the case of pediatric care but in health care generally. For a recent history of institutional review committees, see R. E. Cranford and A. E. Doudera, "The Emergence of Institutional Ethics Committees," *Law, Medicine and Health Care* 12 (Feb. 1984): 13–20.

56. American Academy of Pediatrics, "Principles of Treatment of Disabled Infants," *Pediatrics* 73 (Apr. 4, 1984): 559. These principles for treatment were inspired in part by a number of cases in which Down's syndrome children were not treated on the basis of quality-of-life decisions. See George F. Smith et al., "Commentary: The Rights of Infants with Down's Syndrome," *Journal of the American Medical Association* 251 (Jan. 13, 1984): 229.
57. United States v. University Hospital, No. 83–6343 (2d Cir. Feb. 23, 1984).
58. Pub. L. No. 98–457, 98 Stat. 1749 (1984).
59. Department of Health and Human Services, "Child Abuse and Neglect Prevention and Treatment Program; Proposed Rule. Interim Model Guidelines for Health Care Providers to Establish Infant Care Review Committee; Notice," *Federal Register* 49 (Dec. 10, 1984): 48160–73.
60. Department of Health and Human Services, "Child Abuse and Neglect Prevention and Treatment Program; Final Rule," *Federal Register* 50 (Apr. 15, 1985):14878–901. The final regulations follow the 1984 amendments to the Child Abuse Prevention and Treatment Act and list as exceptions to when withholding of indicated medical treatment would count as child abuse the following circumstances: "(i) The infant is chronically and irreversibly comatose; (ii) The provision of such treatment would merely prolong dying, not be effective in ameliorating or correcting all of the infant's life-threatening conditions, or otherwise be futile in terms of the survival of the infant; or (iii) The provision of such treatment would be virtually futile in terms of the survival of the infant and the treatment itself under such circumstances would be inhumane." Ibid., p. 14888. The regulations thus appear to imply that one is obliged to treat a child aggressively, even if one thought it would die at the age of eighteen months. It seems implausible that the state has general secular moral authority to stop parents from deciding whether they wish to treat their child aggressively only to have it die a year later. For further reflections on these debates, see Earl Shelp, *Born to Die?* (New York: Free Press, 1986); McMillan et al., *Euthanasia and the Newborn;* and A Report of the U.S. Commission of Civil Rights, *Medical Discrimination against Children with Disabilities* (Washington, D.C.: U.S. Government Printing Office, Sept. 1989).
61. Pub. L. No. 98–457, 121, 98 Stat. 1749 (1984).
62. *Current Opinions of the Judicial Council of the American Medical Association—1984* (Chicago: American Medical Association, 1984), p. 10.
63. Ibid., p. 11.

64. Ibid., p. 10.

65. For an overview of some of the implications of the Americans with Disabilities Act for decisions to limit, as well as to ration, health care resources, see David Orentlicher, "Rationing and the Americans with Disabilities Act," *Journal of American Medical Association* 271 (Jan. 26, 1994): 308–14.

66. For an overview of the silent acceptance of infanticide in recent times, see W. L. Langer, "Checks on Population Growth: 1750–1850," *Scientific American* 226 (1972): 3–9. For a study of the generality of the phenomenon of infanticide, see Glenn Hausfater and Sarah Blaffer Hrdy (eds.), *Infanticide: Comparative and Evolutionary Perspectives* (New York: Aldine, 1984).

67. Pope Pius XII, Allocution "Le Dr. Bruno Haid," Nov. 24, 1957, *Acta Apostolicae Sedis* 49 (1957): 1031. English translation from Pius XII, "Address to an International Congress of Anesthesiologists," Nov. 24, 1957, *The Pope Speaks* 4 (Spring 1958): 395–96. For an exploration of the development of the distinction between ordinary and extraordinary means, see James J. McCartney, "The Development of the Doctrine of Ordinary and Extraordinary Means of Preserving Life in Catholic Moral Theology before the Karen Quinlan Case," *Linacre Quarterly* 47 (Aug. 1980): 215–24. As McCartney indicates, the distinction between ordinary and extraordinary care was developed by Soto in 1582 and Banez in 1595. For further information on the distinction, see José Janini, "La operatión quirúrgica, remedio ordinario," *Revista Española de Teologia* 18 (1958): 331–48; Daniel A. Cronin, *The Moral Law in Regard to the Ordinary and Extraordinary Means of Conserving Life* (Rome: Typis Pontificiae Universitatis Gregorianiae, 1958); and Gerald Kelly, "The Duty of Using Artificial Means of Preserving Life," *Theological Studies* 11 (1950): 203–20.

68. The moral significance of the distinction between acting and refraining, and between active and passive euthanasia, has been explored in a number of articles in the philosophical literature and elsewhere. See, for example, Natalie Abrams, "Active and Passive Euthanasia," *Philosophy* 54 (1978): 257–69; Gary Atkinson, "Ambiguities in 'Killing' and 'Letting Die,' " *Journal of Medicine and Philosophy* 8 (May 1983): 159–68; Jonathan Bennett, "Whatever the Consequences," *Analysis* 26 (Jan. 1966): 83–102; Daniel Dinello, "On Killing and Letting Die," *Analysis* 31 (Apr. 1971): 83–86; P. J. Fitzgerald, "Acting and Refraining," *Analysis* 27 (Mar. 1967): 133–39; James Rachels, "Active and Passive Euthanasia," *New England Journal of Medicine* 292 (Jan. 9, 1975): 78–80. These issues are reviewed as well in the very thorough book by Robert Weir, *Selective Nontreatment of Handicapped Newborns* (New York: Oxford University Press, 1984). See also Dennis J. Horan and Melinda Delahoyde (eds.), *Infanticide and the Handicapped Newborn* (Provo, Utah: Brigham Young University Press, 1982).

69. Aristotle, *Politics,* in *The Basic Works of Aristotle,* ed. Richard McKeon (New York: Random House, 1941), 7.6.335b, p. 1302.

70. Sextus Empiricus, *Outlines of Pyrrhonism,* in *Sextus Empiricus,* trans. R. G. Bury (Cambridge, Mass.: Harvard University Press, 1976), 3.211, vol. 1, p. 467. For a criticism of Sextus Empiricus's contention, as well as an acknowledgment of the general acceptance of the father's right to expose children, see A. R. W. Harrison, *The Law of Athens: The Family and Property* (Oxford: Clarendon Press, 1968).

71. Soranus, *Soranus' Gynecology,* trans. Owsei Temkin (Baltimore: Johns Hopkins

University Press, 1956), p. 80. The Roman fathers' right to kill offspring or at least deformed, handicapped, or weak infants was set aside by Constantine in A.D. 318 (*Codex Justinianus* 9.17.1) and again by Valentinian in A.D. 374 (*Codex Justinianus* 9.16.7). These issues are explored by Darrel Amundsen in "Medicine and the Birth of Defective Children: Approaches of the Ancient World," in McMillan et al., *Euthanasia and the Newborn,* pp. 3–22.

72. For a discussion of infanticide and allied issues, see Paul Carrick, *Medical Ethics in Antiquity* (Dordrecht: Reidel, 1985).

73. The Didache, in *The Apostolic Fathers,* trans. Kirsopp Lake (Cambridge, Mass.: Harvard University Press, 1965), vol. 1, pp. 311–13, 2.2.

74. See, for example, the American federal regulations requiring that "no fetus *in utero* may be involved as a subject in any activity covered by this subpart unless: (1) The purpose of the activity is to meet the health needs of the particular fetus and the fetus will be placed at risk only to the minimum extent necessary to meet such needs, or (2) the risk to the fetus imposed by the research is minimal and the purpose of the activity is the development of important biomedical knowledge which cannot be obtained by other means." *Protection of Human Subjects,* 45 Code of Federal Regulations, 46.208(a).

75. See, for example, state laws such as Minn. Stat. § 145, 422–3 (1973) and Louisiana tit. 14 § 87.2 (1973).

76. See, for example, Jerome Kassirer and Marcia Angell, "The Use of Fetal Tissue in Research on Parkinson's Disease," *New England Journal of Medicine* 327 (Nov. 26, 1992): 1591–92; and Daniel Garry, Arthur Caplan, Dorothy Vawter, and Warren Kearney, "Are There Really Alternatives to the Use of Fetal Tissue from Elective Abortions in Transplantation Research," *New England Journal of Medicine* 327 (Nov. 26, 1992): 1592–95.

77. The traditional Christian view, while regarding masturbation as an act that falls short of the mark of a wholehearted focus on God, may regard it within marriage when directed toward reproduction as an understandable accommodation to the fallen character of human nature. See, for example, William Zion, *Eros and Transformation* (Lanham, Md.: University Press of America, 1992), pp. 263–85. Thus, masturbation with a view towards artificial insemination with the husband's sperm may be tolerated, though not ideal.

78. The role of a donor in artificially overcoming the sterility of a couple now includes not just the donation of sperm but of ova as well. In Orthodox Judaism the donation of gametes from unmarried women may constitute less difficulty than the donation of sperm.

79. Mary Warnock, *A Question of Life* (Oxford: Basil Blackwell, 1985), p. 44.

80. These concerns were voiced as the new reproductive technologies were developing. See, for example, Paul Ramsey, "Ethics of a Cottage Industry in an Age of Community and Research Medicine," *New England Journal of Medicine* 284 (Apr. 1, 1971): 700–6; "Shall We Reproduce? I. The Medical Ethics of *In Vitro* Fertilization," *Journal of the American Medical Association* 220 (June 5, 1972): 1345–50; "Shall We Reproduce? II. Rejoinders and Future Forecasts," *Journal of the American Medical Association* 220 (June 12, 1972): 1480–85. For a more general, conservative critique of in vitro fertilization, see Leon Kass, "Babies by Means of *In Vitro*

Fertilization: Unethical Experiments on the Unborn?'' *New England Journal of Medicine* 285 (Nov. 18, 1971): 1174–79. For a general overview of secular moral, legal, and religious concerns, see Office of Technology Assessment, *Infertility: Medical and Social Choices* (Washington, D.C.: U.S. Government Printing Office, May 1988).

81.  Paul Ramsey, *Fabricated Man* (New Haven, Conn.: Yale University Press, 1970), p. 39.

82.  Congregation for the Doctrine of the Faith, *Instruction on Respect for Human Life in its Origin and on the Dignity of Procreation* (Vatican City, 1987), pp. 28, 29–30. For a discussion of *Donum Vitae*, see Lisa Cahill, ''Moral Traditions, Ethical Language, and Reproductive Technologies,'' *Journal of Medicine and Philosophy* 14 (Oct. 1989): 497–522. See also Stanley Harakas, *Living the Faith* (Minneapolis: Light and Life, 1992), especially pp. 133–34.

83.  Joseph Fletcher, ''Ethical Aspects of Genetic Controls,'' *New England Journal of Medicine* 285 (Sept. 30, 1971): 776–83; *The Ethics of Genetic Control* (Garden City, N.Y.: Doubleday Anchor, 1974); *Morals and Medicine* (Princeton, N.J.: Princeton University Press, 1954).

84.  The use of surrogate mothers for in vitro fertilization raises the general problem of creating a contract to govern such endeavors. Though morally such contracts should be binding, they raise a number of important legal issues. See Steven R. Gersz, ''The Contract in Surrogate Motherhood: A Review of the Issues,'' *Law, Medicine and Health Care* 12 (June 1984): 115–17. For a study of surrogate mothers, see Lori Andrews, *Between Strangers* (New York: Harper & Row, 1989).

85.  In general secular morality, it is contracts that will make clear the character of mutual obligations and rights, including obligations to embryos. In the context of general secular morality, the best one can do is to be clear about what is at stake and to make agreements as explicit as possible, given the context and the wishes of the participants. For a statement bearing on some of these issues, see Board of Trustees, ''Frozen Pre-embryos,'' *Journal of the American Medical Association* 263 (May 9, 1990): 2484–87.

86.  Gerald Kelly, *Medico–Moral Problems* (St. Louis: Catholic Hospital Association, 1958), pp. 228–44; and John P. Kenny, *Principles of Medical Ethics*, 2d ed. (Westminster, Md.: Newman Press, 1962), pp. 90–96.

87.  It would be a mistake to understand the traditional Christian appreciation of reproduction and sexuality within the Scholasticism that developed in the West.

Our capacity to control procreation is an expression of our powers of freedom and reason to collaborate with God in the moral order. A human being is viewed not only as a subject which receives passively the ''natural law,'' but also as a person who plays an active role in its formulation. Thus natural law, according to Eastern Orthodox thinkers, is not a code imposed by God on human beings, but rather a rule of life set forth by divine inspiration and by our responses to it in freedom and reason. This view does not permit the Eastern Orthodox Church to conclude that the pill, and artificial contraceptives generally, are in violation of human law.

Chrysostomos Zaphiris, ''The Morality of Contraception: An Eastern Orthodox Opinion,'' *Journal of Ecumenical Studies* 11 (1974): 688.

The Stoic and other Greek accounts of nature that were incorporated into Western

Christian views are not integral to traditional Christianity. As a consequence, "The processes of nature are clearly not inherently sacred and beyond human intervention. Medically there is little difference between processes which interfere to sustain life and those which would interfere to postpone pregnancies or for sufficient reason suppress them entirely." Zion, *Eros and Transformation*, p. 256.

Further, Christianity affirms the eros of marital love. "The ascent to God by way of human love becomes another form of the ascetic way which overcomes self-seeking, the demands for immediate gratification, and the power of death revealed by the movement of time. The power of love to transcend all limitations is a gift of the Holy Spirit." Ibid., p. 361.

88. One might think of proposals to treat individuals as dead on the basis of prolonged asystole, such as discussed in Stuart Youngner and Robert Arnold, "Ethical, Psychosocial, and Public Policy Implications of Procuring Organs from Non-Heart-Beating Cadaver Donors," *Journal of the American Medical Association* 269 (June 2, 1993): 2769–74. The reliance on such so-called non-heart-beating cadaver donors whose brains may be fairly intact may collide with the insights that moved the American Bar Association in 1975 to propose the following brain-oriented definition of death: "For all legal purposes, a human body with irreversible cessation of total brain function, according to usual and customary standards of medical practice, shall be considered dead." President's Commission for the Study of Ethical Problems in Medicine and Biomedical and Behavioral Research, *Defining Death*, p. 117.

89. At the core of traditional Christianity is an affirmation of marriage as a mystery blessed by God and fruitful in pleasure. "A great mystery is being celebrated: forth with the harlots! forth with the profane! How is it a mystery? They come together, and the two make one. . . . They come, about to be made one body. See again a mystery of love! If the two become not one, so long as they continue two, they make not many, but when they are come into one-ness, they then make many. What are we to learn from this? That great is the power of union." St. John Chrysostom, "Homily 12 on Colossians," trans. John Broadus, in *Nicene and Post-Nicene Fathers of the Christian Church*, sermon 1, vol. 13 (Grand Rapids, Mich.: Wm. B. Eerdmans, 1956), p. 318. "As Christ came into the Church, and she was made of Him, and He united with her in a spiritual intercourse. . . . Thinking then on all these things, let us not cast shame upon so great mystery so shamefully. Marriage is a type of the presence of Christ." Ibid., p. 319. "And indeed from the beginning, God appears to have made special provision for this union; and discoursing of the twain as one, He said thus, 'Male and female created He them' (Genesis 1:27)." Chrysostom, "Homily 20 on Ephesians," in ibid., p. 143. "And how become they one flesh? As if thou shouldest take away the purest part of gold, and mingle it with other gold; so in truth here also the women as it were receiving the richest part fused by pleasure, nourisheth it and cherisheth it, and withal contributing her own share, restoreth it back a Man. And the child is a sort of bridge, so that the three become one flesh, the child connecting, on either side, each to other." "Homily 12 on Colossians," in ibid., p. 319. That marriage is a mystery blessed by God, celebrated by the husband and wife and not to be intruded on by others, cannot be understood outside of a particular moral content and context.

# 7

## Free and Informed Consent, Refusal of Treatment, and the Health Care Team: The Many Faces of Freedom

Persons have a fundamental right to be left alone. This right stands at the very center of secular morality, not because it is a good thing to have, but because it is unavoidable and the source of moral authority when moral strangers meet. Because secular morality cannot provide a canonical vision of the good or a canonical content-full account of proper action, the principle of permission is the cardinal source of moral authority. For better or worse, persons are in secular moral authority over themselves and during their consensual activities with others. For those who recognize the concrete values that should guide the good life, secular morality is a wasteland without moral content, without the possibility of moral guidance, and with the possibility of such serious moral failures as suicide and euthanasia. The choices that individuals will be free to make within secular morality will conflict with what people will see within particular content-full moralities. For example, those with strong ideological commitments to egalitarianisms of various sorts will recognize that their aspiration to achieve equality coercively will be without general secular moral authority and go aground on free choice. The centrality of the principle of permission discloses the radical implications involved in recognizing secular morality as the morality of moral strangers. The centrality of the principle of permission discloses the wide-ranging implications of the Enlightenment's failure to establish a canonical, content-full morality. In the failure of reason and in the absence of faith, secular morality is the morality of moral strangers who find themselves bound together and separated by their choices.

Individuals are by default the source of secular moral authority. The right to be left alone simply expresses the possibility of the choice not to give permission. The right to be left alone includes the right not to be hindered when joining freely with willing others. It is those who would interfere who must show their authority. It is around the various expressions of the principle of permission that relations between patients, physicians, and other health care workers take shape. These relations include those of association, dissociation, and nonassociation. Patients and physicians weave a web of commitments, as well as boundaries and borders. The fashioning of a physician–patient relationship involves the building of commitments and the setting of limits. It involves as well the mutual understanding of the commitments and limits, the permissions and refusals, that fashion an actual concrete relationship. In health care men and women create a web of expectations and permissions through agreements to being touched and explored by others, through commitments to confidentiality and the keeping of special trusts, and by fashioning common understandings of goals to be jointly pursued. In health care this includes entrusting certain elements of the care and cure of one's body and mind to some but not to others, usually in part, rarely as a whole. As total commitments are rare in everyday life, the same is the case in health care. Few patients commit themselves without reservation to the care of a physician. Usually something is held back, something is reserved; there is some noncompliance with the instructions of a physician. So, too, most physicians and nurses do not commit all. There are always limits to the dedication of finite beings.

That which creates the substance of this relationship also fashions its limits: the free choices of individual men and women—patients, physicians, nurses, and others. There is no single way in which the relationship must be structured. Different groups will fashion different relationships given their different needs for independence or acquiescence in the care of others. To understand the variations in this relationship, one is brought to the traditional issues of free and informed consent, confidentiality, paternalism, and the rights of patients to refuse treatment or of physicians not to accept a patient. These must be appreciated in terms of the tensions among the various views of the good life that sustain particular ideals of the patient–physician (or patient–nurse) relationship. These views, which are often in conflict, must then be mediated in the general fabric of a peaceable, secular, pluralist society through the agreement of those involved. In short, competing views of beneficence expressed in competing understandings of the patient–physician relationship will need to be fairly accommodated in mutual respect for the persons participating. Fair procedures of negotiation will form the basis for resolving tensions among competing views of proper actions.

Free and informed consent is central to this procedure. Individuals must communicate and appreciate what each party wishes in order to come to an understanding. The physician–patient contract and the understandings between patients

and nurses are the final products of such procedures. These processes of informing and communicating play their central role not simply because they may be
valued in their own right (though they may indeed be highly valued), but also due
to the lack of common understandings among individuals and across communities. Insofar as there is not one authoritative view of the good life and of the
concrete goals of medicine, one will need to create common understandings. Free
and informed consent thus plays its central role not so much out of a commitment
to a liberal ideal, but out of a despair regarding the possibility of discovering a
concrete view of the goals of health care in a secular, pluralist context. In short,
free and informed consent has its cardinal moral significance because of the
conceptual difficulties (i.e., inability of reason to establish authoritatively a particular concrete view of the good life) and historical problems (i.e., the historical
collapse of the Christian, as well as the Enlightenment expectation, for all to
convert to, or by general rational argument to establish, a canonical concrete view
of the good life) that lead to the intellectual problem of gaining moral authority in
a secular pluralist society (a point discussed in chapter 2). When such authority
cannot be discovered, when one cannot decide what must be done, one must ask
the free individuals involved what they want to do and wait for them to come to a
common agreement in order to achieve peaceable action with moral authority.
The appeal to the consent of patients is rooted in the priority of the principle of
permission.

As we will see, the amount and character of required disclosure and formal
agreement is dependent on the extent to which the physician or other health care
professional and the patient share common views of the goals of medicine, the
canons of moral probity, and the character of the good life. The more the physician and the patient are strangers to each other's set of values and goals, the more
necessary it will be to fashion explicit rules to govern free and informed consent,
and for free and informed consent to encompass in detail the matters at stake in
treatment. The more patients and physicians share a common view of the goals
of health care in particular and of life in general, the less necessary elaborate
disclosures need be. However, some disclosures will always be necessary.
Friends need to know, even if only implicitly, the character of their joint endeavors. Friends can disagree and become estranged. In the more serious
endeavors of medicine it will be necessary at least to anticipate such possibilities.

With the authority to consent comes the right to give oneself over to the care of
others and to withdraw from that care, to accept aid and to refuse it. As a result,
the topic of free and informed consent is bound to issues of the moral probity of
suicide and of aiding and abetting suicide, and to the establishment of lines of
authority within the health care team. These various topics are expressions of the
freedom of individuals in health care.

## The patient–healer relationship

The physician and patient are not alone in the patient–healer relationship. In *Epidemics* Hippocrates enjoins the physician:

Declare the past, diagnose the present, foretell the future; practice these acts. As to diseases, make a habit of two things—to help, or at least to do no harm. The art has three factors, the disease, the patient, the physician. The physician is the servant of the art. The patient must cooperate with the physician in combating the disease.[1]

In addition to the physician and the patient in their confrontation with disease, there is also the art. The art, Hippocrates' *technē*, I will read as the medical profession both as a group of individuals and as a body of skills.[2] Professions attempt to set standards as to what will count as canonical problems and proper medical interventions. This sense of profession transcends national boundaries and can exist without a formal organization of physicians such as the American Medical Association.[3] The very idea of the skilled profession thus reaches into the private exchanges of healers and patients, even before and in addition to the intrusions of state authority through laws, regulations, or requirements of licensure.

To understand the position of healers and patients, one must first turn to the ways in which healers are seen as professionals and regard themselves as members of a profession. The idea of a profession carries with it commitments to particular views of beneficence and proper action. Professions are goal oriented.

### The profession

All societies have individuals who play the role of healer, even where the role of healer is not yet fully differentiated from other roles such as that of priest. In societies with an investment in modern science and technology such as ours, the healer often retains magical and priestly roles. This is not unexpected. Healing is sought for concerns that go to the root of human existence: fears of death, deformity, and disability. The healer's role has parallels with that of the lawyer who aids individuals in difficulties with state–recognized powers and that of the theologian or priest who aids individuals in difficulties with the supernatural powers: each is a mediator between individuals and one of the major clusters of potentially adversarial forces. The physician, lawyer, and theologian or priest are engaged in professions that intrude into all elements of human life.

The profession to which the healer belongs is also one of the three traditional learned professions. It is learned in that it requires skill to prevent and control illness, and to forestall death. It is one of the major professions in that pain, deformity, disability, disease, and premature death capture the central attention of both individuals and societies. Such learning and importance set a distance

between the healer and the person seeking care. As the skills become complex
and intricate, requiring deep knowledge of human nature, physiology, and the
mechanisms of disease, a barrier against understanding is erected between the
two. This barrier between the expert professional and the layman cannot be
overcome by a redistribution of knowledge in the same way that a barrier between
the rich and the poor might be overcome in principle by a redistribution of
wealth.[4] The very wealth of knowledge that makes the professional able disables
communication with the person in need of care. In addition, remnants of magical
expectations regarding those who deal with disease and death convey a further
sense of distance and importance usually not ascribed to merely mechanical
interventions.[5]

As a result, the medical profession takes on an esoteric character. It is a domain
of special learning bearing on issues of life and death to which often magical
properties are assigned. In fact, part of the traditional placebo power of the
physician, the ability of the physician to make the patient feel better by the
physician's very presence is tied to this priestly authority of the healer. This
commitment to the esoteric character of the profession is expressed in the Hippocratic Oath where initiates swear to impart the instruction they will be given only
to sons of their teacher and to indentured pupils who have taken the oath, but to
no others. The result is the fashioning of a moral and intellectual elite, a group of
individuals with (1) complex technical knowledge, as well as a special dedication
to (2) aiding those threatened by illness, deformity, and premature death, as well
as (3) preserving and increasing the skill of the professional. The second sustains
a commitment to a set of both moral and nonmoral values. The former values
guide judgments about the proper ways in which patients should be treated, and
the latter values will include understandings of the levels of disability, pain, and
deformity that should be accepted or that should serve as bona fide warrants for
treatment. The third not only supports standards for the use of skills but also
directs the profession to the acquisition of better skills and greater knowledge.
Even without a formal regulatory procedure or membership requirement, the
profession is able to recognize those who belong and who live up to its ideals by
appealing to these goals of beneficence and of knowledge. The health care professions can be self-regulating through appeals to these goals either as (1) groups of
individuals formally organized into societies or (2) groups of individuals informally bound together by commitment to the profession's intellectual and moral
goals.

These goals not only ennoble the health care professions but also are the basis
of moral conflicts as well. Members of the health care professions, as members of
a learned profession, are dedicated to the following sorts of goals, not all of
which are always in harmony: (1) they serve the health care needs and desires
of individuals; (2) they support the health care needs and desires of societies; (3)
they engage in their profession to gain income and prestige (professionals are not

amateurs, individuals engaged in an undertaking without thought of monetary reward); (4) they aid the profession in being self-perpetuating (e.g., in attempting to preserve the art, the members preserve the profession as a special interest group with special privileges and status); and (5) they aim at the acquisition of knowledge. The good of the individual and of society may often be at odds (e.g., reporting requirements with regard to venereal diseases). The pursuit of individual gain not only may financially embarrass individuals and society, but also may lead to undermining the status of the profession. Finally, and here one finds a distinction that marks a learned profession, the pursuit of knowledge may conflict with the interests of the individuals being treated. One might think of the remark often said in derogation, but which is nevertheless instructive: ''The operation was a success but the patient died.'' A learned profession is an intellectual joy even apart from its services to others. There is a pleasure in practicing a learned and difficult skill, even when it cannot be of benefit to others.

The pursuit of knowledge, though in potential conflict with the interests of individual patients, is in potential harmony with the long-range interests of future patients and society generally. The acquisition of better knowledge and increased skill should ensure better-quality treatment for individuals in the future. Such use of current patients for the preservation of the art is necessary even apart from high-technology medicine. Skills must be passed from a learned master to an apprentice healer who while in training may lance a boil, set a bone, or treat a fever with less skill than the teacher. If patients do not come into the hands of young apprentices, the skill will die out. In the medical profession everyone must lance a boil, remove an appendix, or perform a cardiac catheterization for the first time. This investment of the present on behalf of the future is made even more systematic with the idea of medical progress and with a critical regard of claims about the efficacy of standard treatments. The goals of doing the best for patients, and of avoiding unnecessary harms, lead to the practice of systematic medical experimentation and to the healer not only being one who cares for those in need but also one who studies their complaints and their possible cures. The utilitarian (greatest good for the greatest number) understanding of the obligations of the medical profession becomes intertwined with the focus on the often deontological obligations to particular patients.

When a patient confronts a physician (or a nurse or other health care professional), the physician is encountered within the complex context of a profession with diverse goals, only some of which are directed to the treatment and care of that patient. If the patient wants what the profession does not usually give or wants treatments that depart from the standards of the profession, the physician must bear the judgment of the profession in mind. Any negotiation with a particular patient will involve the physician in a possible negotiation with the profession. The profession renders judgments (both formally and informally) about which activities are properly medical, about which violate the standards of the profession, and thus about whether the physician or other health care professional in question is in good standing. Even absent formal regulations, organized professional societies, or licensing procedures, there are important sanctions such as the denial of referrals. Patient requests for particular treatments are thus at once put within the context of a community of health professionals with their views of what actions are proper and what interventions are indicated. The interchanges among patients and health care professionals are defined not only by these two groups of individuals but also by the health care profession itself. Depending on the view of proper practice held by the profession (or groups within the profession), the profession may even support the physician in telling the patient, "If you want to be treated by me, then you will stop asking all these questions and do what I tell you—that way you will get the best treatment and I will have more time to help other patients in need."

Circumstances are, however, complex, for there is not one unambiguous sense of the health care professions or of the medical profession. Postmodernity and the fragmentation of moral narratives touches to the core of the professions. Although there will be the possibility for a general abstract understanding of what it means to be a physician or nurse, a concrete understanding will be available only within a particular community of physicians, nurses, or other health care professionals and their view of the morally proper life and of the good practice of their profession. Thus, as patients negotiate with health professionals about their treatment and care, they will need to determine the professional commitments of those with whom they are about to enter into the agreement for care and treatment. A woman of liberal moral persuasions will need to know, for example, whether the gynecologist with whom she is considering developing a patient–physician relationship holds views against sterilization and abortion. So, too, it will be prudent for someone diagnosed with disseminated cancer to know the physician's views regarding the use of narcotics and other drugs in the control of pain. For example, will the physician be willing to give sufficient pain medication in order to avoid the patient's feeling pain instead of relying on minimal amounts of medication so that the patient must request pain medication and experience pain between doses. Similarly, an individual diagnosed with amyelotrophic lateral sclerosis or Lou Gehrig's disease (a fatal degenerative neurological disease) who does not wish to be preserved to the very end will need to establish a relationship with a neurologist who will support the patient's desires for minimal or no treatment toward the end of the disease's course. In order effectively to fashion a health care contract, the patient will need to know the moral and professional ideals of the physician. So, too, the physician will need to understand the patient's expectations from care.[6]

Physicians will need to take seriously the implications of the plurality of moral visions for the framing of professional moral standards. There is no reason why committed Roman Catholic physicians, for example, should suppose that general secular morality, not to mention the various particular secular moralities, will not place them in circumstances in which they will be invited to engage in seriously sinful matters. Such serious moral differences cannot but in the end invite the development of particular professional organizations framed around their own moral commitments.

### The patient as a stranger in a strange land

Patients, when they come to see a health care professional, are in unfamiliar territory. They enter a terrain of issues that has been carefully defined through the long history of the health care professions. A patient is unlikely to present for care with as well-analyzed and considered judgments as those possessed by health care professionals. Professionals have a community of colleagues to reinforce their views and to sustain them in their recommendations. In addition, the interchange of health care professionals and patients is defined by the language of health care. Pains, disabilities, and even fears are translated into the special jargon of the health care professions. The replacement of the ritual and magic of the shaman by the technology and theory of the scientist-healer may have increased, not diminished, the distance between the healer and the person in search of cure and care.

The patient in this context is a stranger, an individual in unfamiliar territory who does not fully know what to expect or how to control the environment. The patient's usual ways of thinking must be put into abeyance or altered in order to accommodate to the theories and explanations of the healer and the routines of the healer's environment. The stranger must adapt to new and alien cultural patterns and expectations. Things no longer happen as usual; they no longer take place in their taken-for-granted ways. As an outsider in a strange culture, the patient always runs the risk of being a marginal person. The stranger, as Alfred Schutz noted, "has to face the fact that he lacks any status as a member of the social group he is about to join and is therefore unable to get a starting-point to take his bearings."[7] To rephrase Schutz's point so as to focus on health care, the patient as a stranger has difficulty even being oriented in the environment of high-technology medicine, much less wielding authority.

Health care professionals attempt to overcome this distance between the patient and the context of health care by altering the set of expectations held by the patient. This is particularly true when the patient and the healer will be in extended contact, as occurs in chronic illness. In such circumstances, the physician and other health care professionals are usually committed to inducting the patient into the lifeworld of health care. There is an attempt to change and reshape the taken-for-granted expectations of the patient, much as a catechumen is instructed as a part of conversion. To treat chronic illnesses such as hypertension or diabetes, the patient must come to see certain diets as forbidden, as medically unclean, much as individuals entering certain religions must come to appreciate certain foods as ritually unclean. Patients must also be taught to regard changes in their bodies in the same way as do their physicians. Shortness of breath and swelling of the feet after a day's work now become possible signs of medical difficulties that should be reported to the physician. In addition, the patients may learn to measure their own blood pressure and test their urine in order to make inferences about the state of their bodies. Diabetics must calculate their caloric intake, know its source, and administer insulin to themselves in carefully measured amounts. Such activities can be understood only within the system of assumptions and theoretical commitments of the physicians and nurses caring for the patient. Patients with a chronic disease become successful participants in their treatment only insofar as they incorporate into their assumptions the technological and scientific world view of the physicians and nurses who are treating them. Once the patient has moved into and accepted the lifeworld of the healer, compliance with treatment will no longer be alien but a part of the new lifeworld of the patient.

The encounter with the health professional brings profound consequences. To accept a diagnosis is often to be committed to reordering one's very life in terms of the treatments and preventive regimens that the diagnosis warrants. Much of the negotiation between patients and physicians turns on the extent to which a diagnosis should transform a patient's life. In fact, to see a patient with a diagnosis of diabetes as a diabetic, not just a person with diabetes, is an indication of the extent to which a diagnostic label transforms an individual's existence. What is at stake is not simply an external matter concerning how the individual is to be regarded but it touches on how such individuals should regard themselves. The physician may be arguing that such individuals' continued well-being is dependent on their seeing themselves as diabetics. They may want to avoid accepting a diagnostic label that will so thoroughly transform their lives, in part because they do not wish to control their diabetes as strictly as their physician demands, and because the patients do not wish to acknowledge the changes in expectations the diagnosis brings, from the possibility of blindness, impotence, and kidney failure to early death. Health care professionals attempt to transform a patient from a stranger in a strange land into a permanent resident alien in the world of medical expectations and interventions.

## Strangers and friends

Edmund Pellegrino and David Thomasma have argued that the physician and the patient meet as friends dedicated to the good of health.[8] They do this following arguments provided by Plato in the *Lysis*.[9] It is plausible to see the physician (or nurse or other health care professional) and the patient as friends, rather than strangers, only insofar as they are not set apart (1) by the possibly conflicting interests of the health care professions and those of patients, (2) by conflicting views of the goals of health care, (3) by differing understandings of the canons of moral probity, and (4) by differing views of health and disease. Health care professionals may differ from patients (1) in being specially dedicated to the long-range survival and security of their professions and to the development of knowledge for the aid of future patients, (2) in their views regarding the control of pain and the establishment of proper human abilities and form (e.g., how much medication should be given for the control of anxieties), (3) in their judgments regarding the concrete character of the canons of moral probity (e.g., regarding the morality of allowing newborns with severe mental and physical handicaps to die), and (4) in their views of good medical treatment (e.g., regarding what amount of chance for a cure for a patient's cancer is worth what amount of disfigurement).

The more physicians and patients share a common view of the good life, the more plausible it will be that they meet as moral friends. A common view of the good life provides both moral and nonmoral values so that those who share that view know what ought to be done, what risks are prudent, and what actions should be avoided. When individuals share a common view of the good life, they live within a common fabric of mutual understandings and of commitments to common goals. In such circumstances, consenting to common endeavors often requires very little explicit communication, for communication has already taken place through the web of tacit understandings that fashions a common view of the good life. When this occurs, health care professionals and patients do not meet as strangers, but as individuals who are committed to a set of common goals.[10]

Individuals can come from widely differing communities and still be friends. In fact, as Aristotle notes, there may be an advantage to friendship with a foreigner, in that one thus avoids conflicts about personal advancement in the same polis.[11] But friendship with a foreigner is possible only insofar as one does share commitments to certain goals and goods. Aristotle did not have in mind friendship with a barbarian. One way of reading Aristotle's remark for bioethics is that it may be easier for a physician to have a friendship with a patient than with another physician, because physicians are in competition with each other for patients or for advancement within the community of physicians. What is at stake here in distinguishing between moral friends and strangers is the extent to which health care professionals and patients either (1) share a common understanding that does away with the need for a great deal of formal disclosures and consent procedures, or (2) fail to possess such common commitments so that formal procedures of disclosure and consent are necessary to avoid serious misunderstandings.

Much of the formal bureaucratic structure for disclosure and consent in countries such as the United States is a function of the fact that in peaceable, secular, pluralist societies health professionals and patients recurringly meet as strangers.

They are not simply strangers in that they often do not share the same set of professional commitments or scientific and technological understandings. They are strangers as well because their views of the good life are drawn from radically different communities of belief. When devout Roman Catholic physicians encounter Marxist women seeking abortions, or when liberal homosexual physicians encounter conservative Baptist patients in need of advice about treatment for their sexual dysfunctions, much cannot be taken for granted regarding a common understanding of the goals of health care and the canons of civil probity. Pellegrino's proof text passage from Plato for the argument that physicians and patients are friends presumes an unambiguous sense of health.[12] But as chapter 5 has shown, such does not exist. One might even wish to speak of healths in the plural to indicate the diverse views of human well-being that motivate health care from the termination of unwanted pregnancies to the achievement of various sexual lifestyles. The person who would rather have a less invasive resection for carcinoma of the large bowel (in order to avoid a colostomy) rather than the one preferred by the physician (in whose judgment the latter treatment offers a greater chance of long-range survival) engenders a dispute over the goals of health care and the composite sense of health (including physical intactness as well as chances for long-range survival) that should motivate therapeutic interventions.

Bureaucratic mechanisms for disclosure of information by physicians to patients and for the acquisition of free and informed consent are an essential part of the moral life of societies where individuals do in fact meet as strangers in the sense of not sharing the understanding and the moral commitments that often bind friends. Patients do not encounter physicians as they do religious counselors, *pace* Pellegrino.[13] One chooses a religious counselor in great measure because one shares with the counselor a rich web of moral and metaphysical commitments. However, the Southern Baptist may seek an oncologist, not because that oncologist is a fellow believer, but because of the technical abilities of the oncologist. Because physicians and the abilities of medicine are often sought for their efficaciousness as instruments toward the realization of important personal goals, conflicts arise when the goals of individuals do not accord with the value commitments of the physicians and other health care professionals. This is not a problem simply for medicine and the biomedical technologies, but for applied sciences generally, where there are conflicts between those who seek the applications of science and the scientists needed to effect the applications.

Physicians are often cast into a role analogous to those of bureaucrats in a large-scale nation. They must come to terms with the moral commitments and views of individuals from various moral communities while preserving the moral fabric of a peaceable, secular, pluralist society. It is for this reason that Hegel identified civil servants as the universal class (in contrast to this, Marx assigned the role to workers). Civil servants are committed to the general realization of freedom in the nation according to Hegel.[14] Civil servants must provide their services to citizens, whether the citizens are Orthodox Catholics, Roman Catholics, Protestants, Jews, atheists, Marxists, or zealously politically correct liberals.[15] Letter carriers must deliver mail to all on their routes and not discriminate against some on the grounds of their religious or political commitments. The post office should accept the magazines of believers and nonbelievers, magazines of erotica and pamphlets against the reading of pornography, as well as material that aggressively violates the canons of political correctness and material that endorses them. To ensure that this takes place, one may need bureaucratic rules that clearly establish in general what will be done, for whom, and under what circumstances. Physicians and other health care professionals are often in the position of civil servants, in that they must make clear to patients what will be done for them, to them, and under what circumstances. When health care professionals and patients meet as strangers, such disclosures and safeguards must frequently be explicit and often detailed. On the other hand, physicians will need to know what services they have committed themselves to provide. By entering into a particular physician–patient relationship without sufficient warning to the patient about the physician's goals and moral viewpoints, the physician may have made an implicit commitment to provide services in emergency circumstances in ways that conflict with the physician's moral commitments (e.g., a physician who has failed to make such disclosures and who cannot transfer a patient to another physician may be committed in secular morality to perform an abortion to save the life and health of a woman, even if that conflicts with the physician's particular moral commitments). The same will occur, but even in nonemergency circumstances, if the physician joins a health service committed to providing particular forms of health care (e.g., including abortion).

Something is surely lost when patients and health care professionals must meet each other through a maze of bureaucratic rules and formal systems of mutual protection. There is also the danger that such rules and formal constraints will be turned into a fetish through which governments intrude into all elements of the personal life of physicians, nurses, and patients. Such rules and regulations should exist only as protections against individuals' imposing their understandings of the good life on unwilling others. They are not to be sought for their own sake. There are also many areas into which they should not intrude, such as the private choices of individuals about themselves and their willing associates, as well as in decisions of parents regarding defective newborns, as explored in chapter 6. As Robert Burt laments in *Taking Care of Strangers,* there is a price to be paid for government by "laws not men."[16] There are many circumstances in which one should not be a merely disinterested applier of formal rules. Still, in the life lived outside communities constituted out of a common commitment to a concrete view of the good life, one needs a disinterested application of the rules to protect against misunderstandings and to guard against abuses of power.[17] In its place there is much to be gained from the rule of laws, not men.

*Medical care from passing strangers*

A great number of patients do not have personal physicians on whom they rely. They have very little, if any, experience with the idealized physician–patient relationship, often portrayed in terms of the dedicated family practitioner or general practitioner, who knows a patient and the patient's family over the span of a number of years. Instead, patients come to health maintenance organizations, public clinics, or other forms of managed care where the relationship with a particular physician or nurse is often episodic and transitory. In place of a personal physician–patient relationship, patients under such circumstances develop a health care receiver relationship with an institution rather than an individual. Even those who have a personal physician with whom they have a long-standing relationship may still find that in time of serious illness they are examined by numerous consultants. If hospitalized, they may come under the care of residents and attending physicians who rotate through a service on a monthly basis. As a result, even the most affluent patients will share in some of the experiences of the indigent who meet different physicians each time they come for treatment in a clinic or a hospital. Rules and regulations may in these circumstances give a character to an institution. They can indicate to the patient the commitments of the institution from which the patient is seeking treatment. Moreover, in the very fashioning of the rules an institution fashions its character; it comes to understand its commitments and to articulate them for those who come for care.

## Free and informed consent

The practice of free and informed consent is justified both out of respect for the freedom of individuals as well as to achieve their best interests.[18] The practice is a heterogeneous one. It involves gaining permission not only from individuals about to be treated, but also from the guardians of individuals not able to consent for themselves. The first case concerns individuals able freely to choose their own destinies and from whom authority must be gained for common endeavors. The second case concerns those who are in the authority of others.

In the case of competent individuals, one can give a set of justifications for the practice of free and informed consent: (1) it is the way of gaining permission or authority to use others; (2) it respects various views of individual dignity; (3) it endorses various values associated with the liberty or freedom of individuals; (4) it recognizes that individuals are often the best judges of their own best interests; (5) even if they are not the best judges, it acknowledges that the satisfaction of choosing freely is often preferred over having the correct choice imposed by others; and (6) it reflects the circumstance that the patient–physician relationship may often be such as to bring about a special fiduciary relationship that creates an obligation to disclose information. One can thus give justifications for the practices of free and informed consent on the basis of the principles of permission and beneficence. This complex justification leads to moral tensions, since individuals often competently choose in ways contrary to their own best interests. The same obtains in true proxy consent. If an individual appoints a proxy to choose, either according to specific instructions or according to the general instruction, "Do whatever you want," the second individual is a moral extension of the authority of the first. Here one may encounter conflicts between respecting the capricious choices of the designated proxy and securing the best interests of the ward.

Most de facto guardians do not act on the basis of formal advance directives that convey moral authority to and offer instruction to guide a proxy's choice. They are rather next-of-kin who find themselves in the position of needing to make a treatment decision for an incompetent family member. Only a small portion of patients has completed advance directives and those who have have often done so with incomplete instructions to their proxies.[19] Further, when guardians speak on behalf of individuals who have never been competent or who did not, while competent, leave instructions or convey authority to others, the place of the guardian is radically different from an appointed proxy.[20]

Such guardians are not the extension of another individual's freedom. Instead, they may be in authority over their ward as a parent is over an infant by virtue of either having produced that individual or through some moral equivalent of indentured servitude that arises through a minor's receiving parental support while not seeking emancipation. One might think here of parents refusing treatment for their severely defective newborn on grounds of hopelessness, or cosmetic surgery for their ten-year-old child on religious grounds. In addition, such guardians may be in authority to choose particular understandings of an individual's best interests in terms of the values embraced by the community within which the ward lives and to which, it can often be presumed, the ward will or would subscribe. One might think here of Jewish parents requesting that their son be circumcised. Or the guardian may be an authority regarding the incompetent individual's proclivities, interests, and wishes. As such, the guardian becomes a substitute for an expert regarding what would have been the content of directions under an advance directive. One asks the guardian how that individual would want to be treated with the presumption that the guardian may aid in choosing the treatment the individual would have found most appropriate. The guardian attempts to reconstruct what that individual would want. Guardians may at times simply play the role of making needed choices by selecting options from the range of what is acceptable to rational and prudent persons within a particular society when an incompetent individual has left no instructions and is not integrated within a special particular content-full community (e.g., is a devout Christian Scientist). Here one might imagine someone choosing among different treatment options for a ward.

Most proxy choice is made informally without benefit of either a formal advance directive or legislative instruction.[21] Moreover, there are grounds to prefer informal approaches, which can be better adapted to particular clinical needs, as long as there is the possibility of formal oversight. Thus, the Society of Critical Care Medicine states,

Institutions should establish procedures for decision-making for patients without decision-making capacity who are isolated and who lack identified, appropriate surrogates. The procedures should include ethics committee consultation. The goal should be to establish mechanisms so that courts need not routinely be involved.[22]

Indeed, the same statement recommended

If no relatives are available and willing to participate, close associates of the patient should be consulted. These include persons who are available, have been involved with and concerned about the patient, are knowledgeable about the patient's values and preferences, and are willing to apply the patient's values to making the decision.[23]

In all these matters, it is important to recognize that there is evidence that proxy decision makers (including physicians acting on behalf of patients) are poor judges of what patients would really have wanted.[24] As a consequence, the choice of a surrogate decision maker can only up to a point be justified in terms of who is a reliable authority regarding a patient's past wishes. More fundamentally, the status of surrogate decision makers must depend on being placed in authority to make decisions regarding a patient. To gain authorization and to avoid acting without permission or contrary to an individual's wishes, it must be made clear in advance who is likely to be invoked as a surrogate decision maker and under what circumstance.

Proxy consent embraces a composite of practices: (1) the choice by an authorized agent on behalf of an authorizing individual; (2) the choice by parents (or their assignees) on behalf of infants they have produced; (3) the choice by guardians on behalf of unemancipated minors whom they are rearing; (4) the choice by guardians or proxies in terms of the best interests of another as understood within a particular moral community; (5) the choice by a guardian or proxies in terms of the best interests of another as understood with reference to what a rational and prudent person would choose within a particular society; and (6) the choice by guardians or proxies in terms of what that particular person would have wanted.[25] Since proxy or surrogate decision makers are poor judges of the wishes of those for whom they act, it is best to acquire the authority for proxies through their explicit appointment or through their appointment by practices which involve the conveyal of authority or permission to act. Here it is important to note that permission or conveyal of authority can occur by agreeing to enter a practice or institution.

Consider the practice or institution of marriage, which bundles a vast set of consents, permissions, and agreements, and whose secular moral validity does not depend on an explicit rehearsal of the benefits, risks, and range of understandings. Rather, one is put on notice in any society that marriage is a rich and many-faceted institution, which includes the assumption of complex rights and duties, as well as permission to be touched and to be used. In addition, within particular communities, including religious communities, there are special and often asymmetrical relationships created between the husband and wife. To enter into such an institution is to have agreed to accept its obligations. In general secular moral terms, there is no basis to forbid such institutions from putting the burden to be informed on those who enter. Thus, one can imagine the warning, "If you want to get married, be careful to understand the significance of the institution into which you are entering. As with the French Foreign Legion, it is best to be clear as to the status you are acquiring before it is too late." So, too, warnings may be given to would-be patients, "Be on notice. If you have not appointed a guardian or proxy and enter our hospital or enroll in our insurance program, we will consider that you have accepted our practices for appointing guardians and proxy decision makers." We will return to some of these issues later in this chapter.

The various practices of free and informed consent raise questions about what constitutes informed choice (e.g., how likely does a risk need to be to warrant disclosing it to a patient—one chance out of a thousand, a hundred thousand, a million?), who is competent to choose, who is free to choose (e.g., when may adolescents choose their own medical treatment?), who is in authority to choose on behalf of another (e.g., as a designated proxy or through a status such as being a parent), and who is a good judge of the best interests of others (e.g., are parents any better judges of the best interests of their children than dispassionate outsiders?). We will need to examine the rights of individuals to determine their own treatment and the circumstances under which they may determine the medical treatment of others.

## The right to be left alone

One of the ancient presumptions of English law is that individuals should be secure in their bodies against the unauthorized touching of others.[26] This right to the forbearance of others has its roots in ancient pagan Germanic traditions.[27] The presumption against unauthorized touching in the law extends to interventions by physicians from at least the eighteenth century. One finds in a 1767 decision, *Slater v. Baker and Stapleton,* that "it is reasonable that a patient should be told what is about to be done to him, that he may take courage and put himself in such a situation as to enable him to undergo the operation."[28] This decision is not grounded in a view of the patient as the source of authority, but rather in concerns regarding why it would be *useful* to gain consent. However, a bold finding in favor of the patient's right to consent to and refuse treatment based on the patient as the source of authority is found in Justice Cardozo's 1914 opinion in *Schloendorff v. Society of N.Y. Hospital:* "every human being of adult years and sound mind has a right to determine what shall be done with his own body; and a surgeon who performs an operation without his patient's consent commits an assault, for which he is liable in damages.''[29] This opinion can be taken as setting the character of the debate about free and informed consent. The opinion strongly underscores the right of individuals to consent to treatment. Yet it qualifies this right by acknowledging it only in individuals of sound mind and adult years. As we shall see, it was not easy for the courts to accept this right without qualification even for competent adults.

The right to free and informed consent in its most foundational sense within general secular morality includes (1) the right to give uncoerced, undeceived, competent consent to participate in treatment, as well as (2) the right to withdraw from treatment in whole or in part. *Slater v. Baker and Stapleton* underscores free and informed consent as a means for better collaboration between physician and patient in order to secure more effective treatment of the patient. It is only later that the would-be patient's consent as a source of moral authority becomes more central. Justice Cardozo's ruling in *Schloendorff* underscores the role of the patient's consent as the source of authority. This theme becomes prominent in twentieth-century reflections on individual rights and is at times captured simply as the general right to be left alone. One might think here in particular of the dissent written by Justice Brandeis in *Olmstead v. United States:*

The makers of our Constitution . . . sought to protect Americans in their beliefs, their thoughts, their emotions and their sensations. They conferred, as against the Government, the right to be let alone—the most comprehensive of rights and the right most valued by civilized men.[30]

Both Brandeis's opinion and Cardozo's decision raise the issue of whether one need respect all decisions of individuals or only those that appear sound and well reasoned. Need one respect the decisions of competent individuals, even if the decisions themselves appear foolish and ill reasoned? If a decision is competent or authority-conveying only if it is well reasoned from well-established, firm premises, the range of patient wishes to be respected will be markedly restricted. If a decision is competent because it is the free choice of a competent individual (i.e., an individual who generally understands and appreciates the circumstances of the world and the general significance of the decision at hand), then the range of decisions that must be expected will be much greater.

This issue reaches into health care decisions generally. Individuals who hold that the existence of God should be accepted by all rational individuals may conclude that medical and other decisions made on nontheistic presumptions are irrational, moved by passion, prejudice, and ignorance. On the other hand, individuals who do not recognize God's existence or the proper content given through religious faith may conclude that medical decisions made on such theistic presumptions are irrational. This issue was addressed by Chief Justice Warren Burger while a member of the Circuit Court of the District of Columbia when he wrote a dissenting opinion to the denial of a petition for rehearing a request by a woman wishing to refuse a lifesaving blood transfusion on religious grounds. Justice Burger developed his opinion as a gloss on Brandeis's dissent in *Olmstead:*

Nothing in this utterance suggests that Justice Brandeis thought an individual possessed these rights only as to *sensible* beliefs, *valid* thoughts, *reasonable* emotions, or *well-founded* sensations. I suggest he intended to include a great many foolish, unreasonable and even absurd ideas which do not conform, such as refusing medical treatment even at great risk.[31]

According to Burger, individuals should be acknowledged to have the authority to refuse treatment, even if their choices are based on premises and understandings of the world that most would judge to be wrong and foolish.

The principle of permission gives a foundation for a right to be left alone, a right of privacy, a right to refuse the touchings and interventions of others. This right is central to the very notion of a peaceable community bound together by mutual respect as the use of others only with their permission. It sets a boundary against the interventions of others in the sense that they must show their authority to constrain the actions of other moral agents. The sense of this right has been captured in legal decisions that have affirmed the right both to consent and to refuse treatment. The court in *Natanson v. Kline,* for example, gives what is both a gloss on and a development of Cardozo's rule in *Schloendorff:*

Anglo-American law starts with the premise of thorough-going self determination. It follows that each man is considered to be master of his own body, and he may, if he be of sound mind, expressly prohibit the performance of life-saving surgery, or other medical treatment.[32]

The court endorsed a right to be left alone.

To justify successfully in secular moral terms the right to be left alone in one's choices, one need only show that the choice does not involve unconsented-to force against the innocent and that the choice is one of a moral agent: a rational, self-conscious individual, who freely chooses a particular action or omission. To be a choice made by such an agent, the content of the choice need not be rationally grounded or argued for. It is sufficient if the individual understands and appreciates the general circumstances of the choice and in this sense affirms and endorses it. It will be enough if the choice is embraced by the agent within a general context in which choices are freely made and within which the chooser can at least advance the following justification: "I enjoy choosing capriciously, even about risky matters." Such a choice must be one for which the agent knowingly takes responsibility and is responsible. In this sense a choice is a competent choice because it flows from an accountable and therefore competent agent, even if that agent has chosen to choose poorly.

This analysis takes seriously the circumstance that moral agents often choose willfully. They choose in ways that are perverse and morally improper, not simply out of intellectual error, as many ancient Greeks as well as Scholastics thought, but because of a desire to be free of others, and for the immediate exhilaration of breaking free from constraints. Etymologically, capricious actions are goatlike actions. Moral agents at times choose undisciplined frolicking over the careful reflections of a systematically analyzed life. This sense of rebellion for its own sake is captured in the classic statement of Satan's sinful choice in Milton's *Paradise Lost,* "Evil be thou my Good" (4.110). Freedom to choose includes as well the freedom to commit oneself to a particular belief no matter how absurd, or even because it is absurd. One might think here of the phrase, at times attributed to Tertullian, "I believe because it is absurd" (Credo quia absurdum est).[33] The fact that religious individuals commit themselves to beliefs that transcend reason or even conflict with reason does not impeach the competency of the individuals or their right to have their choices respected. The fact that some individuals' choices are for others troublesome, bizarre, and tragic does not of itself mean that one may use force to stop them.

## Three senses of freedom

The notion of choosing freely in free and informed consent includes at least three senses of freedom: (1) being able to choose, (2) being unrestrained by prior commitments or justified authority, and (3) being free from coercion.[34]

FREEDOM TO CHOOSE. For valid consent, the agent must be free in the sense of being able to choose freely as a moral agent. The individual must be able to understand and appreciate the meaning and consequences of the contemplated actions so as to be imputable and responsible for those actions. Given the priority of the principle of permission, all entities that appear as moral agents must be presumed to act with authority over themselves, that is, to be free, unless there is evidence to the contrary. The requirement of understanding and appreciating the significance of one's action is no more than the requirement that the behavior be an action, a behavior undertaken by a moral agent, rather than simply caused by neurological and psychological processes. Choices that fail to meet this by no means severe test include behaviors of the acutely psychotic, the severely senile, the very young, the very drunk, the delirious, at times the very neurotic, and others who are not able to understand their own behaviors or to require others to respect them in the pursuit of their goals.

Even such individuals may be able from time to time to make competent decisions. To borrow a phrase from Heinz Hartmann, there are islands of ego autonomy. Some of these islands may be above the water only at low tide but be completely inundated by the high tides of stress and illness. One must avoid judging individuals to be either fully competent or incompetent. Different individuals in different times and circumstances will be competent or incompetent in different areas and to different degrees.[35] Competence, the ability to understand and appreciate the consequences of one's actions, and thus also the responsibility for one's actions, is neither a global nor a binary phenomenon. However, while partial incompetence may partially excuse, partial competence can be an absolute moral bar against the interventions of others insofar as there is an understanding and appreciation of the significance of refusing such interventions.

UNRESTRAINED BY PRIOR COMMITMENTS OR JUSTIFIED AUTHORITY. There is a second sense of freedom at stake as well: that of being unencumbered by preempting commitments to others. The very freedom of persons allows them to give or barter away their freedom to choose in general and with regard to health care in particular. A requirement for joining an army might be ceding the right to refuse vaccinations, surgical procedures, and other treatments required to maintain battle readiness. In such forms of indentured servitude, individuals transfer to others a right that was theirs. As we noted in chapter 4, something of this sort occurs in the relationship of children with their parents. By accepting parental support and failing to emancipate themselves, children may accept their parents as prima facie authorities regarding their medical best interests. Parents may also make commitments to their children that will preclude the parents' refusal of lifesaving treatment for themselves.

This last issue was raised in the case that occasioned Warren Burger's gloss on Brandeis's dissent in *Olmstead*. The Circuit Court of Appeals of the District of Columbia denied the patient's request to refuse transfusion because, among other reasons, her death would lead her to abandoning her seven-month-old child.[36] One should note that in another case the fact that a parent had financially provided for his children's well-being defeated this consideration.[37] The extent to which being a parent leads to an obligation to support the child will vary from community to community, as will the opportunities to transfer the obligation to other individuals or the community in general. One might note that there are in fact groups who force children to fend for themselves at very early ages. Here the Ik, who were mentioned in chapter 2, may again serve as an example. Ik children are put out of the home and begin to forage for themselves in groups at the age of about three or four.[38]

By committing a crime one may also lose the right to refuse treatment; thus, prisoners in general or those awaiting execution in particular may as a part of their punishment lose the right to refuse treatment. Their commission of the crime would count as their ceding their right to refuse treatment and being kept alive may be part of their punishment. This and other cases show that individuals who are free to consent in the sense of being competent may not be free to choose about themselves because they are restrained by prior commitments or the valid authority of others (e.g., that of parents, military officers, and prison wardens).

FREEDOM FROM COERCION. Finally, even if individuals are able to choose freely and are free of prior constraints, they may still find themselves in coercive circumstances. Since the very fabric of secular morality depends on not using persons without their permission, any agreements extracted under coercion will not be binding. The person who employs coercion to secure an agreement cannot consistently appeal to the notion of a moral community to claim that the person coerced ought to be forthcoming. Valid consent must be acquired without the use of tactics that reduce the consenting individual to a mere means, that is, that set their consent aside. Thus, not only outright threats of violence but deception, threats to break contracts, or the failure to provide information owed will count as unconsented-to and unjustified force against the innocent. Such interventions are forbidden because they violate the principle of permission that supports the minimal notion of the peaceable community. It follows the grounding of secular morality in the authorizing permission of persons that force, deception, and breach of contract are not wrong in and of themselves. They are wrong only when they are used against the unconsenting innocent. Those who employ unjustified force cannot consistently complain when others defend themselves with whatever means necessary, from force of arms to deception.[39] Since in most cases patients must be considered innocent persons, the use of force in medicine is usually forbidden. Still, the use of force or deception is morally justified in order to control a patient who is without warrant threatening health professionals.

One will need in medicine, as in everyday life, to distinguish between acts of coercion and those of peaceful manipulation. If one understands coercive actions as those that place or threaten to place a patient in a disadvantaged state without justification, and if one defines peaceable manipulation as those actions that place or offer to place a patient in an advantaged state to which the patient is not entitled, coercions will be forbidden and peaceable manipulations will be allowed. The first violates the morality of mutual respect grounded in permission by violating the free choice of innocent persons, but the second does not. In fact, peaceable manipulations undergird the very process of peaceable negotiation through which individuals fashion peaceable agreements. People become friends, lovers, marriage partners, in part at least because they please, delight, and satisfy each other.[40] Any and all incentives will in principle be permissible in secular morality, from offering financial inducements and honors to sexual satisfaction and other carnal pleasures, as long as the offer or maneuver does not make rational choice impossible.[41] One may wish in certain communities to avoid particular forms of excessive offers or offers of a particular sort. However, there will not be general arguments to show that such are in principle wrong through violating the very notion of mutual respect, as long as the individual being manipulated can still act, that is, choose, and be held responsible.

Nor will it be possible to understand power differentials as invalidating consent. Imagine the freshman medical student who falls deeply in love with the senior resident in dermatology after she gives a lecture on skin rashes as part of a clinical coordination session integrated into the first semester histology course. Imagine also that the resident has no grading responsibilities for the student, only a chance to give an impressive presentation regarding inflammation of the skin. Can the freshman medical student in general secular moral terms validly consent to sexual dalliance with the resident? Has the thirty-year-old resident taken unfair advantage of the twenty-one-year-old medical student? Are matters changed if the student is eighteen and a day? What if the student is at the undergraduate campus next door? There appears to be no way to regard such differences in power as invalidating consent, at least in general secular terms. The only issue will be whether the student can still knowingly give permission under such circumstances. After all, the twenty-one-year-old student, or indeed the eighteen-year-old student, is accepted as being able to consent validly to dropping out of school, to joining the Marines, the French Foreign Legion, or a Buddhist monastery in Nepal. On the other hand, if the medical school or college is Roman Catholic, it has the secular moral right peaceably to act on its own content-full vision of proper sexual deportment by forbidding its faculty to fornicate with students (or, indeed, with anyone) as a condition of employment. Of course, if the resident's (and the student's) intentions are honorable, all can be resolved by marriage. Once one steps outside of the context of such content-full and structured understandings, one encounters vain and often ludicrous mental gymnastics in the service of assembling shreds of intuitions in order to establish certain consensual carnal conversations as morally illicit. Without a canonical understanding of proper sexual behavior or acceptable inducements, all one can require is that permission be competently given in the absence of coercion. *Mutatis mutandi,* the same is the case regarding general constraints on free choices in health care.

Though the distinction between coercions and peaceable manipulations may on the surface appear clear cut, this is far from the case. As Robert Nozick and others have indicated, what may appear at first to be a peaceable manipulation may under closer examination be shown to be a hidden form of coercion.[42] If, for example, a physician knowingly exaggerates risks and by such deception unduly frightens a patient so that the patient will agree to the form of treatment offered by the physician, coercion has been employed. So, too, if a physician threatens to withdraw promised supportive treatment unless the patient agrees to a particular intervention, which the physician deems to be indicated, coercion is involved. Either instance would be an example of the physician's placing the patient in a disadvantaged circumstance through a form of unconsented-to force (in the first case through force of words, i.e., deception, and in the second case through a threatened breach of contract).[43] These considerations lead to the question of how much information is owed to a patient so that the patient can validly consent.

*Three senses of being informed*

The ability of patients to choose with effective liberty will depend on how much patients know about the likely benefits and risks of the treatment they are considering and its alternatives. Depending on what physicians or other health care professionals disclose to a patient, and how it is disclosed, the patient will be inclined to refuse or to accept a treatment. A physician can make the use of almost any drug appear ill advised, if not risky. For example, the published warnings concerning penicillin include possible fatal allergic reactions, as well as hemolytic anemia, leukopenia, and neuropathies. If the likelihood of these risks is not put in terms of the likelihood of the benefits, a patient may decline a lifesaving treatment.

It is for this last reason that physicians have traditionally been concerned about the disclosure of too much or the wrong information to patients. The fear has been that, as strangers in an alien land, patients are likely to miscalculate the prudent balance of benefits and risks and as a result decline a treatment that would likely be effective with few real costs. Medicine in particular and health care in general are goal-oriented undertakings. They are focused on curing and preventing diseases and on caring for the worries, pains, and anxieties of patients. Only in very particular circumstances has medicine been focused on increasing the freedom of individuals to choose.[44] As the court in *Nishi v. Hartwell* affirmed, "The doctor's primary duty is to do what is best for the patient. Any conflict between this duty and that of a frightening disclosure ordinarily should be resolved in favor of the primary duty."[45]

This dedication to choosing and effecting the best treatment for the patient leads to collisions with the wishes of the patient to understand the nature and risk of treatment. Moreover, the dedication is not a purely altruistic one. Disclosures to patients can be time-consuming and vexatious, in addition to perhaps foreclosing the choice of the treatment deemed best by the physician. These various conflicts of interest between physicians and patients reach into the beginnings of Western medicine. Consider the description given by Plato of the difference in the amount of information disclosed to freemen and slaves.

*Athenian:* . . . You agree that there are those two types of so-called physicians?
*Clinias:* Certainly I do.
*Athenian:* Now have you observed that, as there are slaves as well as free men this kind never gives a servant any account of his complaint, nor asks him for any; he gives him some empirical injunction with an air of finished knowledge, in the brusque fashion of a dictator, and then is off in hot haste to the next ailing servant—that is how he lightens his master's medical labors for him. The free practitioner, who, for the most part, attends free men, treats their disease by going into things thoroughly from the beginning in a scientific way, and takes the patient and his family into his confidence. Thus he learns something from the sufferer, and at the same time instructs the invalid to the best of his power. He does not give his prescriptions until he has won the patient's support, and when he has

done so, he steadily aims at producing complete restoration to health by persuading the sufferer into compliance.[46] (*Laws* 4.720b–e)

Plato endorses a form of respect he takes to be due to free individuals. He also indicates that apart from any consideration of mutual respect, it may be useful to provide patients and their families with that amount of information that will allow patients to be effective collaborators in their treatment. Seen in this light, Plato offers a critique of the attitude of many physicians: informing patients is time-consuming and often complicates effective treatment.

The more difficult issue is coming to terms with patients' demands to know, not simply in order better to cooperate with their physicians, but so that they may choose for themselves, even if those choices undermine what physicians hold to be the best or the most effective therapeutic approach. To what extent are physicians bound to disclose information when they believe that such disclosures are not likely to be useful in the treatment of the patient? One should note here that the right to consent is not equivalent to the right to be informed. Innocent, free individuals have a right not to be forced into being the patients of physicians. But do they have a right to become patients on their terms rather than on the physician's terms? Why may not a physician state, "In return for treatment, you [the patient] must agree to be content with whatever information I judge to be in your best interests"?

Such demands by physicians will not violate the morality of mutual respect. Such demands may be contrary to certain cultural ideals of promoting individual autonomy or encouraging individuals to see themselves, and to be regarded by others, as self-determining. They may increase risks of fraud and duress on the part of physicians and be in violation of legal requirements. They may fail to encourage self-scrutiny on the part of physicians and rational decision making on the part of patients.[47] However, physicians and would-be patients as free individuals may count the goods to be pursued through limited disclosures to outweigh such possible harms. Moreover, patients will always be free to band together and hire physicians whom they can require to provide disclosures to the liking of the would-be patients.

The attempt to articulate the proper balance between physicians' interests in effectively and successfully treating patients versus patient and societal concerns for self-determination has led to various legal standards for sufficient disclosure, each reflecting a particular moral vision. Although there are serious questions to be raised about the authority of the state to impose a particular test for disclosure, the different standards offer concrete portrayals of possible compromises between competing goals and interests.

THE PROFESSIONAL STANDARD. The traditional approach in the law has been to presume that patients should receive that amount of information usually provided by physicians in their community. Physicians were required to make those disclosures of information "which a reasonable medical practitioner would make under the same or similar circumstances."[48] This standard was defended on the grounds that only a physician can accurately determine (1) what amount of disclosure will not have an adverse effect on the patient so as to jeopardize treatment, and (2) what information is actually relevant to the patient's choice. As the Supreme Court of Missouri held in 1965,

> The question is not what, regarding the risks involved, the juror would relate to the patient under the same or similar circumstances, or even what a reasonable man would relate, but what a reasonable medical practitioner would do. Such practitioner would consider the state of the patient's health, the condition of his heart and nervous system, his mental state, and would take into account, among other things, whether the risks involved were mere remote possibilities or something which occurred with some sort of frequency or regularity. This determination involves medical judgment as to whether disclosure of possible risks may have such an adverse effect on the patient as to jeopardize success of the proposed therapy, no matter how expertly performed. . . . After a consideration of these and other proper factors, a reasonable medical practitioner, under some circumstances, would make full disclosure of all risk which had any reasonable likelihood of occurring, but in others the facts and circumstances would dictate a guarded or limited disclosure. In some cases the judgment would be less difficult than in others, but in any event, it would be a medical judgment.[49]

In short, the use of the professional standard was justified on the grounds that the decision about the amount of information disclosed is a medical judgment, one requiring expert knowledge.

Although one might dispute, as other courts have, whether such a judgment is a medical judgment, one can morally defend the professional standard in terms of the principle of mutual respect. Unless otherwise warned, patients may reasonably expect that practitioners will give that amount of disclosure customary for members of that profession, school, or group (e.g., as is given by family practitioners, Jungian psychoanalysts, members of the Libertarian Medical Society, or the association of paternalistic physicians). To give less than that amount of disclosure without prior warning would constitute a form of deception. It may also breach a duty the practitioner has regarding the patient to the profession, school, or group of which the practitioner is a member. To give more than a reasonable medical practitioner would give may presuppose a hierarchy of values different from that endorsed by the profession or school. Such an increased disclosure might require a special warning to the patient of the following sort (appropriately expanded and altered): "I am willing to tell you things that most members of my profession [school or group] hold ought not to be disclosed. The risks of the disclosure are likely to be useless anxiety and worry, all of which may even adversely affect your health. Do you want to hear the information?"

Unless individuals have taken steps to create special expectations and/or special requirements, the professional standard meets the principles of permission and beneficence. It does not violate the morality of mutual respect, as long as the patient knows of the general limits on disclosure. If it is pursued in a reasonable and well-intentioned fashion, the professional standard is also an example of an endeavor to achieve the good of others. The difficulty is that many individuals value self-determination and autonomy more than they do a worry–free and efficient treatment of their diseases. They may value freedom so highly that they will become anxious if they are not allowed to be self-determining. In addition, they may judge that only they can anticipate the likely significance for their lives of different therapeutic choices with their possibly adverse significance. Since there is an important difference between freedom as a value and freedom as a side constraint, the proper ranking to be given to free and informed choice is more to be created than discovered.

In a society where the state does not overstep its secular moral authority, individuals will be able to band together to insure health care consonant with their own moral commitments and other value concerns, including their own views of the proper standard for disclosure in informed consent. Thus, one can imagine the following international health care systems with contracting physicians and hospitals: International Orthodox Jewish Health Care, Papal Magisterial Care, Yuppie International Wellness Cooperatives, Sado-Masochistic Medical Care, Bathhouses International. Each could allow would-be patients to contract into special, content-full standards of disclosure. These health care systems could develop particular practices for the appointment of guardians and proxies. They could fashion their own understandings of futile treatment (i.e., when treatment will be withheld as likely to be "unproductive") and procedures for rationing resources. This is the most defensible approach in the face of moral diversity and limited state secular moral power. When patients band together, they wield economic power that will allow them peaceably to manipulate the compliance of physicians and hospitals, unless all are overborne by the coercive intrusions of the state.

THE OBJECTIVE STANDARD. For more than a decade courts in the United States have been departing from the professional standard in favor of a standard of disclosure based on a duty to explain to a patient the procedure about to be undertaken and "to warn him of any material risks or dangers inherent in or collateral to the therapy, so as to enable the patient to make an intelligent and informed choice about whether or not to undergo such treatment."[50] In order for a patient to make such intelligent, informed choices, it becomes the duty of physicians to acquaint patients with all material risks, where a material risk is understood as a risk that, as the court in *Canterbury v. Spence* held, "a reasonable person, in what the physician knows or should know to be the patient's position, would be likely to attach significance to in deciding whether or not to forego the proposed therapy."[51] The standard for disclosure thus became the need of the reasonable and prudent person for information.

The scope of the physician's communications to the patient, then, must be measured by the patient's need, and that need is whatever is material to the decision. Thus, the test for determining whether a potential peril must be divulged is its materiality to the patient's decision.[52]

Because this standard depends not on what would influence a particular individual, but what would influence reasonable and prudent individuals, it can be termed an objective standard. Instead of relying on the particular subjective concerns of a particular individual, one is to make disclosures on

an objective basis: in terms of what a prudent person in the patient's position would have decided if suitably informed of all perils bearing significance. If adequate disclosure could reasonably be expected to have caused that person to decline the treatment because of the revelation of the kind of risk or danger that resulted in harm, causation is shown, but otherwise not.[53]

These court decisions have made the standard for disclosure that amount of information necessary for the effective choice of a reasonable and prudent person, rather than that amount of information necessary for achieving what would be in the profession's view effective treatment.

This departure from using the judgment of reasonable members of the professional community as the standard to that of reasonable and prudent individuals can be justified if the medical profession is under the moral authority of society. However, in the absence of specific agreements and understandings, that is not the case. Members of a profession are as much entitled to their views regarding proper standards of disclosure as are members of the general public. Moreover, there is no socially or historically unconditioned, atemporal notion of a reasonable and prudent person. Such concepts are in fact always dependent on the particular values of a particular community. A reasonable compromise between the two viewpoints is to be achieved, if at all, through negotiation. Even before the use of the objective standard, the professional standard could be seen as a point of departure for agreements that could bind physicians to make disclosures by an objective or subjective standard.

THE SUBJECTIVE STANDARD. A commitment to certain values of self-determination can lead not only to an objective standard, but also to arguing that physicians should supply whatever information is material to a particular individual's choices. If a patient had a neurotic concern about developing cancer or becoming paralyzed, a physician would be obliged to provide information on these risks, even if they were so remote that they would not count as material considerations for a reasonable and prudent person. Alexander Capron sees the possibility of interpreting the standard embraced in *Cobbs v. Grant* as a subjective standard, since the court held that the physician's duty to provide information ''must be measured by the patient's need, and that need is whatever information is material to the decision.''[54] At law, such an interpretation would constitute a severe burden for physicians who would need to show they had satisfied the worries of particular patients. There would always be the temptation for a patient to consider after the fact that the physician had not dealt with all of the patient's special concerns.

This standard has been embraced in criticism of the objective standard enunciated in *Canterbury v. Spence*.

We therefore hold the scope of a physician's communications must be measured by his patient's need to know enough to enable him to make an intelligent choice. . . . A risk is material if it would be likely to affect a patient's decision. . . . Although the Canterbury rule is probably that of the majority, its "reasonable man" approach has been criticized by some commentators as backtracking on its own theory of self-determination. The Canterbury view certainly severely limits the protection granted an injured patient. To the extent the plaintiff, given an adequate disclosure, would have declined the proposed treatment, and a reasonable person in similar circumstances would have consented, a patient's right of self-determination is irrevocably lost.[55]

This position has been recognized as subjective and depending on what is material to the particular person who need not be a reasonable and prudent person. "Thus, because what is material to a patient's decision is subjective to each patient, objective or general professional standards are ineffective to determine the scope of the physician's duty to obtain an informed consent in a given case."[56]

Even if one concluded on pragmatic grounds that this is not a standard to use in the courts, one might still embrace it as a moral ideal within particular autonomy-oriented views of the good life. If one is concerned with autonomy more than successful treatment, a subjective standard will be morally attractive. Or one might also hold that individuals can effectively choose so as to maximize their best interests, even if they are in part based on special or even neurotic concerns, only if they can determine their own treatment. One might hope that individual physicians would ascertain the special worries and concerns of patients and then disclose to those patients enough information for them to make choices in terms of their special concerns. This would allow even neurotic patients to choose effectively within the context of their obsessions. The extent to which one would see this as desirable would depend on one's comparative ranking of the value and usefulness of self-determination versus objective or professional determinations of effective treatment.

One should realize that the professional standard did not in principle foreclose giving that amount of information that a reasonable and prudent person would want or that a particular patient with special concerns would want. The professional standard was rather premised on the fact that the disclosure of such information was often in fact detrimental to the effective treatment and to the good of the patient, and that it thus ought not to be provided.

THE RIGHT NOT TO BE INFORMED. In developing the objective standard for disclosure, a special subjectively grounded moral exception must be incorporated. Particular patients, if they decline such knowledge, need not be told what rational and prudent individuals (within a particular community with its own particular moral vision) usually need to know in order to make a reasonable decision. Both *Cobbs v. Grant* and *Sard v. Hardy,* for example, explicitly underscore that a physician is not obliged to disclose risks when the patient requests not to be informed.[57] The right to be informed is not an obligation to be informed. Nor does it create an overriding obligation on the part of the physician to inform. It rather requires offering to the patient the opportunity to acquire information. Here again respect of freedom serves as a side constraint, not a value. The goal of free and informed consent should not be to force patients to be autonomous, but rather to afford them the opportunity to be autonomous in their choice of medical treatment.

This underscores the circumstance that different individuals seek different sorts of physician–patient relationships. Some wish to be full collaborators in their treatment, if not directly in control of it. Such individuals see physicians as agents of their already well formed wishes. For such individuals anything but a robust subjective standard of full disclosure may be too weak. On the other hand, many wish to entrust their care to a physician in whom they have faith. Such individuals wish last and least of all to be obliged to listen to all the risks and possible harms to which they may be subjected. They would rather repose their confidence in their initial choice of a physician and see the physician's major duty to be that of shouldering the fears, anxieties, and hesitations that go with making important choices in circumstances of uncertainty. The opportunity to waive disclosure allows patients to fashion a relationship with physicians that will meet the patients' needs. It allows patients to request that the standard of disclosure be the professional standard or one that provides even less information than the reasonable and prudent physician would offer. But what if the physician deems that it is in the patient's best interests to have certain material disclosed anyway? May the physician require the patient to agree to the disclosure as a condition for treatment? Despite the constraints of the law, the physician in secular morality should possess that right in terms of the principles of beneficence and permission, unless the physician through prior agreement has waived the right to require disclosure as the condition for treatment, or has failed to warn the patient in advance of these sorts of requirements so that the patient can engage a different physician.

These matters evoke a special conflict when a well-liberated ecumenical cosmopolitan physician encounters a patient from a traditional society who expects others to make the crucial decisions. Imagine that an affluent widow, a member of the Syrian Oriental Orthodox Church, flies from Damascus with her successful businessman thirty-year-old firstborn son to have a coronary bypass operation performed in a hospital established on a Caribbean island (founded subsequent to

American health care "reform" in order to evade draconian governmental controls), the Adam Smith Memorial Luxury Quaternary Health Care Center. The woman says firmly and with conviction: "God answered my prayer and gave me a son. Let him now answer all your inane questions." The hospital is surely at moral liberty to design a consent form that reads something like the following:

I, ———, appoint ——— as my agent to make any and all health care decisions for me while I am competent or incompetent, except to the extent I state otherwise in this document. I reserve the right to revoke this appointment at any time. Until the revocation of this document, my agent should be given full information concerning my medical condition and concerning the character and nature of contemplated treatment. My agent will have full authority to consent to or refuse treatment on my behalf. It has been explained to me that there are serious risks and dangers in appointing another to speak on my behalf. Understanding these risks full well, I still make this appointment.

Although within particular moralities and visions of how moral agents should take command of their own lives such an appointment may be regarded as inappropriate or immoral, in general secular terms the hospital is at liberty to use such forms.

THE THERAPEUTIC PRIVILEGE. Even court rulings that have upheld the objective standard have recognized circumstances when the disclosure of information would so distress a patient as to make rational choice impossible or in fact seriously to harm the patient. In *Canterbury v. Spence,* for example, the court recognized that "patients occasionally became so ill or emotionally distraught on disclosure as to foreclose a rational decision, or complicate or hinder the treatment, or perhaps even pose psychological damage to the patient."[58] In such circumstances physicians were not to be bound by the objective standard but rather the disclosure could be limited to

that required within the medical community when a doctor can prove by a preponderance of the evidence he relied on facts which would demonstrate to a reasonable man the disclosure would have so seriously upset the patient that the patient would not have been able to dispassionately weigh the risks of refusing to undergo the recommended treatment.[59]

In taking this position the court affirmed a view already developed in the literature,[60] namely, that disclosures that seriously alarm the patient could in fact constitute bad medical practice.[61]

The therapeutic privilege can be interpreted as a form of emergency. Physicians have generally been excused from gaining consent in emergency circumstances when delaying to obtain such consent would lead to death or significant permanent bodily and perhaps mental harm.[62] Instead, they have been allowed to provide that form of treatment that is medically required to save life and limb or avoid permanent bodily harm. Bona fide cases in which the therapeutic privilege is invoked are similar to emergencies if the patient is not able to be consulted because communicating the requisite information would itself make the required choice impossible (i.e., the communication would so distress the patient that competent choice would be impossible). Unless there were some prior agreement or disclosure, the physician may in good conscience provide care according to the standards of the profession, even though it may later become clear that the patient would have wished to be treated differently. If the disclosure is likely to harm the patient, one may similarly presume that the patient would not in fact wish to be harmed, and thus garner a moral justification for the use of the therapeutic privilege.

Moral problems surface if one highly values freedom. Those passionately interested in self-determination may wish to have full disclosure, even if it is likely to harm them. They may value their opportunity to be autonomous more highly than a long life or freedom from pain, deformity, and disability. From a moral point of view, such patients should be free to make agreements with willing physicians to be informed no matter what. Such patients should be able to waive the benefits of the therapeutic privilege.

PLACEBOS AND BENEFICENT DECEPTIONS. There are many circumstances under which individuals implicitly consent to minor deceptions. They may simply be seeking reassurance, even against and despite the facts. We often need a gentle hand that will assure and not necessarily remind us of harsh realities. It would not be morally improper, for example, for a physician to stress the positive aspects of the results of plastic surgery after a serious burn. Under the circumstances, it is unlikely that the patient would expect a physician to do otherwise. The role of the physician here traditionally has been to bolster spirits, not to state bluntly that some will find the patient's appearance distasteful, if not disturbing. On the other hand, the physician should not attempt to convince the patient to enter a beauty contest, if that is not warranted. Nor should a physician fail to speak the unvarnished truth when that would be helpful, the patient is willing to listen, and the physician believes it should be told. To decide where support ends and true deception begins requires not only clinical experience but thorough self-knowledge on the part of the physician. It is easier to be the bearer of good news than of bad news.

Many important social relationships in fact presume other than truthful answers. Some questions, such as "How are you doing?" are not usually meant as invitations for a brief history of one's recent medical problems. Indeed, games such as poker presuppose mutual consent to active deception. Similarly, there may be circumstances under which it is unreasonable to presume that individuals want full disclosure of information. If in an emergency one does not have pain–killing drugs on hand, it is not deceptive to begin an intravenous drip with a glucose solution while solemnly declaring, "As this fluid enters your veins, the pain will begin to diminish." There is a reasonable expectation that the placebo effect will diminish the pain, even though the drip has nothing to do with this directly, but is rather part of the ceremony and ritual through which physicians over centuries have calmed patients and controlled pain. It is not a false statement. It is unreasonable to expect that the patient would want anything but relief of the pain (except in certain bizarre situations in which one might encounter individuals who were known to have committed themselves to truth at all costs and in all circumstances). To provide a preliminary lecture on the placebo effect and ask for permission to employ it would be not only self-defeating but absurd. Not only is such disclosure not required by the principle of permission, but it might very well violate the principle of beneficence.

Emergencies in which a presumptive permission to deceive is clearly available grade into areas where some general explicit consent to deception is required. In programs designed to wean a patient from an addiction through substituting nonactive ingredients, it may be necessary to indicate that unspecified beneficial forms of deception will be integral to the therapeutic regimen. At other times it may be enough simply to state, "If you take this drug, you will begin to feel better and your anxieties will diminish." Again, given the placebo effect, such a statement is not deceptive and in most circumstances further information need not be given unless the patient specifically requests it. Even if the patient requests it, the physician may morally respond, "If you want to be treated by me (or by the Torquemada Detoxification Hospital), take the medicine I give you and trust me."

Negative placebo effects are more problematic. What of drugs that have as possible side effects symptoms that others may suffer as much from suggestion as from the drug? One might think here of nausea, headaches, or impotence. If the physician believes that the patient is suggestible and is more likely to suffer from the symptoms because of the suggestive force of the disclosure than because of the actions of the drug, should a disclosure be made? The answer depends in part on how remote the risks from the drug are and in part on the kind of relationship the physician has with the patient. A close relationship fashioned in trust may enable the physician to know the extent to which the patient would presume that the physician would make such disclosures. On the other hand, if the risks are real and the physician cannot presume such an implicit consent for partial disclosure, then the facts must be stated. Part of being a free competent individual is that one must take the risk involved in the stewardship of one's own destiny. Answers to moral questions about the use of placebos and beneficent deception can be found only in a careful examination of the physician–patient relationship and the moral community in which it develops. All deception and all truth telling are contextual, and medicine is no exception.

FASHIONING THE PHYSICIAN–PATIENT RELATIONSHIP. In general, physicians and patients meet as free individuals. Each by appealing to particular views

of proper action may participate in fashioning the character of the physician–
patient relationship. It is the case that particular patients may be more in need of
the care of a physician than particular physicians will need to provide care to a
particular patient. This is especially true in situations of acute care. But most
physicians and patients meet because of chronic health care needs or because of
the everyday vexations of life that do not require immediate or emergency treatment. Under such circumstances, there are opportunities for patients both individually and in groups to shape the character of health care. In addition, health
care consumers can establish their own insurance plans and delivery networks.
One must remember that it is patients and potential patients who possess the
majority of the resources of all societies. Without recourse to the coercive force
of the state, they can influence the ways in which health care is delivered by
setting standards of disclosure required on the part of physicians who receive
reimbursement through insurance policies, use hospitals owned by particular
communities, or receive salaries through health maintenance organizations supported by particular groups.

One can agree wholeheartedly that a paternalistic medicine, one that decides
what patients should or should not know, may be not only oppressive and vexatious, but in the long run injurious to the health of patients by not encouraging
patient responsibility, and still hold that the use of state force is not justified to
impose either a subjective or objective standard of care. Even apart from constraints on the use of force required by the principle of permission, there may be
advantages to be derived from setting standards for disclosure through multiple
negotiations by various groups of physicians and patients. Individuals vary
greatly in their desires and abilities to shoulder the responsibilities for dealing
with medical decision making. One might imagine a scheme in which subscribers
to insurance programs were asked to check which standard of disclosure they
wished used in their treatment; they might also be asked to review their choices
semiannually or annually. Such agreement could include the acceptance of particular notions of futility (i.e., rules for withholding treatment when it is ''unproductive'') and procedures for rationing.[63]

The principle of permission does not require that individuals be informed, only
that they be given the opportunity to inform themselves. Thus, marriage or
joining the French Foreign Legion can be justified in terms of the principle of
permission in the absence of detailing the benefits and risks. One can be put on
notice to acquire information and this notice can suffice in absence of fraud or
coercion. In addition, prior permission can be acquired when one joins an institution so that in the future explicit permission need not be acquired for particular
interventions. Compare: (1) ''If you join the Legion we will pick what conflicts
we will send you to fight; you do not get to choose,'' and (2) ''If you enroll in
bottom-of-the-line health care services, we will make numerous economically
driven choices among therapeutic and diagnostic interventions, which will save

you money (that is why our enrollment fees are so low), but it will expose you to particular risks of death, disability, and suffering. In order further to save money (and therefore offer you services at a reduced fee), we will not invest time in explaining these choices to you. If you want more information, we have a 952-page pamphlet describing our procedures in detail, which can be purchased for $120.'' This approach will surely offend against particular laws in many countries, as well as against particular content-full understandings of beneficence, but it cannot be condemned in general secular moral terms. The opportunity to consider in advance and review whether one wishes either to be autonomous in decision making or to convey trust to a physician or institution may best allow patients to realize with freely cooperating physicians, nurses, and others one's own views of a proper health care provider relationship.

## Making choices for others: three forms of paternalism

The *Oxford English Dictionary* defines paternalism as ''the principle and practice of paternal administration; government as by a father; the claim or attempt to supply the needs or to regulate the life of a nation or community in the same way as a father does those of his children.'' Patients often regress under the stress of disease and want to be treated as children by health professionals. Informal requests for paternalistic care occur as a matter of course in health care because patients are in a strange environment. Like many travelers in unfamiliar lands where the language is in part a barrier to communication, they may look for others to lead them. Consider the ways in which individuals who visit foreign countries as part of a package tour embrace a form of paternalism. They trust the tour guide and company to have selected the reasonable places to see and places to eat. In a similar fashion, patients often look to their physician for guidance and direction.

Often, given particular value commitments, paternalism should not be avoided. One must treat infants in a paternalistic fashion. The very senile must be similarly treated, often leading to tensions as children and parents radically reverse their social roles. The moral issue is the extent to which paternalism in health care is allowable and desirable. To address this issue one must first recognize the different forms of paternalism, each of which raises different moral issues.[64]

PATERNALISM FOR INCOMPETENTS. In the case of individuals who have never been competent, such as infants, young children, and those profoundly or very severely mentally retarded from birth, paternalism is unavoidable. Others must choose on their behalf. Others must determine their best interests. Paternalism in which parents protect and foster the best interests of their incompetent children is a good example. It is justified in terms of the principle of beneficence and unconstrained by the principle of permission. This form of paternalism also plays a role in the choices made on behalf of individuals who were once competent and who failed to direct in advance how they were to be treated, should they become incompetent. In the absence of specific instructions, others must choose on their behalf either by appeal to a standard of a reasonable and prudent person (within a particular moral community), or by an appeal to a standard articulated by a particular community of individuals committed to a particular set of standards and values. As we will see, each standard has its own problems. The more one attempts to establish the best interests of a ward by appeal to what a reasonable and prudent individual would choose, the less content such standards have. On the other hand, the more one appeals to concrete understandings of best interests fashioned in particular moral communities, the more divergent judgments become.

One is then pressed to ask who should determine which standard to use, and on what basis. These two points are obviously closely intertwined. If one allows a guardian to choose in terms of the guardian's particular moral community (e.g., as an Amish, Jehovah's Witness, or Christian Scientist), one has already decided to allow the pursuit of a particular interpretation of best interests. If one constrains the guardian to choose as a reasonable and prudent person would choose, to what sense of reasonableness and prudence ought one to appeal? One returns here to the problems raised in chapters 2 and 3 with regard to discovering concrete standards for proper beneficent actions. There will also be conflicts about who is in authority over an incompetent and thus free to choose the standard. As has already been argued, parents come to be in authority over the infants they produce. Similarly, absent prior agreements, individuals who care for and nurture formerly competent people come to be in authority over them, for such persons can no longer possess themselves and therefore can come into the possession and authority of others. Within certain restrictions, which we will explore further in the section on proxy consent (as well as those already examined in chapters 4 and 6), those in authority can be accepted as proper judges of the best interests of their wards because they have a form of property right in their wards as masters have in their indentured servants. As we saw in chapter 4, humans who are not persons cannot possess themselves. They are most plausibly held to be possessed by those who produced them or care for them. As a result, those in authority over others may choose for their wards not simply to achieve their best interests, but also in order to control and direct their lives. For example, many of the choices made by parents for their children are made not to achieve the best interests of the children (nor necessarily in order to thwart their best interests), but in order to achieve parental goals and values not directly related to the children's care. If no one is an authority, beneficence may dictate choosing a guardian who appears best able to determine the ward's interests. When the ward is a member of a particular community, the choice is generally properly made by an appeal to that community's standard, especially if those deciding have no strong and overriding view of the good, not to that of reasonable and prudent persons generally, whatever that might mean. This is particularly the case when the person was previously competent. The best-interests standard of the previously competent person's community most likely represents that individual's prior preferences.

FIDUCIARY PATERNALISM. The appointment of another individual to choose on one's behalf justifies paternalistic actions in terms of mutual respect. The appointed individual may determine the best interests of the ward, not simply because the proxy is a good judge of those interests (which may or may not be the case), but by virtue of having been placed in authority by the explicit choice of the ward. Fiduciary paternalism occurs in two forms.

1. *Explicit fiduciary paternalism.* Patient–physician relationships are often explicitly paternalistic. When a patient tells a physician, "You decide what you think is the best form of treatment," authority is conveyed to the physician and a paternalistic relation is created. If this request is accepted, the physician must then attempt to use professional judgment to determine what forms of therapeutic intervention would maximize the patient's best interests. The physician must then determine by whom and by what standards the patient's best interests should be defined. In the case of physicians in such a context, the standard invoked is often that of the profession. Still, the criteria must be clarified.

To some extent, all patient–physician relationships that involve complicated and technical interventions require such a fiduciary paternalism, unless the patient is also a physician expert in that area. Otherwise, even physicians who are patients must repose their faith in another. The liberty of the physician to choose on behalf of the patient will be determined by the patient's wishes in the matter, including the extent to which the patient has formed a judgment regarding the issues at stake. "Doctor, I wish I could make up my mind whether to have a coronary bypass operation. But I can't. I really would rather you tell me what you would do in this circumstance."

The extent to which it is sensible to speak of advance directives establishing a fiduciary paternalism will depend on the extent to which paternalism requires that another determine the best interests of the ward. Thus, it might seem implausible to speak of explicit advance directives appointing a particular individual to effect them as creating a fiduciary paternalism. Not all agents act paternalistically on behalf of the individuals who appoint them. Rather, because authorized agents effect the wishes or carry out the orders of those who appoint them, those who appoint them are not simply wards, even when they are no longer competent. However, when an individual is appointed to care for another and is given latitude in deciding the criteria for proper care, a paternalistic relation has been established. One might imagine such being effected through an instrument establishing a durable power of attorney. The most extreme example of explicit fiduciary paternalism would be the instruction, "Please do what you think best over the course of the treatment, even if I lose heart and ask you to stop. You just keep doing what you think is right." Only in special circumstances, with particular people, can an advance directive be sufficiently concrete and content-full to direct choices. If one is treated within the embrace of a particular moral community, little may need to be specified. For example, if one is receiving care as a Pius Xth Roman Catholic within the St. Peter of Verona Holy Inquisitor Hospital, one may be at peace having treatment specified by hospital rules and policies. A simple advance directive may suffice. In any case, it is difficult to anticipate the range of issues that will be confronted in treatment so that it is useful to appoint someone to choose in gray areas or in unforeseen circumstances.

One may also effect a Ulysses contract. Imagine that one decides to experience what it is like to have dental work without local anesthesia. One tells the dentist to forgo local anesthesia and to drill no matter how much one screams to the contrary. Imagine also that the dentist, Doc Holliday, agrees. He ties the patient down and begins to drill. The patient screams in pain. "This is a big mistake! Stop and give me anesthesia!!!" Is Doc Holliday obliged to do so in general secular moral terms? The answer is no. Yet he may, if he so wishes. The patient has transferred to Doc Holliday the right to treat without anesthesia. If Doc Holliday continues to treat despite the patient's desperate screams, he has not violated the morality of mutual respect. Neither has Doc Holliday acted against the principle of beneficence if Doc Holliday holds that he is proceeding in accord with the patient's long-term best interests (e.g., that, after the procedure is over, the patient will say, "I am glad you forced me to go through this as we agreed. I am a better person as a result."). Nor does Doc Holliday violate the principle of beneficence if he believes according to his own standards that the patient will be better off. But Doc Holliday is not obliged not to use anesthesia once the patient requests him to provide it. In general secular morality, there can be neither duties to oneself nor laws against Ulysses contracts. The principle of permission gives one authority over oneself. It is simply that in this case authority has been transferred to Doc Holliday, who is at liberty but not obliged to recognize the patient's change of mind. The patient has given Doc Holliday the right to treat without anesthesia, but there is no one whose directive Doc Holliday is obliged to follow, once the patient asks for anesthesia. At that point Doc Holliday may give anesthesia.

2. *Implicit fiduciary paternalism.* Even though patients have not explicitly appointed others as their surrogate decision makers, it is often argued that there is an implicit presumption that others will make certain sorts of decisions on their behalf.

Minor, *short-term* paternalistic interventions are often justified on the ground that reasonable and prudent individuals would not mind and do in fact want such interventions if they are undertaken when there is some doubt whether the individuals are competent or well informed. These forms of intervention are often seen as instances of the weak paternalism justified by John Stuart Mill.

Again, it is a proper office of public authority to guard against accidents. If either a public officer or any one else saw a person attempting to cross a bridge which had been ascertained to be unsafe, and there were no time to warn him of his danger, they might seize him and turn him back, without any real infringement of his liberty; for liberty consists in doing what one desires, and he does not desire to fall into the river. Nevertheless, when there is not a certainty, but only a danger of mischief, no one but the person himself can judge of the sufficiency of the motive which may prompt him to incur the risk; in this case, therefore (unless he is a child, or delirious, or in some state of excitement or absorption incompatible with the full use of the reflecting faculty), he ought, I conceive, to be only warned of the danger; not forcibly prevented from exposing himself to it.[65]

In such paternalistic interventions the right of individuals to choose capriciously, indeed, recklessly, is not denied. Rather, it is assumed that individuals would wish to be protected against errors that are not integral to their plans or choices when such protection involves only a minor intrusion.

Such considerations may in general secular morality morally justify not only preventing suicide when it is not clear that an individual is truly incompetent, but also in fact civilly committing individuals for a brief period of time to allow for an evaluation of their mental health. For example, California enacted a code to allow civil commitment for seventy–two hours in order to evaluate individuals thought to be mentally ill and a danger to themselves.[66] The code also provided for an additional fourteen-day commitment when there is an imminent threat of an individual's committing suicide.[67] The extent to which such further commitment would be morally justified will depend on how seriously one doubts the competence of the would-be suicide.

One should note that requiring greater certainty of competence when an individual's choices are likely to be dangerous is a form of weak paternalism. If a patient consents to a standard treatment with few and negligible risks and with a considerable promise of benefit, physicians or nurses rarely question the validity of the consent, even if the patient is only marginally aware of the significance of the choice.[68] This may be justified on the principle that most individuals choose what rational and prudent persons choose and that consent, however enfeebled, suggests that the individual in question has no objections. In addition, where there is little risk and much good to be achieved, there appear to be few grounds to intervene to protect the best interests of the patient by special determinations of competency. So, too, if a patient refuses a treatment when there is little chance of success or of significant benefit, there is little ground for not accepting the patient's apparent competence. For instance, if terminal patients appear fairly competent, there is little ground for a careful assessment of competence prior to accepting their decision to refuse treatment. However, when the patient wishes to choose a risky treatment or refuse clearly beneficial treatment, physicians should establish clearly that the patient is competent. Such patients can be seen on the analogy of Mill's individual approaching the bridge and may be hindered in their decisions until it is clear that they are choosing competently. When there are no well-founded doubts concerning competence, one may not interfere in bizarre and risky undertakings of others without offending against the principle of permission. When there is a significant risk of a false positive determination of competence, or when a false positive determination of competence would lead to significant harms to a patient, one should not accept a patient's directions without some investigation. Otherwise, fastidious assessments of competence will rightly appear out of place.

Some have also argued that citizens of a society have implicitly agreed to paternalistic interventions as a form of insurance against unwise or dangerous actions.[69] This view is impossible to defend if one takes freedom of individuals seriously, that is, distinguishes between freedom as a value and freedom as a side constraint. Even if one held that many agreed to such interventions, individuals while competent could explicitly declare their nonparticipation in such paternalistic insurance schemes.

BEST-INTERESTS PATERNALISM. This form of paternalism is also termed strong paternalism: the contention is that under certain circumstances one may override the competent refusal of an individual in order to achieve the best interests of that individual. Since this is the most morally problematic form of paternalistic intervention, some have this form of paternalism in mind when they speak of paternalism in general. Thus, Bernard Gert and Charles Culver provide the following five conditions, which they take to be necessary and sufficient for paternalism (i.e., best-interest paternalism or strong paternalism in our terminology):

A is acting paternalistically toward S if and only if A's behavior (correctly) indicates that A *believes that:*

(1) his action is for S's good
(2) he is qualified to act on S's behalf
(3) his action involves violating a moral rule (or doing that which will require him to do so) with regard to S
(4) he is justified in acting on S's behalf independently of S's past, present, or immediately forthcoming (free, informed) consent
(5) S believes (perhaps falsely) that he (S) generally knows what is for his own good.[70]

There are difficulties with this analysis.[71] The central moral difficulty lies in the problem of establishing the priority of duties of beneficence over duties under the principle of permission. As chapter 3 has shown, outside particular moral communities, where individuals have already agreed to a particular ordering of goods and harms that will place successful medical intervention higher than liberty interests, it will be moraly blameworthy to engage in such paternalistic actions.

*Proxy consent and the emancipation of minors*

As we saw in the beginning of the section on free and informed consent, individuals may plausibly claim on quite different grounds to have the right to choose on behalf of others: (1) a guardian may have been explicitly authorized by the ward while the ward was still competent; (2) guardians may be in authority over the ward because they produced the ward (i.e., parents); (3) a guardian may be in authority over the ward because of the indentured servitude that develops between parents and children, that is, between those who care for others and those who agree under those circumstances to accept their care; (4) a guardian may be a good judge of the best interests of the ward as seen within the community to which the guardian and ward belong; (5) a guardian may be a good judge of the best interests of the ward in terms of what reasonable and prudent persons would choose. In the first three cases guardians claim the right to choose because they are in authority, not necessarily because they are good authorities, as in the last two cases.[72]

Children come into their own possession incrementally, as they gain the capacity to understand and appreciate the significance of their actions and as they assume authority over and support of themselves. There are no sharp boundaries between competence and incompetence, or between being under one's parents' authority and being free of it. The concept of the mature minor underscores the circumstances under which minors, though they are not emancipated through living apart and supporting themselves, are partially freed from parental authority in areas where they understand and appreciate the significance of decisions having substantial bearing on the future character of their lives (e.g., reproductive choices) and which decisions do not require parental subvention. It is plausible to hold that children in different circumstances and different areas may thus come partially into their own possession by being morally responsible for such choices. In such circumstances (e.g., concerning decisions bearing on the future existence of the child) either the scope of the indenture to parents may not include ceding the right to choose in such important areas affecting one's future life, or even if it does involve such a cession of rights, the state may not be interested in protecting parental rights because of the costs involved in affording such protection (e.g., the difficulty of determining the extent to which such rights have plausibly and competently been ceded to parents).

How is one to balance the right of those in authority to choose and the interest of authorities to protect the best interests of wards? How is one to strike a balance between the right of guardians to be left alone in making their choices regarding their wards, and the right of wards to be free to make choices in areas where they have an emerging authority to control their own lives. Given the arguments to this point, it seems plausible to state the principle for intervention on behalf of a ward and against the wishes of a guardian in the following fashion.

---

PRINCIPLE FOR INTERVENTION ON BEHALF OF A WARD

Out of consideration of violations of the principle of permission and/or the principle of beneficence as the principle of nonmalevolence, one may use (but, because of countervailing significant costs, not be obliged to use) force to rescue a ward from a guardian in authority, if and only if:

    i.   The child asks for rescue, is competent, and the guardian's actions or omissions injure the body or mind of the ward to a degree significantly contrary to the best interests of the ward, as determined by the standard of the rescuer, and the rescuer pays any costs imposed on the guardian; or

   ii.   The ward's actions or omissions are malicious, that is, malevolent; or

  iii.   The actions or omissions are contrary to agreements made with the ward before the ward became incompetent; or

  iv.   The actions of the guardian are such as are very likely to be interpreted as direct injuries by the ward and the ward is competent.

---

The principle sets the limits of a guardian's authority and establishes the realm of a rescuer's authority.

Whatever values a rescuer might hold, that individual will need to determine that the goods to be achieved outweigh the costs involved in the rescuer's intrusion. To warrant a rescue where the person is not competently asking for aid nor where the injury is in violation of a prior agreement, the injury must be malevolent and, to justify the costs of the intrusion, involve significant and direct physical or mental harm to the future person. One is not constrained, absent prior agreements or a special view of the good life and beneficence, to live in ways that will maximize the advantage of present, much less future, persons. As has already been observed, it is impossible to justify protecting future individuals from being used as means. Also, to satisfy the fourth condition, circumstances must be clear in order to show that a guardian is using a future person as a means *merely,* that is, in ways such that it is clear that the person will not consent. To be at the mercy of the wisdom and vision of past persons is the unavoidable predicament of future persons. Future persons have the right to expect that past persons will not have acted in ways that directly use force against them in ways it seems nearly certain they would reject. Because interpreting an outcome as an injury depends on a complex set of values and understandings of the world, one will need to be very certain that the ward will in fact interpret the guardian's interventions as an injury. One runs the risk of falsely interpreting as a harm what will be received as a beneficence and therefore groundlessly interfering with the proper actions of actual persons. Besides, parents always have the following powerful rejoinder: ''We have not acted malevolently. In fact, we have acted benevolently within the context of our particular ideological or religious vision. Moreover, we would never have had any children (or, in the case of wards, raised and cared for these individuals) if we could not raise them in our ideology (or faith). Our children can only complain if nonexistence itself would be worse than the life we will give them.'' This retort is powerful and likely undermines most attempts at rescue under the fourth condition except those that would involve prearranged injury or death in the event of the apostasy of a ward from the moral vision of the guardian. Given such apostasy, such actions would be clearly against the consent of those injured. Moreover, the notion of ''injury'' would not depend on a particular vision of the good life, but on the unconsented-to character of the use of another person.

It is very difficult to make clear and certain judgments in these matters. The rearing of children and the caring for wards take place in the embrace of visions of the good life and of beneficence. The very vitality of the visions often leads to conflicts that are insoluble, TEYKU.[73] What, for example, ought one to make of ritual or other mutilations of the bodies of incompetent individuals? One might think here of male circumcision, which rarely has medical indications and which is usually performed for religious or vaguely traditional reasons.[74] The foregoing analysis shows that it is clearly permissible under the assumption that the act is benevolent and it is not clear that the individual will object when he in the future becomes competent. This assumption is an especially well grounded one in the context of a religious community. The same argument will support the tattooing and scarification of individuals that are a part of the tradition of particular communities.

In the end, the best interests of individuals can only be understood concretely within particular moral communities. There is no understanding of parenting or guardianship that does not involve a particular vision of beneficence, of which there are many. The need for content can be met only at the price of taking a particular moral stance or perspective. In order to dispel avoidable confusions, persons should be put on notice that they will be treated according to the standards of the best interests of the communities within which they live. If they live outside of communities with sufficient moral content, or if they live within the fragmented remains of competing moral visions, they must be informed of who will serve as their guardians and by what standards decisions will be made.

The difficulty lies with those who have never been competent; that is, never in any of the areas of their lives have they been persons in the strict sense of moral agents. When individuals have not in advance stipulated their desires for care, these analyses, for better or worse, lead to a great but not absolute latitude of choice for parents and other guardians of incompetents. For example, when a guardian wishes to choose a course of action that will lead to death, as for example when a Jehovah's Witness refuses blood transfusions for a child, how can one speak of a future possible concurring permission as required by the principle of proxy consent? It might be suggested that one should examine the extent to which adult Jehovah's Witnesses are true to their faith, even to the point of refusing blood transfusions and dying. However, that would be to miss the point. If a Jehovah's Witness refuses a blood transfusion for an infant, that child never becomes a future person to be injured. In addition, the general secular moral obligations of beneficence due to sentient nonpersonal life will protect only against malevolent acts and thus will not serve to forbid infanticide for which nonmalevolent grounds are given in justification. Where it is implausible that the actions are nonmalevolent, one may use force to protect the infant.

In exchange for treatment in hospitals and clinics supported by communities not in agreement with the Jehovah's Witnesses or similar beliefs, one could envisage such hospitals and clinics, and their physicians, making any care conditional on the acceptance of whatever care is required to preserve life and limb. However, if Jehovah's Witnesses were like the Amish or the Yanomamo and retreated into communities closed off from the rest of society in order to ensure that their children would receive only that amount of health care consistent with their religion, or to establish their own hospitals, there would be no grounds for intervention, except to rescue competent children who wished treatment.[75]

### Research involving human subjects

Research is integral to medicine as a science. It is a part of the disciplined knowing of the health care professions. All health care professions, as has already been observed, treat patients not only for their own good, but for the good of the profession. At the very minimum, skills must be passed on from one generation of practitioners to another, and the patient serves as a medium. As members of learned professions, physicians and nurses seek not just to maintain their skills, but also to increase them. A systematic scrutiny of the encounters between health care practitioner and patient is needed in order to learn more so as to be able to treat better. The result is a tension between the health care professional's roles as healer and scientist. This conflict between roles has been at the root of traditional criticisms of human experimentation. In the late Middle Ages, increased experimentation by physicians and surgeons led to warnings by the Christian Church.[76] Bartolomaeus Fumus, in his *Summa Armilla* of 1538, stated that physicians sin "if they supply a doubtful medicine for a certain one, or do not practice in accord with the art, but desire to practice following their own stupid fancy, or make experiments and such like, by which the patient is exposed to grave danger."[77] A similar suspicion that experimentation was equivalent to rash treatment of the patient continued even in American law until recently.[78]

These hesitations have been combined with a view that experimentation on human subjects involves a morally questionable use of persons. As Hans Jonas argues,

[The] compensations of personhood are denied to the subject of experimentation, who is acted upon for an extraneous end without being engaged in a real relation where he would be the counterpoint to the other or to circumstance. Mere "consent" (mostly amounting to no more than permission) does not right this reification. Only genuine authenticity of volunteering can possibly redeem the condition of "thinghood" to which the subject submits.[79]

On the basis of these concerns, Jonas sets very stringent criteria for authentic volunteering and equates most consent with a form of conscription.[80] Jonas endorses these high standards to overcome what he contends is a central moral problem in research using human subjects. "What is wrong with making a person an experimental subject is . . . that we make him a thing—a passive thing, merely to be acted upon."[81] These general concerns regarding the moral probity of research involving human subjects have been vindicated at least in part by the history of the abuse of humans in experimentation. Though the atrocities reviewed at Nuremberg may come most quickly to mind, there were considerable abuses before the Second World War, as Jay Katz's review of experimentation indicates.[82] The Tuskegee syphilis study in the United States also demonstrates the need for the special protection of human research subjects.[83] One would need to add that the mere publication of codes and laws does not appear to be sufficient to protect human subjects. As Hans-Martin Sass has shown, quite exacting and in many respects progressive rules for the protection of human subjects were in fact enacted in Germany in 1931 and were theoretically in force until 1945.[84]

The use of human subjects in research is thus tied to the need to afford special protection for free and informed consent so as to ensure that adequate knowledge is communicated and that consent is free of coercion. Because of the conflicts between roles, subjects may often confuse research without benefit for them with treatment that could in fact improve their health. Moreover, students, prisoners, and other special populations may be both overtly and covertly coerced to participate in human research. The principle of permission requires that, as a condition of mutual respect, individuals be protected against both deception and coercion. The principle of beneficence requires that there be a net benefit to others. Here one must note that biomedical research is directly and indirectly tied to benefits for patients. Indeed, one's moral concerns regarding the practice of human experimentation will in part depend on one's view of the safety of health care in the absence of rigorous research. One need not only fear the reckless use of humans in medical research. One should also fear the costs of reckless treatment—treatment not based on adequate research. The other side of the concern to protect human subjects is the concern to protect patients against untested, poorly tested, and ill-founded treatments.

RESEARCH AS BENEFICENCE.    People have an impulse to do things to help those in need. Throughout history and across cultures individuals have devised various means to prevent illness and cure disease. The difficulty is that a great number of these interventions, from trepanning and bleeding to blistering, purging, and clystering, usually do more harm than good. Much of the history of well-intentioned medical treatment is the history of useless suffering. Even the most superficial analysis of that history would suggest that more individuals by many magnitudes have suffered from ill-founded treatments than have suffered from the side effects of research. If one abandons the notion that standard or accepted treatments are good simply because they are standard and accepted, one is confronted with the recurring question whether any of the accepted modalities of medicine do more harm than good.

This question has been a part of the development of modern scientific medicine. One must recognize the chaotic state of the materia medica until quite recently.[85] It was a collection of various treatments, only some of whose uses were well founded. As a result, there was a search for a *methodus medendi,* a methodical or systematic approach to treatment. Such an approach requires research involving humans. As Thomas Sydenham put it, one needed a system of care "approved by numerous experiments."[86] The advances in modern medicine came both through developments in the basic medical sciences, as well as through systematic and statistical assessments of standard means of treatment. They depended on a growing skepticism regarding traditional means of treatment. One might think here of the classic study by Louis in 1835 to show that bloodletting did not in fact have, as was supposed, a beneficial effect on inflammatory diseases.[87] One is brought to a general suspicion of all treatment that has not been systematically assessed. One has substantial grounds for fearing that untested treatments will do more harm than good.

Research bears in different ways on the possible treatment of actual patients. One can distinguish among (1) research that is likely to be of direct benefit to the subject; (2) research likely to benefit individuals with the same disease or disorder as the subject; (3) research that is likely to establish whether particular treatments are on balance beneficial or harmful; (4) research focused on developing new treatments; and (5) fundamental research directed to basic understandings of biology and the disease processes. All five forms of research lead, whether directly or indirectly, to the abandonment of previously established treatment modalities when they are shown to provide more harm than benefit compared with alternative treatments or with no treatment at all. Systematic and careful research in medicine is integral to controlling and directing the impulse to cure so that it does less harm and more good. Research is integral to a beneficent medicine. Research is not simply a part of the knower's interest in knowing, nor is it simply tied to a pursuit of some future state in which there will be perfect treatments for all diseases and disorders. It focuses, in addition, if not first and foremost, on particular patients who may be benefited, as well as contemporary individuals who will be aided in the future by the abandonment of old treatments and the establishment of better treatments. The risks involved in the use of subjects in human experimentation can be realistically assessed only against the background of the risks involved in a medicine unguided by systematic research. One finds here yet one more application of the Socratic adage that the unexamined life is not worth living, namely, that medicine unexamined through systematic research may be a danger to patients. In this light, the role of the consenting research subject is not that of a "thing" co-opted into the service of alien goals, but of an individual collaborating in an important social goal that may be of importance to that individual as well.

RESPECTING SUBJECTS, PROTECTING SUBJECTS, AND TOLERATING DARE-DEVIL RESEARCH. Because of the misunderstandings that individuals are likely to have about the nature and significance of medical research, researchers will usually have a moral obligation to use special care in gaining the consent of would-be subjects. One will need to avoid all forms of deception to which the subject does not consent, and one will need to eschew all forms of coercion. A good example of the attempt to achieve such protection is found in the American Code of Federal Regulations for the Protection of Human Subjects. There, informed consent is clearly spelled out in terms of the need to warn would-be subjects of the circumstances of the research and of the opportunities for both refusal and participation. Research subjects are strangers in a strange land and, like patients, will need to be shown how to orient themselves in order to choose freely, that is, in order not to be deceived or otherwise coerced.

However, the review of research for approval generally attends not only to the character and completeness of disclosures in gaining consent, but also limits dangerous research or research to which subjects agree primarily out of concern for payment. Such restrictions are not required by the principle of permission, or by the principle of beneficence if a high value is given to liberty. Such restrictions rather express a particular governmentally endorsed understanding of the proper conduct of research endorsed by governments. For example, if it is morally proper for individuals freely to volunteer for service in the armed forces, it should be morally proper as well to volunteer for service in research forces. In fact, one might very well imagine why it would be useful to have a stable population of individuals highly paid and highly motivated to participate in human research.[88] Such individuals might be forbidden by their contract from withdrawing from particular forms of research, just as individuals, once they have joined the armed forces, have ceded their right to decline to participate in or to withdraw from certain activities. Such an approach to research would be in violation of current regulations.

There is also a wide range of research endeavors that is unlikely to be approved by the institutional review boards established to review research in institutions receiving federal research support, but which research would not be in violation of the principles of permission and beneficence.[89] Here one would find research ranging from that which is extremely dangerous to that for which high rates of pay are offered. Outside of a particular vision of beneficence, there is no basis for forbidding individuals to volunteer freely for risky research, especially if it promises great benefit to others. Many approve of such research in the case of autoexperimentation. One might think here of the Nobel Prize winner Werner Forsmann, who catheterized his own heart.[90] As we have seen from the examination of the nature of peaceable manipulation, there is also nothing wrong with offering individuals as much money as is required to attract their services, as long as the offer does not itself render them incompetent. So, too, there will be no grounds in principle for forbidding research that most would think to be both boonless and harmful. One might think here of advocates of nonorthodox approaches to health care, privately funding and conducting trials of their therapies. Such endeavors need not and ought not be supported by those who hold them to be harmful or ill advised. However, if the individuals involved understand and appreciate the risks, their choices should be tolerated. One should be as tolerant of martyrs for unconventional understandings of science as one is of martyrs for what others may hold to be unconventional religious viewpoints (e.g., an adult Jehovah's Witness deciding to die rather than accept a blood transfusion, or a devout Roman Catholic deciding to die rather than accept a direct abortion to protect her from heart failure due to the strain on her heart with serious mitral valve disease).

RESEARCH ON SPECIAL POPULATIONS. To a great extent we have already explored the moral limits to experimentation on humans who are not persons in the strict sense. Fetal experimentation has already been discussed in chapter 6, and in the previous section we have examined the range of allowable proxy consent. Although the principle of proxy consent gives fairly broad moral latitude to the guardian, particular moral visions drive particular concerns for the good of wards that have limited the amount of risk to which incompetent subjects may be exposed. One might think of the requirement by the Code of Federal Regulations that federally funded research involving children not involve greater than minimal risk to the subjects if it has no prospect of directly benefiting the individual subject, unless it is likely to yield generalizable knowledge about the subject's disorder or condition.[91] Even then, such research is not allowed unless the risk represents only a minor increase over a minimal risk, except in circumstances where the research offers an opportunity to understand, prevent, or alleviate a serious problem affecting the health or welfare of children.[92] But how is one to understand "minimal risks"? Consider the view that minimal risks are understood as those that "are not greater, considering probability and magnitude, than those ordinarily encountered in daily life or during the performance of routine physical or psychological examinations or tests."[93] How does one understand minimal risks for the family from motorcycles, hang-gliders, and treks through the Amazon forest? It is unlikely that the character of current restrictions can be sustained in general secular terms.

Questions of consent to research arise as well with regard to individuals who agree to participate under coercive circumstances. One must include here not only prisoners but also students, who may fear that their future will be determined in part by their willingness to participate in research programs. Given the history of the exploitation of prisoners, there is much to be said for the protection afforded by federal regulations to prison populations.[94] These restrictions, which for practical purposes forbid using prisoners in any federally funded research not directed to the treatment of individual prisoners or the understanding of diseases and conditions bearing on prisoners, also remove the prisoners' opportunity to contribute to society and to recapture a sense of moral dignity through such altruism. In so completely protecting prisoners against coercive pressure to participate in research, one further undermines the dignity and moral capacity of prisoners. Finally, one must observe, as Hans Jonas has indicated, that there is nothing intrinsically wrong with forcing prisoners to participate in human experimentation, if it is a part of their punishment.[95] Aside from concerns about the possible abuse of such an opportunity to use prisoners, and the change in ethos such activities might entail, the central question is whether such compulsion has clearly been made part of the punishment. One might imagine punishments for various crimes including specified periods of serving as a subject of research of a particular sort. Committing the crime would entail consenting to the research. Here one also finds part of the secular moral answer regarding the use of students as subjects. Unless participation in research is part of a course elected by a student, special protections against coercion may be needed.

DECEPTION IN RESEARCH. As we have seen, there is a moral impetus to do research in order to protect individuals from well-intentioned interventions that will in fact do more harm than alternative treatments and in some cases than no treatment at all. It is hard to know truly in medicine because of (1) the problem of random remissions and spontaneous cures; (2) the remembrance by physicians of their therapeutic triumphs more clearly than their failures, thus distorting their judgment of a treatment's efficacy;[96] (3) the placebo effect, which aids even intrinsically inefficacious treatments in benefiting patients; and (4) the psychology of discovery that leads individuals to see what they anticipate.[97] As a result, it has been hard to determine when conservative versus surgical treatment of coronary artery disease offers greater benefit,[98] or if radical mastectomies offer a greater chance of survival than simple mastectomies.[99] Although one might think that such a clear outcome as being alive or dead after a period of time would lead to easy assessment, the various distortions of observer bias have made judgment difficult.

Much of modern medical research depends on not disclosing to subjects what drugs they are actually receiving, or which treatment they will receive, in order to compensate for distorting forces. For example, often both the investigator and the subject-patient are not informed which of a set of drugs the subject-patient is actually receiving. Instead, the investigators and the patients involved in the study are informed that the subjects will be receiving one of two or more drugs through a random assignment in order to compare their relative efficacy. Such double-blind random clinical trials, which are employed because of the history of observer bias, are not immoral for employing such deception unless the prospective subjects are not warned of the deception. Here again the model of poker is instructive. In playing the game, the participants agree to certain forms of mutual deception but not others (e.g., poker bluffs but not hidden cards). So, too, in random clinical trials subjects must be informed (or at least be offered information about) what kinds of information will not be disclosed, what form of randomization will occur, why it will take place, what information will be provided, and when. Since the amount of certainty required to hold that a trial has been completed is arbitrary, subjects should not be deceived regarding when and under what circumstances codes will be broken to indicate that one treatment has been shown to be more useful than others.[100] What is essential is that subjects not be misled regarding the risks and benefits of a research protocol. The principle of mutual respect does not require that individuals be protected against deception, but only that they not unwittingly be subjected to deception.[101] There is no violation of the principle of beneficence either, if in the end the good is accomplished.

THE DEMOCRATIZATION OF SCIENCE AND THE PARTNERSHIP OF KNOWLEDGE. To recognize individuals as free and able to consent or refuse to participate in research is to see science as the collective endeavor of a great number of free men and women. Those who govern its course are not only scientists, physicians, surgeons, and nurses, but patients and research subjects. Medicine will not be able to extend its skills from one generation to another if current patients are not willing to allow their bodies and minds to be explored by students and young physicians and nurses who are acquiring the skills necessary to care for and, if possible, cure the complaints of patients yet to come. So, too, when patients and others freely participate in research, they join in the collective endeavor of individuals concerned to avoid treatments that do more harm than good and to acquire treatments that cure better and with fewer costs, as well as in the general cultural aspiration to the better understanding of man and the human condition. The principle of permission defines the character of this interaction; the principle of beneficence supports the altruistic dedication of some to the good of all.

## Confidentiality

The fabric of health care is sustained by trust. Patients bare their bodies and minds to physicians, and physicians treat patients in all of the vulnerable moments of their lives, from copulation and birth to disease and death. In order to ensure adequate care for the concerns of patients, physicians need to know what is bothering them and how they understand their problems. As a result, a bond of confidentiality has protected physician–patient relationships since the beginnings of modern Western medicine. One might think here of the famous passage from the Hippocratic oath, "And whatsoever I shall see or hear in the course of my profession, as well as outside my profession in my intercourse with men, if it be what should not be published abroad, I will never divulge, holding such things to be holy secrets."[102] As a matter of fact, communications to either priests or physicians are not as secure as the client–lawyer privilege, which is near to being absolute. In theory, priests can be compelled to testify in many jurisdictions regarding supposedly confidential disclosures made in the confessional.[103] In addition, physicians have a special duty to inform public authorities that their patients have contracted sexually transmitted diseases, have sustained gunshot wounds, have abused children, or otherwise have been associated with problems regarding which the state demands disclosure. For instance, there has been an increasingly recognized legal duty of health care professionals to disclose to third parties a possible danger from a patient under treatment.[104]

The principle of permission makes it morally permissible to create such special exclaves secure against such requirements for disclosure. The particular individuals who might be benefited by the disclosure have no general secular moral right to the physician making a disclosure that will protect them, even though they may have a moral claim on the patient for such disclosure. Moreover, the fact that a priest or a physician comes to know that an individual is dangerous (e.g., is infected with the AIDS virus and may infect others) does not in itself increase the dangerousness of the individual. Silence on the part of the priest or physician is not itself a direct injury against those who may be the individual's victims. Holding oneself out as an individual to whom one can speak in absolute confidentiality does not in and of itself constitute an injury against others just because one might come to know of possible dangers to others. In addition, there may be special advantages from both priests and physicians offering strict confidentiality. The capacity of physicians or priests to function in their special roles, which have social value, may be undercut by the notion that compelling state interests could force disclosure of their private communications. Priests provide a secure exclave where one may speak without hindrance or hesitation about one's sins and guilt. So, too, the Hippocratic commitment to confidentiality offers an opportunity to speak fully of one's medical concerns, which may also be tied to sins and legal infractions. This not only may lead to a more adequate treatment of patients, but also will underscore the special value of recognizing exclaves of privacy secure against state intrusion.

Arguments such as the latter lie behind the client–lawyer privilege, which is nearly absolute. This privilege has been justified, inter alia, on the grounds that a defendant has the right to at least one confidant who will champion that individual's interests against the powers of the state.[105] One need not stand alone against the state. The same considerations support a privilege for both physicians and priests. A physician is often an individual's sole confidant in defense against the blind forces of illness. So, too, priests are seen as an individual's special refuge from personal guilt and for defense against the wrath of the Almighty.

Whether it will on balance be desirable to endow the patient–physician or the priest–penitent relationship with the absolute confidentiality usually given to the lawyer–client relationship will depend on the usefulness of the role. One must note that even the history of the priest–penitent relationship shows that an un-qualified seal of confession did not always exist, at least in the West. Many argued, for example, that those who confessed heresy need not be guaranteed any such special privilege.[106] In the end, the notion of an absolute obligation to maintain confidentiality developed even to the point of protecting the disclosure of sins one intended to commit in the future. The priest could at best give a general warning to those endangered, but could not disclose the identity of the sinner.[107] The ground for this absolute protection lay in the fear that any excep-tion to the seal of confession would deter individuals from shriving and thus saving their souls.

The same argument is available against the legal duty of physicians to report to the state or third parties the fact that a particular patient has either a sexually transmitted disease or constitutes a possible danger to others and where treatment will not increase the risk to others. It should be noted that the treatment of patients with AIDS contrasts with the current treatment of sexually transmitted diseases such as gonorrhea and syphilis. With such diseases, treatment decreases the likelihood of transmission to spouses and others. But the treatment of patients with AIDS may increase their likelihood of living longer, without decreasing their infectivity, at least until there is a way to kill or remove the virus. Treating an infected individual may therefore increase the risk to others, if the patient does not agree to warn those who are likely to be infected (e.g., sexual contacts). However, it is important to distinguish real risks to others versus inconsequential concerns (e.g., infected psychotherapists transmitting the infection to their pa-tients in the course of counseling).

The more one has grounds for suspecting that such disclosures prevent indi-viduals from seeking treatment or hinder them from seeking treatment in a timely fashion, without increasing the risk to others, the more one will suspect that the requirements of disclosure will do more harm than good. It is considerations such as this that have traditionally led physicians to underreport sexually transmitted diseases even when required, and to the establishment of clinics in some cities, which have treated sexually transmitted diseases with a commitment to absolute confidentiality, given the danger of disclosure for the careers of such patients, even prior to the AIDS epidemic. So, too, it might be one thing for physicians to agree to disclose child abuse discovered in the course of treating children, and another thing to require physicians to disclose such abuse when the parents seek treatment for it. The clear and certain threat of disclosure is likely to hinder such parents from seeking timely treatment, thus leading to further abuse and injury to their children. Even current requirements to disclose abuse discovered in the course of treating a child brought by a parent who is then willing to receive treatment may be unwise. Similarly, a careful examination of the costs and benefits involved in requiring disclosure to third parties that a patient is possibly dangerous may show that once this requirement is well known, dangerous patients who could have been adequately treated will not seek treatment in a timely fashion. The fact that a particular disclosure of a patient's dangerousness could have saved the life of a particular third party should not obscure the fact that a general rule requiring disclosure may in fact lead to the deaths of more individuals. If such costs are involved, a rule providing for such disclosure is not the sort that prudent men and women ought to adopt. One may be brought to establishing the same absoluteness for patient–physician communications as for client–attorney communications. But even the ill-considered actions of free men and women must be tolerated. Some may weigh the possible danger to identifiable individuals greater than the danger to statistical individuals, leading to a rule for disclosing danger to identifiable third parties, even when such a rule will harm more individuals in the long run. Indeed, there is no reason why health professionals, like ministers of different religions, might not decide to offer different commitments to confidentiality. There is, after all, no one universal content-full moral narrative concerning confidentiality.

One should recognize how widespread different formal and informal rules for disclosure are. Physicians in the armed forces, company physicians, or physicians employed by schools may have special duties to disclose information to third parties in ways unassociated with the treatment of a patient. As a result, there are numerous areas for possible conflict between the goals of treatment with patient confidentiality and the special goals of the organizations employing the physicians. In principle, this conflict is no different from the conflict between the physician as healer committed to confidentiality and the physician as public health officer committed to reporting sexually transmitted diseases. It should receive the same solution. Students, workers, and members of the armed forces should be given notice of the extent to which such physicians will depart from the usual practices of physician–patient confidentiality. If individuals generally come to know that the disclosure of information will not be protected by confidentiality, there is no violation of the principle of permission and perhaps not even the principle of beneficence, given the special weighting of the harms and benefits.

Finally, one must stress the complexity of health care relationships and the difficulties of maintaining confidentiality. Even in the private physician's office, the confidentiality of communications may be eroded when the patient applies for insurance or in other circumstances voluntarily releases information. Most patients often underappreciate the extent to which they are disclosing personal information to third parties not directly involved in their care. Individuals may need to act collectively to seek ways of persuading life insurance carriers and others to accept more limited access to patients' records. Such limitations will surely not be without cost to those seeking insurance under such conditions. As regional and national patient data banks are created as parts of national health care systems, especially with electronic storage, it will be ever more difficult to maintain confidentiality or be treated anonymously. If all treatment is paid through a governmental insurance system that requires a patient insurance identifier number, and individuals are denied access to private health care on a cash basis, it will be nearly impossible to be treated anonymously.

Restrictions on the disclosure of information will become more desirable from the point of view of patients as medicine is able to determine distant future risks of developing diseases, including diseases in the workplace. Otherwise, employers and schools may not hire or admit individuals with a high future probability of developing a serious disease. A better understanding of the genetics of illnesses and occupational diseases will increase the need to protect the confidentiality of medical records. However, many forces work against the preservation of confidentiality. The very enterprise of coherent health care in a large hospital setting, including the dedication to high-quality health care, presupposes that many individuals, not just physicians, see the records of patients. The protection of confidentiality requires systematic commitments, not only to guarding information in general, but to sequestering particular areas of information. The content of particular, appropriate policies cannot be discovered in advance. Such content must be created through particular choices. There will be numerous alternative possibilities and there is no reason why only one choice should predominate, as long as individuals are put on notice regarding the character of confidentiality that will be afforded.

## Suicide, euthanasia, and the choice of a style for dying

Just as a particular content-full policy regarding confidentiality cannot be discovered, so, too, it is impossible in general secular terms to discover an appropriate content-full secular policy regarding choices at the end of life. Secular morality is in principle blind to the content-full moral issues at stake in choices about the good death, for it is a content-less morality for moral strangers. The principle of permission sustains the secular moral right of free individuals for better or worse to choose their own ways of living and dying. In fact, the principle of beneficence, from the general perspective of secular ethics, gains content only in terms of such choices, for such choices fashion concrete visions of meaning and purpose.

Death requires choices. The good death, as the good life, requires forethought and planning. It is unlikely to happen by chance. There was much made of this in the late Middle Ages in the *ars moriendi* literature.[108] This concern can be captured in contemporary terms. One must write one's deathbed speech while in good health, for it is unlikely that one will have the opportunity to write it in the modern intensive care unit. Such forethought may include the use of advance directives, through which competent individuals can plan for their treatment in the future when they may be seriously ill and incompetent.[109]

The modern era has departed in radical ways from traditional views of death. The medieval Western Christian prayed, "A subitanea et improvisa morte, libera nos, Domine" (From a sudden and unprovided-for death, deliver us, O Lord).[110] Many members of contemporary societies hope, instead, to die without warning, painlessly in their sleep. Since such painless deaths are not the rule, even we in contemporary societies must fear an unprovided-for dying, one that will occur under circumstances that will vex us and boonlessly use our resources. Technologies that can save our lives and postpone death underscore the need to decide when to accept death and prolong dying no longer. They raise the ancient question of whether and when individuals should take their own lives or be aided in their suicides. Just as there is less general agreement regarding moral content and ultimate meaning, new medical technologies have increased our effective range of free choice and have here, as elsewhere, called out to us to act in responsible ways in new circumstances.

Responsibility in these matters is frequently avoided by asserting that one should maximally treat so as to extend human life as far as possible, under the supposition that medicine has been traditionally obliged to save life at any cost. This supposition, however, is false. Medicine traditionally avoided treating hopeless cases. The unrestrained commitment to treat individuals at any cost in order to save life of any quality (as exemplified, for instance, in the particular ideology of the Americans with Disabilities Act) is a modern peculiarity without classical roots.[111] One might think here of Seneca's remark that no one can complain of life or of suffering, because if the pains are too great, suicide is always available.[112] If one suffers, according to Seneca, it is no one's fault but one's own. In this vein, we are led to deciding which lifesaving treatment to accept, which to refuse, and when if ever suicide is a morally appropriate option.

To raise these questions is to recognize how issues of death and dying must be reconsidered at the end of the Christian age. Outside of a particular moral perspective, there will be no guidance as to what suffering should be borne, when death should be accepted, or when suicide should be undertaken. Choices in these matters require a content-full understanding of the purposes of life and death. For the West, this had been provided from the Christian synthesis that developed during its Middle Ages. Within this Christian understanding, suffering had a purpose, pain had a redemptive meaning, and death was recognized as not the end of personal existence. Moreover, suicide could not be undertaken, because it was acknowledged that the death of an innocent individual could not be directly intended, even if that death was one's own.

The proscription of directly intending the death of an innocent individual led to the widespread application of the principle of double effect when treating pain and limiting treatment (see also the comments on the principle of double effect in the previous chapter). This principle, originally fashioned primarily for moral judgments in wartime (e.g., in a just war foreseeing but not intending the death of innocent noncombatants could excuse one from moral blame in their death), came to be applied to medical issues as well.[113] The principle held that one could engage in actions likely to harm or even kill another, as long as (1) the physical evil was not intended (e.g., a good Roman Catholic soldier could shoot arrows over a city's walls, foreseeing but not intending that innocent civilians might be killed); (2) the good sought from the actions did not follow directly from the harms (e.g., the city would not be brought to surrender because of the death of the innocent civilians); (3) the action was not in itself intrinsically evil (e.g., one could indirectly kill noncombatant children, but not commit adultery in order to take the city); and (4) there was a proportionate good to be derived (e.g., the likely benefits would outweigh likely harms).[114] This principle allowed devout Roman Catholics not only to engage in actions that have as their foreseen but not intended effect sterilization and contraception, but also to provide a basis for discontinuing lifesaving treatment or providing pain control likely to bring an earlier death.

One could properly decide that further investment of resources in prolonging life is not obligatory because it constitutes an inordinate, disproportionate, or extraordinary drain on the resources of a family or society. Ordinary means for preserving life are defined as "all medicines, treatments, and operations, which offer a reasonable hope of benefit for the patient and which can be obtained and used without excessive expense, pain or other inconvenience."[115] "Ordinary" is not used here to indicate simply what is usual, but what is appropriate, proportionate, or ordinate. Here the term in medical ethics captures a now obsolete meaning of the word, namely, "temperate," which approximates one of the prime meanings of "ordinatus," namely, well ordered. An ordinary treatment is one that corresponds to well-ordained, customary treatment, which is to take into account not just considerations of costs, but quality of outcome (e.g., that health could be regained), as well as reasonable quantity of life.[116] Costs include such social concerns as the need to leave one's native town or village in order to seek treatment in a distant city.[117] Indeed, Roman Catholic theologian Gerald Kelly, S.J., once held that providing digitalis or intravenous glucose for a comatose ninety-year-old with cardiorenal disease would be extraordinary treatment.[118] Within this content-full, concrete moral vision, Roman Catholic theologians are thus able to understand the duty to treat as being inversely proportional to the costs of treatment and directly proportional to the length and quality of success.

Indeed, the Roman Catholic bioethical tradition will allow a patient to discontinue mechanical ventilation as an undue burden and to be provided with sufficient analgesia so as not to suffer pain, distress, and air hunger. What is essential is that death not be directly intended and that the amount of analgesic used not be such as simply to kill.

The principle of double effect permits individuals to engage in actions that they foresee would lead to death as long as they do not intend the death. Double effect, combined with the principle of ordinary versus extraordinary treatment, sets limits to the obligation to provide expensive care. The principle of double effect also allows giving pain-controlling medication that is likely to increase the chance of the patient's dying earlier, as long as the death is not intended, the pain is not controlled through killing the patient, and there is a sufficient or proportionate reason (e.g., severe pain). In short, Roman Catholics with very conservative moral viewpoints may both limit life-prolonging treatment and engage in activities that will likely hasten death. This position should not be unexpected. If one believes in an afterlife, it would be morally incongruous to employ all available resources to cling tenaciously to this life. Indeed, within many religious perspectives, the attempt to save life at all costs would be a form of idolatry of physical life.

It may not be an accident that the ethos of providing every chance of clinging to this life emerged as religious belief and the certainty concerning an afterlife waned. One must wonder whether the determination of some to prolong life at any cost does not spring from the loss of a theodicy of suffering and of a belief in an afterlife. They seem in many respects like Fyodor Pavlovich in *The Brothers Karamazov,* who "does not believe in God, but is afraid of hell. He 'intends to remain on the earth as long as possible.'"[119] Some appear to have concluded that, if one lives only once, life is worth saving at any expense. One should note how this view contrasts with that of the believer who sees this life as a journey to a final destiny with God. Communities that construe the right to life as a duty to stay alive under all circumstances may suffer from confusions consequent on the collapse of the Christian vision that has directed the West since the Middle Ages.

Outside of a particular moral or religious context in which directly intending the death of an individual is immoral, distinctions between intention and foresight, as well as between active and passive euthanasia, as well as between killing and letting die, cease to have intrinsic moral significance. In general secular morality, they may take on moral weight from different possible consequences in different circumstances. However, outside of a particular moral vision, all else being equal, it becomes impossible to make out what would be wrong in directly intending to kill one's self or to aid another in suicide in order to avoid intractable pain and suffering. The point is that, without reference to a moral and/or metaphysical account of pain and suffering, it is difficult if not impossible to explain why such should be endured, or why consensual killing would be in itself wrong.

In general secular moral terms, proscriptions of suicide, assisted suicide, and euthanasia become but one more taboo,[120] a complex of hesitations grounded in ethical considerations from our past, whose moral commitments one no longer takes seriously.[121] In such a context, the roots of proscriptions are forgotten and access to assisted suicide becomes a plausible constitutional right.[122]

It is only within a concrete content-full moral vision that one recognizes the meaning of suffering and the character of the good death. Consider the following prayers and how they contrast with a general secular understanding of pain and difficulty: "I acknowledge and believe, O Lord, that all trials of this life are given by Thee for our chastisement, when we drift away from Thee, and disobey Thy commandments."[123] Suffering and disease are recognized as one's due and as an opportunity for repentance: "I know, O Lord, that I justly deserve any punishment Thou mayest inflict upon me for I have so often offended Thee and sinned against Thee, in thought, word, and deed. . . . Grant that my sickness may be the means of my true repentance and amendment of my life according to Thy will, that I may spend the rest of my days in Thy love and fear."[124] For the nonbeliever, such confidence in suffering and in prayer is at best puzzling, and at worst misplaced.[125] The nonbeliever is very unlikely to accept the notion that suffering should be borne patiently, for, all else being equal, there is no purpose that such an individual recognizes to be achieved in such submission. Such an individual does not see the framework within which submission to God's will would make sense.

The difficulty is that in the ruins of a collapsing Judeo-Christian moral vision it is difficult for individuals to assemble coherent moral intuitions regarding how one should approach life and death decisions. Once moral sentiments are disarticulated from the content-full moral and metaphysical framework in which they had once been embedded, they no longer can provide reliable guidance. On the one hand, in general secular terms it will appear as if there is nothing morally improper in assisting suicide or supporting voluntary euthanasia. On the other hand, since this life will appear to be all there is, it can take on an absolute significance. Previous moral concerns regarding murder and in favor of the respect of human life may be transferred to a particular content-full moral assertion regarding the importance of saving lives at all costs. However, even in secular terms, individuals may have values that outweigh their concerns to preserve their own lives. In the absence of a coherent, content-full moral vision, there will be at best a confusion within which the only general secular guidance will be that derivable from the consent of those involved.

*The right to be left alone and deciding to die*

If moral authority in secular context is derived from individuals, then the right of consent, of giving permission, will have moral centrality. Further, if one has the right to consent, it follows that one has the right to refuse treatment, even lifesaving treatment. The ruling in *Natanson v. Kline* captures this point of general secular morality. The court stated that "Anglo-American law starts with the premise of a thorough-going self determination. It follows that each man is considered to be master of his own body, and he may, if he be of sound mind, expressly prohibit the performance of lifesaving surgery."[126] The recognition of the right to be left alone, not to be touched without one's permission, to be allowed to refuse clearly lifesaving treatment, has been accepted only after some controversy. Although in most cases the request to refuse treatment has been honored, where the individual refusing treatment was neither pregnant nor the guardian of dependent minors,[127] some courts have held that such refusal could be tantamount to suicide, which if not illegal was at least against public policy.[128]

Opposition to the refusal of lifesaving treatment when death is not immanent is closely bound to the Christian condemnation of suicide, which came to be incorporated in Western law. In Anglo-American law suicide was traditionally forbidden because "the suicide is guilty of a double offence; one spiritual, in invading the prerogative of the Almighty, and rushing into his immediate presence uncalled for; the other temporal, against the king, who hath an interest in the preservation of all his subjects."[129] Opposition to suicide came to be expressed in a wide range of concerns by the state for the would-be suicide and for third parties. The state's right to prevent suicide came to be derived from compelling state interests to (1) prevent citizens from committing an offense against God and/ or good public morals, (2) protect the state's interests in the productivity of its citizens, (3) preserve respect for life because of the utility of this attitude in assuring decent care for individuals, (4) enforce the obligations of individuals to support their dependents, discharge their debts, and to fulfill their contracts, and (5) protect individuals from imprudent choices, even when they harm only themselves.[130]

Given the arguments in chapter 4 regarding the limited authority of states, and those in chapter 3 regarding the rights of individuals to noninterference under the morality of mutual respect, the contentions in favor of state force weaken. A secular state does not have a secularly defensible right to employ force to protect the rights of God, nor to establish a particular concrete moral point of view beyond those enforcements that depend for their justification on the principle of permission and the general commitment to beneficence (i.e., the restriction of certain malevolent acts and the achievement of those goals of beneficence for which there is permission). This is not to say that God has no rights. It is simply that God's rights and one's duties to Him are not visible in a secular context.

The contention that one may forbid the refusal of treatment because it would undermine the sanctity of life has generally been rejected. Competent individuals possess a secular moral right to pursue peaceably as far as is possible with consenting others the realization of their particular view of the good life and the good death. With this right comes the right not to join with others. If such in fact leads to a lower evaluation of life, one has discovered one of the prices of freedom, not grounds for compelling cooperation. Free individuals, at least in general secular terms, are not responsible for the free actions of others, though they must live with the consequences of others' free choices. The world might in general be better if people had married spouses other than the ones they chose. From that, no state interest follows to compel individuals to marry only ideal partners at ideal times. So, also, free individuals should be able to die as they choose, even if they do not choose ideal times.

The objection to suicide or the refusal of lifesaving treatment on the basis of enforcing contracts carries the greatest weight. A state may properly use force to compel an individual to pay debts or discharge obligations before quitting this life. The armed forces might require officers to promise not to refuse lifesaving treatment or to commit suicide, save under very delimited circumstances. Other contracts, which may not be as explicit, would need to be examined in great detail and with great care. It is plausible that dependent children would have a right to veto the suicide of their parents, insofar as those parents have promised support of a certain sort. The extent of such commitments would clearly vary from culture to culture and family to family. Individuals should be able to circumvent such restrictions by acquiring special suicide insurance to allow them, should they ever choose, to commit suicide and to create an endowment for their children's support. Such policies could be conceived as insurance against the cost of being in a circumstance where suicide is a reasonable option. One might note that many insurance policies pay even with suicide, once they have been in force for a certain period of time. As long as such policies were engaged early in life, and as long as the frequency of suicide were not too high, the costs would not be great. Finally, one must note that the more it becomes likely that the individual refusing treatment and choosing suicide will in any case die, or the more disabled the individual is, the less plausible it is that enforced continuance of life will lead to the discharge of duties.

The contention that the state has a general secular moral right to protect free individuals from their own misguided choices finds little support from the arguments in this volume. The treatment of paternalism in section two of this chapter and of the limited authority of the state in chapter 4 supports the strong autonomy rights that were sketched in chapters 2 and 3. Being free means having the right to choose tragically and in a misguided fashion. On the other hand, individuals may establish special paternalistic relations. Individuals who are concerned about their reactions in times of despondency would be well advised to establish some form of advance directive to compel treatment or to impede suicide under specified circumstances. Finally, one must stress that the duty to respect freedom does not include a duty to respect the unfree choice of death by mentally ill persons. When an individual does not competently choose to refuse treatment or to commit suicide, there is no freedom to respect and one is instead directed by the principle of beneficence to achieve the good for that person, rather than to conform to statements that reflect mental illness, not free choice. These reflections lead generally to supporting the right of individuals to refuse treatment, even lifesaving treatment, and to commit suicide.

*Advance directives, proxy consent, and stopping treatment on the incompetent*

If competent individuals may personally refuse treatment, there should be no secular moral objection in principle against their doing so through an agent or through an advance directive. Persons now are in full secular moral authority over themselves and may fashion agreements with others that will bind indefinitely (*pace* contemporary law) unless they themselves again become competent to act to void such agreements (see the treatment of Ulysses contracts earlier in this chapter). Such is the moral foundation of both durable powers of attorney and other forms of living wills, which function as instruments for individuals to control their treatment when they are no longer competent. From a secular moral point of view, one should be able not only to appoint others to choose among treatment options as reasonable and prudent custodians of one's future treatment, but also appoint them to choose in special ways or simply capriciously (a liberty that appears at present unavailable), even to the point of refusing lifesaving treatment. The need for such directives is found in the precarious nature of life, fraught as it is with the risk of being incompetent and debilitated for a considerable period before death. Moreover, given the conflicting views of best interests in the face of serious illness and debility, it is important to establish who is in authority where it is often very difficult to establish who is a reliable authority regarding best interests. Given the cardinal place of the secular moral principle of permission, individuals have the secular moral right through an oral or written directive to forgo lifesaving treatment, even when they are not suffering from a terminal disease.

In establishing such directives, one must determine whom to place in authority and the extent to which the individual selected is an authority regarding one's own wishes. On the one hand, there are good grounds for providing as much instruction to proxies and others as possible. On the other hand, the opacity of the future and the difficulty of applying general principles to particular contexts argue in favor not simply of giving directions, but also of appointing an individual (perhaps guided by some general directions or instructions) as in authority to make decisions on one's behalf.

In the absence of an advance directive, it may be very difficult to determine who is in authority to make decisions for an incompetent individual. Such circumstances of ambiguity may lead to conflicts among family members about who is in authority regarding an incompetent's best interests. A spouse may choose not to treat, but a guilt-ridden estranged child may insist that all treatment be provided. To avoid such difficulties it may be best to establish clearly at law who is presumptively uniquely in authority: a spouse, the older parent, the oldest child. Individuals may always defeat such presumptions by a specific advance directive establishing the authority of a different individual. If such lines of presumptive authority are not established, the hesitations of family members may lead to an agonizing prolongation of the process of dying. The financial, psychological, and social costs may make it appropriate to give insurance discounts for those who enact a living will.

Here one must stress that prolonging life is not always in an individual's best interests. Even in the absence of an advance directive or previously established views on the matter of terminating treatment, the circumstances of life may be so difficult as to justify refusing treatment because it would be more of an injury than a benefit. However, any judgments in this matter depend on a particular content-full moral vision and such is not available in general secular contexts. Individuals in particular moral contexts can understand what is worth doing and what is not. In general secular terms, one can only create arbitrary public standards that may most easily be articulated in terms of cost considerations and the likelihood of success. In any event, the right to refuse treatment does not imply a right to demand treatment. Communities can without inconsistency affirm the right to refuse treatment, while limiting the treatment that can be demanded at communal expense.

Most accounts of beneficence will likely take the position that costs, as well as the likelihood of failure, defeat duties of beneficence. For example, the traditional distinction between ordinary and extraordinary care (which is shaped by moral assumptions at odds with the ideology of the Americans with Disabilities Act) provides a general rubric that can guide guardians in limiting care. This can be put schematically (repeating from chapter 6).

$$\frac{\text{Strength of the duty}}{\text{of beneficence}} = \frac{\text{Chance of success} \times \text{Quality of life} \times \text{Length of life}}{\text{Costs}}$$

One's concerns for individuals that are not and will not be persons in the strict sense may be less, in general secular moral terms at least, than for persons in the strict sense. Absent agreements to the contrary, such considerations may guide guardians.

In the absence of a particular guiding content-full moral vision, guardians may morally not only make quality-of-death decisions, but quality-of-life decisions regarding irreversibly incompetent wards, who have never competently expressed a contrary view.[131] For the most part, courts have seen the first to be a proper province of proxy decision makers. Yet they have retreated from allowing quality-of-life decisions. Still, the claim that one may not make quality-of-life judgments requires a particular canonical moral vision that will not be present in a general secular context for individuals who cannot invoke respect under the principle of permission.

## Death in an age of disbelief

In a number of circumstances, merely refusing treatment may not be enough for many people who think this life is all there is, or who are unconstrained by traditional Judeo-Christian morality. The decision to stop treatment in order not to prolong the process of dying may not lead to an easy death. Even if pain can be controlled, the various debilities consequent on disease and the treatment of disease, ranging from anal and urinary incontinence to exhaustion, may make further life unacceptable. For the person without religious guidance, euthanasia or suicide may then appear to be the most reasonable choice, and the aid of others may be needed. An example is provided by the death of Sigmund Freud. After sixteen years of struggling with cancer, and after thirty-three operations, he lay on his deathbed in London at the age of eighty-two. When he saw that prolonging life would in fact be boonless, he asked his personal physician to ease his way. "My dear Schur, you remember our first talk. You promised me then you would help me when I could no longer carry on. It is only torture now and it has no longer any sense."[132] Ernest Jones, Freud's biographer, records: "The next morning Schur gave Freud a third of a grain of morphia. For someone at such a point of exhaustion as Freud then was, and so complete a stranger to opiates, that small dose sufficed."[133] Freud had evidently considered such a remedy from the time of the first diagnosis of his illness.[134] A similar judgment was made by the physicist-philosopher and Nobel Prize winner Percy Bridgman (1882–1961). In July 1961, he had a disseminated malignancy and faced the possibility of considerable pain and the loss of what he had in his youth termed intellectual integrity.[135] He wrote, "I would like to take advantage of the situation in which I find myself to establish a general principle, namely, that when the end is as inevitable as it now appears to be, the individual has a right to ask his doctor to end it for him."[136] On August 20 of the same year he took his own life and left the following note: "It isn't decent for Society to make a man do this thing himself. Probably this is the last day I will be able to do it myself. P.W.B."[137]

These actions reflect a well-established secular moral view that rational suicide is not only allowable but in certain circumstances laudable. As Seneca argued in his letter on suicide, "Living is not the good, but living well. The wise man therefore lives as long as he should, not as long as he can. . . . He will always think of life in terms of quality, not quantity."[138] Thus Seneca argued that when "one death involves torture and the other is simple and easy, why not reach for the easier way? . . . Must I wait for the pangs of disease . . . when I can stride through the midst of torment and shake my adversaries off?"[139] Seneca, who took his own life in a famous scene recorded by Tacitus, could see no justifiable grounds against suicide where a prolonged and tortuous death awaited.[140] The philosopher David Hume even saw it as a duty to oneself. "That suicide may often be consistent with interest and with our duty to ourselves, no one can question, who allows that age, sickness, or misfortune may render life a burthen, and make it worse even than annihilation."[141]

Those following the views of Seneca and Hume must be tolerated in terms of the principle of permission. One might think here of the fact that up until 1973 the use of force against a rational suicide or the aiders of a rational suicide would have counted as assault and battery in the state of Texas. Texas, which unlike other Anglo-American jurisdictions never forbade suicide, did not criminalize aiding and abetting suicide until 1973. The argument was that if suicide was not a crime, it could not be a crime to aid others in a noncriminal activity. In taking this position, Texas departed from most, if not all, American jurisdictions.

It may be a violation of morals and ethics and reprehensible that a party may furnish another poison or pistols or guns or any other means or agency for the purpose of the suicide to take his own life, yet our law has not seen proper to punish such persons or such acts.[142]

Here it is useful to read the Texas court as distinguishing between the moral authority of Texas as a peaceable, secular pluralist state, and the moral commitments of particular communities, which might recognize the evil in suicide and in aiding and abetting suicide. It will be very difficult for a secular, peaceable, pluralist state to interfere with secular moral authority in the free choices of individuals and of those who assist them in refusing treatment or committing suicide.

Given the arguments in this book, the central secular moral evil in murder is not taking the life of an individual, but taking that life without the individual's permission. Old Texas law can furnish another example. In the first days of the republic, neither suicide nor aiding and abetting suicide nor dueling was a crime.[143] In this the republic took seriously the notion that with consent there is no harm, *volenti non fit injuria*.[144] This view was not shared by the Judeo-Christian heritage, which recognized the evil of taking all human life, especially innocent life. In general secular morality, individuals are secure in their rational choices with themselves and consenting others, no matter how reprehensible or ultimately misguided they may be.

One might even raise the issue of whether there can be a duty to die—a duty not only to refuse treatment, but under certain circumstances to have one's death expedited. One can imagine special circumstances where, for example, joining an espionage organization obligates one to agree to commit suicide in order to avoid compromising a mission. One can create special circumstances in which one promises to take one's life so that one would have a secular moral obligation to do so. In secular morality one is at liberty to make promises that one can within a particular moral perspective understand to be opprobrious. The moral foundations for this position become clear when one (1) distinguishes freedom as a constraint on human actions from freedom as a value and (2) recognizes the content-less character of general secular morality. In contrast, for example, Kant condemned suicide because he saw it as a rejection of the basis of the moral community. ''To destroy the subject of morality in his own person is tantamount to obliterating from the world, as far as he can, the very existence of morality itself; but morality is, nevertheless, an end in itself.''[145] Kant here confuses the conceptual conditions for the possibility of being blameworthy or praiseworthy with the material conditions for having a moral community. If all rational agents decided to commit suicide, they would not be choosing in a way that would contradict the very *concept* of a community based on mutual respect, though they may be setting aside the possibility of the *existence* of a moral community. Further, it is not possible, *pace* Kant, to use oneself as a means merely, for one always consents to the uses one makes of oneself.[146] The character of Kant's argument leads him to hold that he can in general secular terms justify forbidding not only suicide but masturbation,[147] as well as selling or giving one's organs to another, because such would involve using one's self as a means merely. Kant contends that ''to give away or sell a tooth so that it can be planted in the jawbone of another person . . . [is] partial self-murder.''[148] The analyses in this volume of the principle of permission undercut this line of argument and lead, as we have seen, to holding that murder is a moral offense primarily because it involves taking the life of another individual without that individual's consent. Competent suicide or taking another's life at that person's request does not violate the secular moral principle of permission, unless there are prior agreements to the contrary (e.g., agreements not to commit suicide or engage in dueling or obligations to discharge debts).

Whether suicide or killing another at that person's request violates the principle of beneficence will depend on the ranking of harms and benefits to which one appeals. When the individual to be killed is in severe pain, secular beneficence-based arguments may indeed construe it as morally laudatory, if not obligatory, to hasten death. If the individual is ill and debilitated, obligations to support dependents or discharge debts may have become moot and no longer plausibly hinder the choice to die. Consider Hume's suggestion that suicide under certain circumstances would be an act of social responsibility. ''But suppose that it is no longer in my power to promote the interest of society; suppose that I am a burthen to it: . . . In such cases my resignation of life must not only be innocent but laudable.''[149] One might imagine a patriotic citizen with a debilitating terminal disease committing suicide in order not to encumber further the Medicare fund. Failing to take the time to leave instructions for others about the level of treatment one wishes should one become irreversibly and seriously demented may count as a form of moral and social truancy, insofar as such unclarity commits family and society to forms of treatment the individual would not have wanted. For those who do not appreciate the immorality of direct killings, it may even seem obligatory to leave instructions regarding the circumstances under which one ought to be killed.

The prospect of an ever-developing technological capacity to extend life under circumstances that are costly and at times of little enjoyment to the individual underscores the issues of refusal of lifesaving treatment, suicide, and voluntary euthanasia. Although for many these issues necessarily raise the specter of a dictatorial state enforcing involuntary euthanasia, there is little to support this concern in the absence of a statist culture. The fact that Texas, which for over 130 years had no law against suicide or against aiding and abetting suicide, while easily avoiding dangerous slippery slopes to state-imposed euthanasia, shows that such policies do not necessarily lead to abuse, if by abuse one means involuntary euthanasia. What is key to preventing such abuse is whether the society takes seriously the limits of secular state power.[150]

This secular concern with abuse as state-mandated suicide or euthanasia (or with suicide and euthanasia effected through the coercion of relatives or others) contrasts with the traditional Western concern since the Middle Ages: that individuals not be tempted to end their own lives. When this is no longer understood as a moral danger, one has stepped outside of the Christian moral vision which has fashioned Western European and American policies bearing on choices regarding death and dying. For those who live within the Judeo-Christian moral vision, they will regard the allure of suicide and voluntary euthanasia as one of the major temptations for the future. In a world of scarce resources and expensive technologies, it will appear only too reasonable that one should treat maximally and then freely effect death when treatments fail and pain and suffering become intolerable. Such will become the most reasonable secular use of resources. The use of euthanasia, both directly and through advance directives, will appear as a responsible and appropriate individual choice. There will be immense pressures driven by economic concerns and fears of pain, suffering, and disability that will make suicide, assisted suicide, and euthanasia as reasonable and as acceptable as prenatal diagnosis and abortion. Outside of a particular content-full moral vision, it will be impossible to recognize anything wrong in such choices.

Here it is necessary to emphasize that a secular moral defense of the right of competent individuals to refuse treatment or take their own lives is not an endorsement of tolerating suicide generally.[151] The majority of individuals who seek to commit suicide do so because of mental difficulties. They should receive psychiatric treatment, not aid in committing suicide. In addition, a great proportion of the competent individuals who choose suicide may do so on ill-considered grounds or because of circumstances that can be remedied through the kindness and compassion of others. Such individuals should be the subject of peaceable persuasion aimed at preventing suicide. However, when one has excluded all such individuals from consideration, there are individuals with debilitating diseases or in the final stages of decrepitude who may not be able to see the evil of direct killing. How can one explain to the agnostic yuppie that one should live out the last few weeks or months of a death from cancer complicated by multiple metastases and multiple organ difficulties. Such individuals may not wish to spend their final days in nursing homes or other long-term nursing facilities. Such considerations will return many to the pagan context that existed before the framing of the Western Christian moral synthesis. In that regard, one must note that the so-called Hippocratic oath, which was more likely written by a group of neo-Pythagoreans than by Hippocrates, did not represent Greco-Roman medical practice as a whole.[152] Many physicians of that time probably did give advice regarding how to achieve a quick and painless death.[153]

Assisted suicide and euthanasia would require revisions of the laws bearing on suicide and murder. Even under the old law of the state of Texas, which tolerated aiding and abetting suicide, death had to be effected by the person committing suicide. If another pulled the trigger or placed poison in the suicide's mouth, that person became a murderer, not an abettor of suicide. For many individuals with severely debilitating diseases, more help would be required than the old law allowed, and which the new Texas law completely proscribes.[154] Such individuals might want to be assisted in dying, but because of disease and disabilities would need not simply passive facilitation but active help. Although such individuals have the secular moral right to be assisted by those who agree to help them, they would not have a right to commit suicide, to be assisted in suicide, or to receive euthanasia in institutions morally opposed to such endeavors. Nor would the principles of permission or beneficence require either physicians or institutions to recommend an alternative provider to a patient seeking such services. Such a requirement would depend on a particular moral vision of beneficence.[155]

These issues will be inescapable as we extend life expectancy without a dramatic compression of morbidity in old age, and as the remnants of the Christian age are abandoned. The risk of growing older, only to be severely mentally and physically debilitated, may be more than secular society in general or many individuals in particular will wish to bear. In the future there will be an ever-increasing risk, as more individuals live beyond the age of eighty-five, not only of suffering the minor debilities of old age, but of spending months, if not years, requiring comprehensive nursing care. That risk can be avoided if individuals are allowed to direct that they should be painlessly killed under certain specified circumstances. Such individuals would not need fear growing old to the point at which life would be an indignity to them and a burden to others. Not only would such a policy remove this fear, but it would also free resources to protect the health and augment the pleasures of life when it still can be lived with full indulgence.

## Euthanasia

If there is no difference in principle between intending someone's death and merely allowing it, there will be no absolute moral bar against killing an individual on request. Indeed, the principle of permission does not bar terminating the life of an individual who was once competent and (1) who is not competent and (2) will not again be competent, (3) where it appears by clear and convincing evidence that the person would have wished not only to be allowed to die but to have death expedited in the circumstances in question. Only involuntary euthanasia, not nonvoluntary euthanasia (i.e., euthanasia that is not explicitly refused, but can be presumed to be in accord with a now incompetent individual's past wishes), can be forbidden by an appeal to the principles of permission or beneficence. Permission is not violated and one appears to be acting in the person's best interests.

In this secular moral context, the old distinctions between foresight and intention become irrelevant. One can no longer understand what would be improper in directly intending or effecting an innocent individual's death. The focus is then on consent, on whether there is truly voluntary suicide (i.e., the individual competently chooses self-killing), truly voluntary assisted suicide (i.e., the individual assisting does so with the free invitation of and without coercing the person who wishes to commit suicide), and truly voluntary or at least not involuntary euthanasia (i.e., competent persons are killed only at their request, and incompetent individuals only if it can be presumed that this is in accord with their wishes). Distinctions between active and passive euthanasia cease to have any intrinsic moral significance. Nor does the distinction between passive euthanasia and letting die (which depended on the presence or absence of the direct intention to kill) carry moral weight. In our increasingly post-Christian context, such distinctions will appear as reflections of outworn taboos. When one has lost the guidance of a canonical moral vision regarding how one should live and how one should die, moral authority can only be derived from permission, from consent. This, then, becomes the central focus of secular moral concern in decisions regarding the cessation of treatment or the direct killing of individuals. For many, this will be all to which they can appeal, not only with moral strangers, but also with moral friends. *O tempora! O mores!*

## The health care team

The character of health care is defined by a web of exclusions and inclusions shaped by the various values that direct the free choices of patients, physicians, nurses, and allied health professionals. Decisions to be treated, to be helped, to be left alone, to refuse treatment, or to be less than fully compliant with medical recommendations, as well as requests for care, cure, and support, reflect often competing views of good health care. So, too, do decisions of physicians and nurses regarding what care they will provide and under what circumstances. Provision of coherent care is complicated by the number of men and women involved. They determine the character of health care through numerous free choices. In addition, the decisions of governments, insurers, hospitals, and other third parties shape the character of care. But even in terms of the physicians involved, the matter is complex. When a patient is admitted to a hospital, there may not only be an admitting physician, but also an attending physician, a resident, and an intern, who may change every month. In addition, consultants will be engaged to provide opinions regarding specific problems or particular forms of treatment. The greatest continuity of care may be achieved by the nurses involved with the patient.

To speak of this coterie of individuals as a health care team may suggest more coherence and organization than often exists. Allied to the problem of organization is a problem of deciding who directs the team and with what authority. Traditionally, the attending physician has been seen as the captain of the team. Here one might recall stronger metaphors, such as the notion of the physician as the captain of the ship.[156] Such metaphors have been weakened by the increasing independence, and in some cases independent licensure, of nurses, as well as by the increased emphasis on the rights of patients. If authority to treat the patient comes from the patient directly or through the patient's family, is the patient more the captain of the ship, and the physician the pilot? Insofar as patients or their families want to take charge of the course of treatment, they can come to be those centrally responsible and accountable for the direction of care. They may insist that consulting physicians report not simply to the attending physician, but to the patient and/or family. Insofar as patients or their families pay consultants directly or through their insurance, such is a powerful request. Patients and their families may insist that they themselves direct the treatment. Insofar as patients control the funding of health care, it is not unreasonable to suppose that radically patient-centered changes can be realized. Though such changes could be achieved, they would involve major alterations in the ways in which physicians have traditionally supported and cared for patients and their families. An activist pursuit of patient autonomy will be undertaken at the price of the traditional trust, reliance, and comfort afforded by putting oneself or one's family in the hands of a worthy physician. Those involved will need to judge for themselves what benefits should be pursued and what costs avoided.

The more medical care is given outside such a personal relationship, the more one will need explicitly to spell out one's wishes in order to give direction to care-givers. One will need to indicate in some detail what kind of care one will want, should one become incompetent and no longer be a self who can authoritatively give and withhold permission. Again, the sparse character of advance directives is rarely sufficient to indicate adequately what treatment is to be provided or forgone.[157] Indeed, the less one lives within the embrace of traditional communities and personal relationships, the more one may need to make understandings explicit. Not out of some legal concern, but to avoid feelings of guilt and misunderstandings on the part of family members, it may at times be useful for relatives to be special supernumerary witnesses to an advance directive as a moral commitment to honor the requests of the patient. When the patient is sent to a referral hospital where physicians may rotate monthly in providing care, the patient and family will need to take special steps to ensure that the wishes of the patient (and of the family of an incompetent patient) are clearly known and understood. Formal written directives may offer the only reliable safeguard against being provided treatment or being resuscitated against one's wishes because a new attending physician, resident, or intern did not know of the prior decisions of the patient or family. Patients and their families must captain the direction of health care if such outcomes are to be avoided. Still, even when patients take such an interventionist role (which many patients may not wish to shoulder), the physician remains inescapably the pilot, the individual who knows where wishes can go aground and hopes be shipwrecked. The physician is the one who knows the intimate geography of possibilities in setting a course through dangerous waters.

The structure of the health care team will depend on the extent to which patients seek to captain their destiny and the extent to which physicians, nurses, and others believe that charting a particular course is necessary for good health care. Physicians may insist that consultants report to them, not directly to the patient. They may insist that nurses not inform patients of their judgments regarding care and prognosis but defer to physicians in this matter. Whether consultants speak directly to patients or primarily to the attending physician, whether nurses will have independent areas in which they can communicate decisions regarding the treatment and prognosis of the patient, or the extent to which nurses and other allied health care professionals function as physician assistants will in the end depend on the agreement or peaceable acquiescence of all involved. The circumstance that the profession of physician's assistants[158] developed as nurses withdrew from being physician extenders may show that there is a persistent and important role for individuals who assist physicians as their agents.[159]

The meaning and significance of the health care professions and the ways in which they collaborate one with the other do not reflect the deep structure of reality. They are the outcomes of human choice. Until now, much of the change has been incremental. Now, however, against a background of increasing moral diversity and the weakening of traditional expectations, much has been brought into question and very likely much will be reshaped as human expectations and financial reality change.

## Consent, moral diversity, and health care policy: why does everything have to be uniform?

The secular moral character of health care is to be created, not discovered. There is no single secular canonical ranking of values that should dictate the role of physicians, patients, nurses, and others. Each can surely withdraw or refuse to participate. However, none may compel the uncritical services of the other. No one may independently and unilaterally fashion the concrete character of health care. Each depends on the free agreement of the others to participate in the complex endeavors of health care. Patients and others should be at liberty to create opportunities for the realization of particular moral visions in health care policy. Which is to say, associations and institutions should be able to create their own health care policy, reflecting their own moral visions. This is an issue to which we will turn in the next chapter. Here it is enough to note that, just as there are hospitals established by Seventh Day Adventists and Roman Catholics, one may establish special libertarian or paternalist hospitals that can allow the patients to have the special moral character of care they seek.

The emergence of ethics committees may be motivated in part by the need to secure moral direction in a cultural context where content-full guidance is absent. In religious hospitals with content-full moral commitments, such committees face the challenge of applying well-framed understandings in new contexts. In other hospitals, committees must often (1) frame moral policy so as (2) to educate staff, (3) provide consultations, and (4) mediate conflicts. Religious hospitals must often respond to threats to their institutional moral integrity (e.g., how should a traditional Christian hospital react if a requirement for licensure is that the hospital provide abortion, support sexual activities outside of the marriage of a man and a woman, or allow euthanasia on its premises?).[160] Hospitals without a content-full moral commitment must often decide what guidance they can provide beyond charting the lines of permission and refusal among the various parties to bioethical controversies. Such hospitals must hope that their ethics committees can help them frame an institutional morality. Given the diversity of moral visions, the role of hospital ethics committees and the policies they create need not, indeed should not, be uniform across hospitals.

If states and other groups refrain from using secularly unjustifiable coercive power, there will be opportunities for various associations to support diverse moral visions peaceably. Such associations could sustain various parallel health care systems built around particular content-full moral visions. Many would understand the moral evil involved in abortion and euthanasia. Others might provide special insurance discounts for those agreeing to prenatal diagnosis and abortion, as well as euthanasia under defined circumstances. Yet others may simply wish to contract for cheaper health care, although they recognize that this will expose them to some increased risk of suffering and death. To allow individuals to agree to morally diverse visions of health care will require taking moral diversity seriously, as well as the secular moral authority that individuals have to collaborate freely with consenting others.[161] To allow individuals to agree to cheaper health care at some increase of risk of dying and suffering will require recognizing that all reality is a gamble and that health care choices are properly made by free individuals in the face of uncertainty. After all, if mile for mile one is one-tenth as likely to die flying in a commercial jet as driving in a car, it would be quite sensible to purchase flights on an airline at half the usual price and twice the likelihood of crashing.

The possibility of such liberty, as well as the defense of important moral values that are understandable only within particular moral communities, is contingent on restraining various passions towards equality and uniformity in health care access that would eliminate moral diversity through the coercive imposition of particular understandings of justice and fairness. As was seen in chapter 4, coercive state commitments to particular visions of fairness, equality, and justice are without secular moral authority. The character of health care is in the end determined not only by the free choice of those who participate, but also by the coercive intrusions of those who would impose by force their own visions of beneficence and fairness.

## Notes

1. Hippocrates, *Epidemics* 1.12.1O–15, in *Hippocrates,* trans. W. H. S. Jones (Cambridge, Mass.: Harvard University Press, 1962), vol. 1, p. 165.
2. The body of skills and knowledge possessed by members of a learned profession constitutes a conceptual structure that guides and defines the community. See, for example, Karl Popper's treatment of ideas as a world of quasi-Platonic objects: Karl R. Popper and John C. Eccles, *The Self and Its Brain* (New York: Springer, 1977), pp. 36–50.
3. At the time of Hippocrates (ca. 460–377 B.C.) there was no formal association or lobby group such as the American Medical Association. There was also little formal control of the medical profession. See, for example, the Hippocratic treatise *Law.* However, there were avenues for the equivalent of malpractice suits against physicians in ancient times. Darrel W. Amundsen, "The Liability of the Physician in Classical Greek Legal Theory and Practice," *Journal of the History of Medicine and Allied Sciences* 32 (Apr. 1977): 172–203; "The Liability of the Physician in Roman Law," in H. Karplus (ed.), *International Symposium on Society, Medicine and Law* (New York: Elsevier, 1973), pp. 17–30: "Physician, Patient and Malpractice: An

Historical Perspective,'' in S. F. Spicker et al. (eds.), *The Law-Medicine Relation: A Philosophical Exploration* (Dordrecht: Reidel, 1981), pp. 255–58.

4. Alfred Schutz provides a very helpful treatment of the problems associated with the social distribution of knowledge and how this bears on the differences among experts, laymen, and well-informed laymen. Alfred Schutz and Thomas Luckman, *The Structures of the Life-World,* trans. R. M. Zaner and H. T. Engelhardt, Jr. (Evanston, Ill.: Northwestern University Press, 1973), pp. 304–31.

5. There is a certain awe involved in interventions with powerful mechanical devices, such as the space shuttle. There may be a special sense of awe or respect for those who repair such devices, which in part depends on the complexity of the mechanism being repaired.

6. An exploration of the problem that patients face in anticipating the moral and professional commitments of physicians is provided by Alasdair MacIntyre, "Patients as Agents," in S. F. Spicker and H. T. Engelhardt, Jr. (eds.), *Philosophical Medical Ethics: Its Nature and Significance* (Dordrecht: Reidel, 1977), pp. 197–212.

7. Alfred Schutz, "The Stranger: An Essay in Social Psychology," in Arvid Brodersen (ed.), *Collected Papers* (The Hague: Martinus Nijhoff, 1964), vol. 2, p. 99.

8. Edmund D. Pellegrino and David C. Thomasma, *A Philosophical Basis of Medical Practice* (New York: Oxford University Press, 1981), pp. 64–66, 72, 86, 187, 200; see also Pellegrino and Thomasma, *For the Patient's Good* (New York: Oxford University Press, 1988).

9. Plato discusses the issue of the patient being a friend to the physician for the sake of health in *Lysis,* 218d–219d.

10. Pellegrino and Thomasma's interpretation of this passage is dependent on Plato's assumption that there is a univocal sense of health and that both the physician and the patient have a common understanding of the good of health to be achieved through medicine.

11. Aristotle, *Magna Moralia,* 2.12115–16.

12. "The sick man, as we just now said, is a friend to the physician. Is he not? He is. On account of sickness, for the sake of health? Yes." Plato, *Lysis,* 218e, in Edith Hamilton and Huntington Cairns (eds.), *The Collected Dialogues of Plato* (Princeton, N.J.: Princeton University Press, 1969), pp. 162–63.

13. Pellegrino and Thomasma, *Philosophical Basis of Medical Practice,* p. 72.

14. G. W. F. Hegel, *Hegel's Philosophy of Right,* trans. T. M. Knox (London: Oxford University Press, 1965), sec. 303.

15. Ibid., sec. 270 Zusatz. In this section Hegel criticizes the anti-Semites of his day and gives what can be interpreted as an argument for a religiously neutral-tolerant state. For an exploration of Hegel's commitments to a limited tolerant state, see H. T. Engelhardt, Jr., "Sittlichkeit and Post-Modernity: An Hegelian Reconsideration of the State," in H. T. Engelhardt, Jr., and Terry Pinkard (eds.), *Hegel Reconsidered: Beyond Metaphysics and the Authoritarian State* (Dordrecht: Kluwer, 1994), pp. 211–24.

16. Robert A. Burt, *Taking Care of Strangers* (New York: Free Press, 1979), p. 19.

17. Even within communities bound together by a concrete view of the good life, there is

a place for the rule of law, not that of men: the law should always be a source of protection for persons against unconsented-to force. In many communities this will not require bureaucratic rules. The more the community is a face-to-face community, the less need there will be for elaborate formal regulations.

18. For a review of some of the issues raised by free and informed consent in the law, see Alexander M. Capron, "Informed Consent in Catastrophic Disease Research and Treatment," *University of Pennsylvania Law Review* 123 (Dec. 1974): 340–438; Donald G. Hagman, "The Medical Patient's Right to Know: Report on a Medical-Legal-Ethical, Empirical Study," *UCLA Law Review* 17 (1970): 758–816; Leslie J. Miller, "Informed Consent: I," *Journal of the American Medical Association* 244 (Nov. 7, 1980): 2100–2103, "Informed Consent: II," *Journal of the American Medical Association* 244 (Nov. 21, 1980): 2347–50; "Informed Consent: III," *Journal of the American Medical Association* 244 (Dec. 5, 1980): 2556–58; "Informed Consent: IV," *Journal of the American Medical Association* 244 (Dec. 12, 1980): 2661–62; Marcus L. Plante, "An Analysis of 'Informed Consent,'" *Fordham Law Review* 36 (1968): 639–72; J. R. Waltz and T. W. Scheuneman, "Informed Consent to Therapy," *Northwestern University Law Review* 64 (1970): 628–50. See also Paul Appelbaum, Charles Lidz, and Alan Meisel, *Informed Consent: Legal Theory and Clinical Practice* (New York: Oxford University Press, 1987); Ruth Faden and Tom Beauchamp, *A History and Theory of Informed Consent* (New York: Oxford University Press, 1986); President's Commission for the Study of Ethical Problems in Medicine and Biomedical and Behavioral Research, *Making Health Care Decisions,* 3 vols. (Washington, D.C.: U.S. Government Printing Office, 1982); and Stephen Wear, *Informed Consent: Patient Autonomy and Physician Beneficence within Clinical Medicine* (Dordrecht: Kluwer, 1993). These articles provide an introduction to some of the legal issues raised by this volume's analysis of free and informed consent. The reader should note that *The Foundations* focuses on conceptual issues, not directly on issues raised in the law.

19. A. W. Broadwell, E. V. Boisaubin, J. K. Dunn, and H. T. Engelhardt, Jr., "Advance Directives on Hospital Admission," *Southern Medical Journal* 86 (Feb. 1993): 165–68.

20. Natalie Abrams, "Medical Experimentation: The Consent of Prisoners and Children," in Spicker and Engelhardt, *Philosophical Medical Ethics,* pp. 111–24. See also Loretta Kopelman and John Moskop (eds.), *Children and Health Care: Moral and Social Issues* (Dordrecht: Kluwer, 1989).

21. Mary Ann Cutter and Earl E. Shelp (eds.), *Competency* (Dordrecht: Kluwer, 1991); see also Becky White, *Competence to Consent* (Washington, D.C.: Georgetown University Press, 1995).

22. Task Force on Ethics of the Society of Critical Care Medicine, "Consensus Report on the Ethics of Foregoing Life-sustaining Treatments in the Critically Ill," *Critical Care Medicine* 18 (Dec. 1990): 1439.

23. Ibid.

24. A. B. Seckler, D. E. Meier, M. Mulvihill, and B. E. Cammer, "Substituted Judgment: How Accurate Are Proxy Predictions?" *Annals of Internal Medicine* 115 (July 15, 1991): 92–98; and Marion Danis, Joanne Garrett, Russell Harris, and Donald L.

Patrick, "Stability of Choices about Life-sustaining Treatments," *Annals of Internal Medicine* 120 (Apr. 1, 1994): 567–73.

25. The dominant ideology will usually determine, for better or worse, what is considered a reasonable and prudent choice within a particular society.

26. The Magna Charta (June 15, 1215) gave a general protection against unjustified governmental use of force against individuals. "No freeman shall be taken or imprisoned, or disseised, or outlawed, or banished, or any ways destroyed, nor will we pass upon him, nor will we send upon him, unless by the lawful judgment of his peers, or by the law of the land" (sec. 39).

There were also grounds for action against individuals who beat others without justification. Thus, William Blackstone gives the following commentary regarding battery:

The least touching of another's person wilfully, or in anger, is a battery; for the law cannot draw the line between different degrees of violence, and therefore totally prohibits the first and lowest stage of it: every man's person being sacred, and no other having a right to meddle with it, in any the slightest manner. And therefore upon a similar principle the Cornelian law *de injuriis* prohibited *pulsation* as well as *verberation;* distinguishing verberation, which was accompanied with pain, from pulsation, which was attended with none.

William Blackstone, *Commentaries on the Laws of England* (1765), Book 3, p. 120. Blackstone originally published his work between 1765 and 1769. Earlier commentaries give a more restricted notion of battery, as that provided by Thomas Wood (1661–1722): "A *Battery* is any Injury done to the Person of another in a Rude or Angry Manner; as by Striking, Pushing, Jostling, Catching by the Arm, Filliping upon the Nose, Spitting in the Face, Pulling of a Button in a Rude and Insolent Manner, etc." *An Institute of the Laws of England* (London: Nutt and Gosling, 1724; repr. 1979), p. 423. This might be compared with the Texas penal code, which holds that a person commits the offense of assault if he "intentionally or knowingly causes physical contact with another when he knows or should reasonably believe that the other will regard the contact as offensive or provocative." *Texas Penal Code Annotated,* sec. 22.01(a) (3) (Vernon Supp. 1982). Modern codes have developed the views of Cornelian law regarding assault and battery, to which Blackstone alluded.

27. Free individuals were immune under ancient Germanic law from the torture regularly used in the Mediterranean world and later in the Inquisition of Western Christendom. It was a crime to use violence against a free individual. Consider the following passage from a classic treatise on torture: "For the cringing suppliant of the audience chamber, abjectly prostrating himself before a monarch who combines in his own person every legislative and executive function, we have the freeman of the German forests, who sits in council with his chief, who frames the laws which both are bound to respect, and who pays to that chief only the amount of obedience which superior vigor and intellect may be able to enforce. . . . This personal independence of the freeman is one of the distinguishing characteristics of all the primitive Teutonic institutions." Henry Charles Lea, *Torture* (Philadelphia: University of Pennsylvania Press, 1866; repr. 1973), pp. 24–25. There was in general a disinclination to subservience of any kind. Consider, for example, the account given by Dudo of St. Quentin (ca. 970–1043) of an encounter between Rollo, the first duke of Normandy (r. 911–

32) and Charles the Simple (r. 898–929), king of France. Rollo was asked to do homage to the king by kissing his foot, whereupon the duke asked one of his men to perform the obeisance on his behalf. The man did so by lifting the king's foot to his mouth, upending the king on his back. Peter Foote and David M. Wilson, *The Viking Achievement* (London: Sidgwick & Jackson, 1980), p. 79.

28. Slater v. Baker and Stapleton, 2 Wils. 359, 95 Eng. Rep. 860 (Kings Bench 1767). There were significant limits to the amount of information required to be disclosed for patient consent. Consider Justice Oliver Wendell Holmes's remark: "the patient has no more right to all the truth than he has to all of the medicines in the physician's saddlebags." Quoted in Eugene M. Hoyt, "Mandatory Disclosure Standards or Informed Consent—Texas Style," *Texas Medicine* 79 (Oct. 1983): 56.

29. Schloendorff v. Society of N.Y. Hospital, 211 N.Y. 125, 105 N.E. 92, 93 (1914). This decision was anticipated, for example, by Mohr v. Williams, where the court ruled that a procedure undertaken by a physician without a patient's consent should count as a tort. Mohr v. Williams, 95 Minn. 261, 104 N.W. 12 (1905).

30. Olmstead v. United States, 277 U.S. 438, 478 (1928) (Brandeis, J., dissenting).

31. In re President & Directors of Georgetown College, Inc., 331 F.2d 1000, 1017 (D.C. Cir.) *cert. denied*, 337 U.S. 978 (1964) (Burger, W., dissenting) (emphasis in original).

32. Natanson v. Kline, 186 Kan. 393, 404, 350 P. 2d 1093, 1104 (1960).

33. The attribution to Tertullian (?/160–ca. 230) of the phrase, "Credo quia absurdum est," which is not found in any of his extant writings, is discussed by Etienne Gilson in *History of Christian Philosophy in the Middle Ages* (New York: Random House, 1955), p. 45. Similar passages can be found. Tertullian said with regard to the death of Christ, "Prorsus credibile est quia ineptum est" (It is straightforwardly believable because it is silly) and with regard to the Resurrection, "Certum est, quia impossibile est" (It is certain because it is impossible). *De carne Christi*, sec. 5. There are similarities with Augustine, who argued that one must believe in order to understand. *De Trinitate* 8.5.8 and 9.1.1. As Blessed Augustine stated in *In Ioannis evangelium tractatus* 40.8.9, "Non quia cognoverunt crediderunt, sed ut cognoscerent crediderunt. Credimus enim ut cognoscamus, non cognoscimus ut credamus." (They have not known because they have believed, but so that they might know they have believed. For they believe in order to know, they do not know in order to believe.) These writings provide an example of the position that only through the special grace of belief is true knowledge of the important goals of life and the truths of existence available. Outside of such grace, belief often will seem to be folly in the eyes of the Greeks and scandal in the eyes of the Jews (1 Corinthians 1:23).

34. The first sense of freedom is that of being able to be self-determining. It does not include the strong condition that one must be rationally self-determining, as Kant requires for autonomous choice. The second sense identifies being at moral liberty to act in a particular sphere, where moral constraint is grounded in the principle of permission. The last sense recognizes that, if one coerces the permission of another, then one sets aside the basis to claim a right to what the coerced person agrees to provide. When the absence of enabling conditions and the presence of third–party

CONSENT, REFUSAL OF TREATMENT, AND THE HEALTH CARE TEAM    363

coercion, however unfortunate, are not attributable to the individuals directly involved, such circumstances do not invalidate agreements given, except insofar as the
circumstances render impossible the discharge of a duty.
35. Baruch A. Brody and H. Tristram Engelhardt, Jr. (eds.), *Mental Illness: Law and
Public Policy* (Dordrecht: Reidel, 1980).
36. In re President & Directors of Georgetown College, Inc., 1008. The court held that
the duty was not directly to the infant but to the community regarding the infant: "The
patient had a responsibility to the community to care for her infant. Thus the people
had an interest in preserving the life of this mother." The court was correct in holding
that individuals ought not to create new burdens for the community. On the other
hand, insofar as communities allow parents to place their children for adoption or as
state wards, and one circumscribes that right simply because the individual wishes to
exercise it so as to refuse lifesaving treatment, that circumscription may involve
coercively imposing a particular set of moral values. In addition to the community's
interest in the child and the society's interest in not being subjected to undue financial
burden, there is also the question of the obligation of the parent to secure the well-
being of the child.
37. In re Osborne, 294 A.2d 372, 374 (D.C. 1972).
38. Colin M. Turnbull, *The Mountain People* (New York: Simon and Schuster, 1972),
p. 121.
39. The reader should note that this view of lying departs radically from the Kantian
understanding. See, for example, Immanuel Kant, *The Metaphysics of Morals*, AK
VI 429–31. Kant argues for the immorality of lying on the grounds that it violates
one's duty to oneself considered as a moral being, as well as making that individual
responsible for all of the unforeseen consequences of the lie. The significance of lying
changes when one distinguishes between freedom as a value and freedom as a side
constraint. If the freedom at stake in the morality of mutual respect is freedom as a
side constraint, freedom as the source of permission, as I have argued in chapter 3,
then individuals may free themselves of duties to themselves. In addition, the moral
significance of lying changes when it is seen as a justified use of defensive force. The
same arguments that Kant employs to justify defensive force (and for that matter
retributive force) will justify defensive lying and deception. An individual who acts
against the very possibility of mutual respect loses grounds for consistently protesting
against defensive force, including lying. Those who use defensive force cannot be
held to have violated the notion of mutual respect, in that they have treated the
violator in a way consistent with the violator's expressed moral principles. Not only
does the individual using defensive force (including lying) have a warrant for its use,
but the individual who occasions its use through imperiling an innocent individual is
the one most reasonably to be held accountable for the consequences of the means of
defense. Among other things, this argument shows that spies in a just war may not
only kill the enemy but also deceive them.
40. William H. Masters and Virginia E. Johnson, *The Pleasure Bond* (Boston: Little,
Brown, 1970). On this point, consider the poem of William Blake, "The Question
Answer'd":

> What is it men in women do require?
> The lineaments of Gratified Desire.
> What is it women do in men require?
> The lineaments of Gratified Desire.

Insofar as relationships are based at least in part on the satisfactions of desires, not simply on rational considerations, they are open to being structured by peaceable manipulations of the sort, "I will do this for you if you do that for me."

41. If one agrees with Frankfurt, one might hold that a manipulation is peaceable, even if the person manipulated can no longer turn down the inducement offered as long as the manipulated individual affirms the state of affairs. Even if the manipulation moves the individual who is being manipulated so that the person's first-order volitions compel agreement, the action is still free if it is affirmed by second-order volitions. An example of this might be an experimenter offering a would-be research subject a million dollars to participate in a risky experiment. Even if the individual is so interested in the money that it would be impossible to decline the offer, the choice is still free, to develop Frankfurt's suggestions, if the individual affirms this state of affairs. Compare "I wish he hadn't offered me that money: I wish I could turn it down, but I just can't," and "I'm glad she offered me that money: I couldn't turn it down if I wanted to, but I would never want to turn down such an offer: I'm very glad it was made." H. Frankfurt, "Freedom of the Will and the Concept of a Person," *Journal of Philosophy* 68 (1971): 5–20; "Coercion and Moral Responsibility," in T. Honderich (ed.), *Essays on Freedom of Action* (London: Routledge, 1972), pp. 72–85; and H. Frankfurt and D. Locke, "Three Concepts of Free Action," *Proceedings of the Aristotelian Society*, supp. vol. 49 (1975): 95–125. See also Irving Thalberg, "Motivational Disturbances and Free Will," pp. 201–20, and Caroline Whitbeck, "Towards an Understanding of Motivational Disturbance and Freedom of Action," pp. 221–31, in H. T. Engelhardt, Jr., and S. F. Spicker (eds.), *Mental Health: Philosophical Perspectives* (Dordrecht: Reidel, 1978).

42. Robert Nozick, "Coercion," in S. Morgenbesser et al. (eds.), *Philosophy, Science, and Method* (New York: St. Martin's Press, 1969), pp. 44–72; Joel Rudinow, "Manipulation," *Ethics* 88 (1978): 338–47.

43. It should be evident to the reader that the term force in phrases such as "the use of unconsented-to force against the innocent" is employed in an extended sense to include all violations of the principle of mutual respect, of using persons without their permission. Such violations will include not only the use of direct violence but also attempts to intervene in the lives of others by means of deceptions, threats, or duress. One should note also that failing to honor a contract is not simply an omission but a form of intervention in that it depends on the prior creation of a contract. Interventions will not include the failure to provide goods needed by another, but not due to another through prior contracts or possession. Without the existence of a prior set of understandings, such omissions cannot be regarded as forms of intervention. The term force underscores the border crossing involved in the use of violence, the threat of violence, the breach of a contract, or the employment of deception. In such circumstances one uses a means to compel another individual so as to control or interfere with that individual in ways to which that individual may not have given permission.

There will be some circumstances in which unconsented-to force can be used against an individual who is in a strict sense innocent. Imagine that one is sitting at the bottom of a building with a shoulder–launchable surface-to-air missile. An innocent individual has just been pushed from the top of the building. One does not have enough time to run away so as to avoid being seriously injured if not killed by the impact of the falling individual. However, one has sufficient time to fire the surface-to-air missile. The firing is justified because the falling individual, innocent or not, willing or not, is in fact threatening the person at the bottom. The falling individual is about to engage in an unauthorized border crossing, willing or not. Were we dealing with cases such as this in some detail, we would be committed to a more ample analysis of "innocent person" and "proper defense against unjustified force." Here it is enough to suggest that in some circumstances compulsory vaccination may be like the use of a surface-to-air missile. If others are likely to contract a disease if left unvaccinated and spread it to innocent individuals who cannot vaccinate themselves or otherwise protect themselves, force may be justified to require vaccination in order to protect individuals who otherwise would be brought into contact with the disease without their consent, without an opportunity to avoid the contact, and without an opportunity to avoid contracting the disease. There will be the problem of how much energy innocent third persons must invest in avoiding contact or in avoiding the development of the disease, before one may vaccinate others in order to protect the unvaccinated group. One must note that if the individuals who make contact with the disease do so in part of their own free choice, they may totally defeat their claim that others must vaccinate themselves or otherwise take precautions. As a consequence, this argument may support compulsory vaccinations against highly contagious diseases, such as smallpox (in order to protect those who cannot be vaccinated in time), but not against diseases such as AIDS, which can usually be contracted only through positive actions that are already generally known to carry certain risks, including that of AIDS. It is hard to step out of the way of highly contagious diseases such as smallpox, but easy to step out of the way of diseases such as AIDS. Hemophiliacs are in the unhappy position of needing a good from others (blood products) to which they have no prior rights. In the terms of chapter 8, if they contract AIDS in such circumstances, it is highly unfortunate, but not unfair.

44. An exception may be certain forms of psychoanalysis, which are focused on increasing the capacity to choose freely and/or responsibly. See, for example, Thomas Szasz, *The Ethics of Psychoanalysis* (New York: Basic Books, 1965). I have analyzed some of the issues raised by such value-infected approaches in H. T. Engelhardt, Jr., "Psychotherapy as Meta-ethics," *Psychiatry* 36 (Nov. 1973): 440–45.
45. Nishi v. Hartwell, 473 P 2d 116, 119 (Hawaii 1970), quoting Watson v. Clutts, 136 S.E. 2d 617, 621 (N.C. 1964).
46. Plato. *Laws*, trans. A. E. Taylor, in Hamilton and Cairns, *Collected Dialogues of Plato*, pp. 1310–11.
47. Capron, "Informed Consent in Catastrophic Disease Research and Treatment," 364–76.
48. Natanson v. Kline, 186 Kan. 393, 404, 350 P.2d, 1093, 1106 (1960).

For a discussion of the strong support of the professional standard by British courts, see George J. Annas, "Why the British Courts Rejected the American Doctrine of Informed Consent," *American Journal of Public Health* 74 (Nov. 1984): 1286–78.

49. Aiken v. Clary, 396 S.W. 2d 668, 674–75 (Mo. Sup. Ct. 1965).

50. Sard v. Hardy, 397 A. 2d 1014, 1020 (Md. 1977).

51. Canterbury v. Spence, 464 F.2d 772, 797 (D.C. Cir. 1972).

52. Cobbs v. Grant, 8 Cal. 3.d 229, 245; 502 P. 2d 1, 11; 104 Cal. Rptr. 505, 515 (Calif. 1972).

53. Canterbury v. Spence, 464 F. 2d 772, 791 (D.C. Cir. 1972).

54. Capron, "Informed Consent in Catastrophic Disease Research and Treatment," pp. 407, 416.

55. Scott v. Brandford, 606 P. 2d 554 (Okla. 1980) at 558 and 559.

56. Spencer v. Seikel, 742 P. 2d 1126 (Okla. 1987) at 1129.

57. Cobbs v. Grant, 502 P. 2d 1, 12 (Calif. 1972). Sard v. Hardy, 397 A. 2d 1014, 1022 (Md. 1977).

58. Canterbury v. Spence, 464 F. 2d 772, 789 (D.C. Cir. 1972).

59. Cobbs v. Grant, 8 Cal. 3.d 229, 246; 502 P. 2d 1, 12; 104 Cal. Rptr. 505, 516 (Calif. 1972).

60. Hubert W. Smith, "Therapeutic Privilege to Withhold Specific Diagnosis from Patient Sick with Serious or Fatal Illness," *Tennessee Law Review* 19 (1946): 349–60.

61. Natanson v. Kline, 350 P. 2d 1093, 1103 (1960).

62. The therapeutic privilege can be interpreted as the acceptance of one among many content-full views of proper professional medical conduct.

63. Mark A. Hall, "Informed Consent to Rationing Decisions," *Milbank Quarterly* 71 (1993): 645–68. For a more encompassing study see E. Haavi Morreim, *Balancing Act: The New Medical Ethics of Medicine's New Economics* (Washington, D.C.: Georgetown University Press, 1995).

64. For an introduction to the literature concerning paternalism, see Joel Feinberg, "Legal Paternalism," *Canadian Journal of Philosophy* 105 (1971): 113–16; Allan Buchanan, "Medical Paternalism," *Philosophy and Public Affairs* 7 (1978): 370–90; Charles M. Culver and Bernard Gert, "The Morality of Involuntary Hospitalization," in Spicker et al., *The Law-Medicine Relation*, pp. 159–75; and James F. Childress, *Who Should Decide? Paternalism in Health Care* (New York: Oxford University Press, 1982).

65. John Stuart Mill, *On Liberty*, ed. G. Himmelfarb (New York: Penguin, 1982), pp. 165–66.

66. Calif. Welf. & Inst. Code, sec. 5150 (West 1972 & Supp. 1982).

67. Ibid., sec. 5260.

68. James F. Drane, "Competency to Give an Informed Consent," *Journal of the American Medical Association* 252 (Aug. 17, 1984): 925–27.

69. Gerald Dworkin, "Paternalism," *Monist* 56 (1972): 6–84.

70. Charles M. Culver and Bernard Gert, "Paternalistic Behavior," *Philosophy and Public Affairs* 6 (1976): 49–50.

71. Childress, *Who Should Decide?* pp. 237–41.

72. I borrow here, as elsewhere, from the distinctions between being in authority and being an authority, which are summarized by Richard E. Flathman, "Power, Authority, and Rights in the Practice of Medicine," in George Agich (ed.), *Responsibility in Health Care* (Dordrecht: Reidel, 1982), pp. 105–25.

73. As I indicated in chapter 3, I have borrowed the Talmudic term TEYKU to indicate matters that cannot be decisively resolved by rational argument. See Louis Jacobs, *TEYKU* (New York: Cornwall Books, 1981).

74. Edward Wallerstein, *Circumcision: An American Health Fallacy* (New York: Springer, 1980). For a recent review of some of the controversies regarding female circumcision, see Stephen A. James, "Reconciling International Human Rights and Cultural Relativism: The Case of Female Circumcision," *Bioethics* 8 (Jan. 1994): 1–26. See, also, Loretta Kopelman, "Female Circumcision/Genital Mutilation and Ethical Relativism," *Second Opinion* (Oct. 1994): 55–71. In developing arguments against female circumcision, the difficulty is to avoid developing arguments against male circumcision, so that religious circumcision of infant sons would become a form of child abuse. Given the history of the atrocities against the Jews, this is not a mean consideration.

75. These views lead to tolerance, in general secular moral terms, of the actions by the defenders of Masada, which included taking the lives of children, insofar as all participating who were competent agreed to the mutual suicide. One might note that there is some evidence of compulsion; see Flavius Josephus, *Wars of the Jews,* 7.9

One might note how difficult it is to decide whether parental decisions show malevolent disregard of the welfare of a child. Individuals are generally ready to intervene to provide treatment for the children of parents who refuse treatment due to religious commitments to a non-mainline religion. Consider the report of an Italian couple who declined surgery and radiotherapy for their child diagnosed as having Ewing's sarcoma, and instead took the child to Lourdes. The child experienced a spontaneous remission (or miraculous cure!). Eugene F. Diamond, "Miraculous Cures," *Linacre Quarterly* 51 (Aug. 1984): 224–32.

The view of toleration to which the arguments in this volume lead (no matter how unpleasant such conclusions may be) are similar to the position of Ohio, at least through 1983, regarding the right of parents to forgo standard medical care for their children and to rely instead on prayer. "Nothing in this section shall be construed to define as an abused or neglected child any child who is under spiritual treatment through prayer in accordance with the tenets and practice of a well-recognized religion in lieu of medical treatment, and no report shall be required as to such child." Ohio's Juvenile Code 2151.421. The conclusions may not be as radical as they appear at first blush.

76. Darrel Amundsen, "Casuistry and Professional Obligations: The Regulation of Physicians by the Court of Conscience in the Late Middle Ages" (Part I), *Transactions and Studies of the College of Physicians of Philadelphia* 3 (1981): 22–39; "Casuistry and Professional Obligations: The Regulation of Physicians by the Court of Conscience in the Late Middle Ages" (Part II), *Transactions and Studies of the College of Physicians of Philadelphia* 3 (1981): 93–112.

77. Ibid., part I, p. 35.

78. Brown v. Hughes, 94 Colo. 295, 30 P. 2d 259 (1934); Carpenter v. Blake, 60 Barb., 488 (N.Y., 1871).
79. Hans Jonas, "Philosophical Reflections on Experimenting with Human Subjects," in P. A. Freund (ed.), *Experimentation with Human Subjects* (New York: Braziller, 1969), pp. 3–4.
80. Ibid., pp. 16–17.
81. Hans Jonas, "Philosophical Reflections on Experimenting with Human Subjects," *Daedalus* 98 (1969): 235.
82. Jay Katz, "Prologue—Experiments Prior to 1939," in Jay Katz, *Experimentation with Human Beings* (New York: Russell Sage Foundation, 1972), pp. 284–92.
83. J. H. Jones, *Bad Blood: The Tuskegee Syphilis Experiment* (New York: Free Press, 1981).
84. Hans-Martin Sass, "Reichsrundschreiben 1931: Pre-Nuremberg German Regulations Concerning New Therapy and Human Experimentation," *Journal of Medicine and Philosophy* 8 (May 1983): 99–111.
85. See, for example, William Cullen, *Treatise of the Materia Medica* (Philadelphia: Mathew Carey, 1808).
86. Thomas Sydenham, preface to "The History of Acute and Chronic Disease," in *The Entire Works of Dr. Thomas Sydenham,* ed. and trans. John Swan, 3d ed. (London: E. Cave, 1753), p. xiii.
87. P. C. A. Louis, *Recherches sur les effets de la saignée dans quelques maladies inflammatoires* (Paris: Baillière, 1835). See also the first treatise on the use of confidence levels in medical statistics, J. Gavaret, *Principes généraux de statistique médicale* (Paris: Bechet jeune et Labe, 1840).
88. I am indebted to Hans-Martin Sass for his discussions of this issue with me.
89. For an attempt to set out general moral principles for research, see the National Commission for the Protection of Human Subjects of Biomedical and Behavioral Research, *The Belmont Report* (Washington, D.C.: U.S. Government Printing Office, 1978, DHEW [OS] 78-0012). As the reader will notice, this report defends a principle of justice, in addition to principles of autonomy and beneficence. The analyses in this volume indicate that the principle of justice can in fact be reduced to the principles of permission and beneficence. The two appendices to this report offer an introduction to the philosophical issues bearing on the use of human research subjects.
90. *Nobel Lectures, Physiology or Medicine, 1942–1962* (Amsterdam: Elsevier, 1964), p. 511.
91. *Protection of Human Subjects,* 45 Code of Federal Regulations, 46.406.
92. Ibid., 46.407.
93. Ibid., 46.102(g).
94. Ibid., 46.301–6.
95. Jonas, "Philosophical Reflections on Experimenting with Human Subjects," p. 246n.
96. Arthur Elstein, "Human Factors in Clinical Judgment," in H. T. Engelhardt, Jr. et al. (eds.), *Clinical Judgment* (Dordrecht: Reidel, 1979), pp. 17–28. Michael Scriven, "Clinical Judgment," in ibid., pp. 3–16.

97. Norwood Hanson, *Patterns of Discovery* (Cambridge: Cambridge University Press, 1961).

98. See, for example, J. S. Carey, "Veterans Administration Coronary Cooperative Study," *Journal of the American Medical Association* 241 (June 29, 1979): 2791–92; R. G. Hoffman et al., "The Probability of Surviving Coronary Bypass Surgery," *Journal of the American Medical Association* 243 (Apr. 4, 1980): 1341–44; M. L. Murphy et al., "Treatment of Chronic Stable Angina," *New England Journal of Medicine* 297 (Sept. 22, 1977): 621–27.

99. See, for example, G. Crile, Jr., "The Breast Cancer Controversy," *Transactions and Studies of the College of Physicians of Philadelphia* 41 (1974): 243–53; J. A. Urban, "Treatment of Primary Breast Cancer," *Journal of American Medical Association* 244 (Aug. 22, 1980): 800–803; and U.S. Department of Health, Education, and Welfare, *The Breast Cancer Digest* (Bethesda, Md.: NIH Pub. 80–1691, 1979), pp. 26–35.

100. A random clinical trial is usually halted when the data show that there is only a very small likelihood, say five times out of a hundred, or one time out of a hundred, that the results are likely to be due to chance rather than to a true relation. How certain ought one to be before one stops a trials? The sooner one stops, the likelier it is that the findings were due only to chance. The longer one continues the trial, the longer individuals who would benefit from the new treatment must wait for a final decision to be made. There are no answers that can be discovered for such questions, since they represent a balance among various possible harms and benefits. Answers must be created by the contract made with subjects when they agree to participate. It is only such agreements that can establish when subjects should be informed of the implications of studies and of when studies should be considered appropriately to be terminated. For an excellent study of many of these issues, see Baruch Brody, *Ethical Issues in Drug Testing, Approval, and Pricing* (New York: Oxford University Press, 1995).

101. The reader should recognize that deception plays a major role in psychological studies. Here the same moral principle should apply as I have outlined in the body of the chapter. Individuals should be warned that they will be subjected to deceptions. Where the risks from the deception are minor, it can usually be presumed that a general disclosure with few details will adequately serve the purpose of respecting the freedom of the would-be subject (e.g., "Over the next few weeks you will be subjected to certain minor deceptions in order to study the process of learning"). Finally, researchers need not provide more information than is ordinarily provided in everyday life. Thus, participant researchers who actually take on a bona fide role need not disclose that they are also psychologists. Here as elsewhere there may be a divergence of law and morals.

102. Hippocrates, *Oath,* in Hippocrates, vol. 1, p. 301.

103. One should note that it is highly unlikely that courts would attempt to break priest–penitent confidentiality, even in jurisdictions where there is no legally recognized privilege.

104. For an analysis of the development of the legal duty to disclose to third parties the dangerousness of the patient, see William J. Winslade, "Psychotherapeutic Discre-

tion and Judicial Decision: A Case of Enigmatic Justice,'' in Spicker et al., *The Law-Medicine Relation*, pp. 139–57.

105. Monroe H. Freedman, *Lawyers: Ethics in an Adversary System* (Indianapolis: Bobbs-Merrill, 1975). See also Stephen Toulmin, "The Meaning of Professionalism: Doctors' Ethics and Biomedical Science," in H. T. Engelhardt, Jr., and D. Callahan (eds.), *Knowledge, Value, and Belief* (Hastings-on-Hudson: Institute of Society, Ethics and the Life Sciences, 1977), pp. 254–78.

106. Henry Charles Lea, *A History of Auricular Confession and Indulgences in the Latin Church* (New York: Greenwood Press, 1968), vol. 1, p. 444. For a general account of the commitment not to disclose sins confessed, see Bertrand Kurtscheid, *A History of the Seal of Confession* (London: Herder, 1927).

107. Lea, *A History of Auricular Confession*, p. 445.

108. Nancy Lee Beaty, *The Craft of Dying* (New Haven, Conn.: Yale University Press, 1970).

109. A somewhat dated but still useful review of recent law and public policy regarding both treatment refusal and the use of advance directives is provided in President's Commission for the Study of Ethical Problems in Medicine and Biomedical and Behavioral Research, *Deciding to Forego Life-Sustaining Treatment* (Washington, D.C.: U.S. Government Printing Office, 1983). For a recent study, see Nancy M. P. King, *Making Sense of Advance Directives* (Dordrecht: Kluwer, 1991).

110. *Rituale Romanum* (Tours: Typis Mame, 1952), pp. 233–57.

111. Darrel W. Amundsen, "Prolonging Life: A Duty without Classical Roots," *Hastings Center Report* 8 (Aug. 1978): 23–30.

112. Seneca, "On the Sadness of Life," in *The Stoic Philosophy of Seneca*, trans. Moses Hadas (New York: Norton, 1958), p. 205.

113. Joseph T. Mangan, "An Historical Analysis of the Principle of Double Effect", *Theological Studies* 10 (Mar. 1949): 41–61. See also Richard McCormick, *Ambiguity in Moral Choice* (Milwaukee: Marquette University Press, 1973).

114. For a review of issues raised by the principle of double effect, see Richard McCormick and Paul Ramsey (eds.), *Doing Evil to Achieve Good* (Chicago: Loyola University Press, 1978).

115. Gerald Kelly, *Medico-Moral Problems* (St. Louis: Catholic Hospital Association, 1958), p. 129.

   The tradition required treatment only if there was hope of health (*si sit spes salutis*) or where hope of recovery appeared (*ubi spes affulget convalescendi*). Also, one was never required to engage in futile treatment (*nemo ad inutile tenetur*) or even treatment when it could only postpone death or briefly blunt the illness (*parum pro nihilo reputatur moraliter*). In addition, the very aversion to a form of treatment (*horror magnus*) could defeat the obligation to accept treatment by constituting an undue burden. It is worth noting that one Jesuit theologian determined in the 1940s that the maximum amount of money that even a rich individual was obliged to invest in his own treatment was two thousand dollars. Gerald Kelly, "The Duty of Using Artificial Means of Preserving Life," *Theological Studies* 11 (1950): 203–20.

   One should note that similar constraints on the obligation to treat were recognized by Jewish scholars. One of the most interesting analyses comes from the Talmud account of the death of Judah the Prince. "Rabbi's handmaid ascended the roof and prayed: 'The immortals desire Rabbi [to join them] and the mortals desire Rabbi [to remain with them]; may it be the will [of God] that the mortals may overpower the immortals.' When, however, she saw how often he resorted to the privy, painfully taking off his tefillin and putting them on again, she prayed: 'May it be the will [of the Almighty] that the immortals may overpower the mortals.' As the Rabbis incessantly continued their prayers for [heavenly] mercy she took up a jar and threw it down from the roof to the ground. [For a moment] they ceased praying and the soul of Rabbi departed to its eternal rest." *Kethuboth* 104a (Soncino edition).

One should note that the Orthodox Jewish position allowed treatment to be limited only when the patient was terminal and in the imminence of death, or more properly, "Goses" (i.e., when death was expected within three days). Immanuel Jakobovits, *Jewish Medical Ethics* (New York: Bloch, 1962), p. 121. In contrast, the Roman Catholic position allowed a patient whose life could be saved to decline lifesaving treatment out of a consideration of financial, psychological, social, and other costs. The Roman Catholic position, in obliging one to accept treatment only if it could restore health, gave weight to quality-of-life considerations.

116. Daniel Cronin, "The Moral Law in Regard to the Ordinary and Extraordinary Means of Conserving Life," dissertation for Pontifical Gregorian University, Rome, 1958. See also H. T. Engelhardt, Jr., and Thomas J. Bole, "Entwicklungen der medizinischen Ethik in den USA: Die Verführung durch die Technik und der Irrtum einer Lebenserhaltung um jeden Preis," *Arzt und Christ* 36 (1990): 113–21.

117. Kelly, *Medico-Moral Problems*, p. 132.

118. Ibid., p. 130.

119. Fyodor Dostoevsky, *The Brothers Karamazov* (New York: Norton, 1976), p. 779.

120. An index of the extent to which opposition to physician-assisted suicide (PAS) and voluntary active euthanasia (VAE) is considered to be a function of a taboo is shown by a recent article that advances ways to empower patients to "control their own destiny without requiring physicians to reject the taboos on PAS and VAE that have existed for millennia." James Bernat, Bernard Gert, and R. Peter Mogielnicki, "Patient Refusal of Hydration and Nutrition," *Archives of Internal Medicine* 153 (Dec. 27, 1993): 2723. For an exploration of the moral costs and benefits of legalizing voluntary active euthanasia, see Dan W. Brock, "Voluntary Active Euthanasia," in *Life and Death: Philosophical Essays in Biomedical Ethics* (New York: Cambridge University Press, 1993), chap. 8, pp. 202–32. It is interesting to note that the public support for voluntary active euthanasia is at around 62 percent, a level of support that appears to have remained stable since at least 1978. See, for example, Jeremiah Suhl, Pamela Simons, Terry Reedy, and Thomas Garrick, "Myth of Substituted Judgment," *Archives of Internal Medicine* 154 (Jan. 10, 1994): 90–96.

121. Jack Kevorkian, "The Last Fearsome Taboo: Medical Aspects of Planned Death," *Medicine and Law* 7 (1988): 1–14.

122. See, for example, Michigan v. Kevorkian, no. 93-11482, 1993 WL 603212 (Mich. Cir. Ct. Dec. 13, 1993). The ignorance of the court regarding Christian morality is interesting to note, for it quotes as an authority an opinion that Christians did not

come to consider suicide a crime until the sixth century, a clearly false assertion. Indeed, by the fourth century there were detailed reflections regarding the circumstances under which a funeral service could be provided to someone who had committed suicide because of insanity. See Question 14 of the 18 questions of Pope Timothy of Alexandria in Sts. Nicodemus and Agapius (eds.), *The Rudder of the Orthodox Catholic Church,* trans. D. Cummings (1957; repr. New York: Luna Printing, 1983), p. 898. However, in a general secular context, the evil of physician-assisted suicide and voluntary euthanasia will not be appreciated. See, for example, Compassion in Dying v. State of Washington, 850 F. Suppl 1454 (WD Wash., 1994).

123. "A Prayer in Time of Trouble," in *A Pocket Prayer Book for Orthodox Christians* (Englewood, N.J.: Antiochian Orthodox Christian Archdiocese, 1990), p. 21.
124. "A Prayer of a Sick Person," in ibid., pp. 22–23.
125. The traditional believer need not be committed to a painful death and can gladly accept an easy exit if God provides it. The following prayer occurs frequently in Orthodox Catholic religious services: "A Christian ending to our life, painless, blameless, peaceful; and a good defense before the dread Judgment Seat of Christ, let us ask of the Lord." Ibid., p. 82. Indeed, the Office at the parting of the soul from the body includes a petition that God allow death to occur with dispatch. "Therefore we pray unto Thee, the Father Who is from everlasting, and immortal, and unto Thine Only-begotten Son, and unto Thine all-holy Spirit, that Thou will deliver N. from the body unto repose." *Service Book of the Holy Orthodox-Catholic Apostolic Church,* trans. Isabel Hapgood, 6th ed., (Englewood, N.J.: Antiochian Orthodox Christian Archdiocese, 1983), pp. 366–67.
126. Natanson v. Kline, 186 Kan. 393, 404, 350 P. 2d 1093, 1104 (1960).
127. For instances of Jehovah's Witnesses being allowed to refuse lifesaving treatment, see In re Estate of Brooks 205 N.E. 2d 435 (Ill. 1965); In re Milideo 390 N.Y.S. 2d 523 (Sup. Ct. 1976); for a case where the right to refuse treatment was upheld, even if it were tantamount to suicide and suicide were a crime, see, Erikson v. Dilgard, 252 N.Y.S. 2d 705, 706 (Sup. Ct. 1962).
128. Contra, J.F.K. Mem. Hosp. v. Heston, 279 A. 2d 670, 672–73 (N.J. 1971).
129. Blackstone, *Commentaries on the Laws of England* (1765), book 4, p. 189.
130. H. T. Engelhardt, Jr., and Michele Malloy, "Suicide and Assisting Suicide: A Critique of Legal Sanctions," *Southwestern Law Journal* 36 (Nov. 1982): 1003–37. For a general review of some of the philosophical issues raised by suicide, see M. Pabst Battin, *Ethical Issues in Suicide* (Englewood Cliffs, N.J.: Prentice-Hall, 1982), and M. Pabst Battin and David J. Mayo (eds.), *Suicide: The Philosophical Issues* (New York: St. Martin's Press, 1980).
131. Though guardians will enjoy such secular moral freedom, there will often be the danger of coercive governmental intervention, as under the Americans with Disabilities Act.
132. Ernest Jones, *The Life and Work of Sigmund Freud* (New York: Basic Books, 1957), vol. 3, p. 246.
133. Ibid.
134. Ibid., pp. 144–45.

135. Percy W. Bridgman, "The Struggle for Intellectual Integrity," *Harpers Magazine* 168 (Dec. 1933): 18–25.

136. Gerald Holton, "Percy Williams Bridgman," *Bulletin of the Atomic Scientists* 18 (Feb. 1962): 23.

137. Ibid.

138. Seneca, *Stoic Philosophy of Seneca,* p. 202.

139. Ibid., pp. 204–5.

140. Tacitus records how Seneca committed suicide with his wife when faced with the alternative of suicide or an execution by Nero. "Then by one and the same stroke they sundered with the dagger the arteries of their arms. Seneca, as his aged frame attenuated by frugal diet, allowed the blood to escape but slowly, severed also the veins of his legs and knees. Worn out by cruel anguish, afraid too that his sufferings might break his wife's spirit, and that, as he looked on her tortures he might himself sink into irresolution, he persuaded her to retire into another chamber. Even at the last moment his eloquence failed him not; he summoned his secretaries and dictated much to them which, as it has been published for all readers in his own words, I forbear to paraphrase." Moses Hadas (ed.), *The Complete Works of Tacitus* (New York: Random House, 1942), pp. 391–92.

141. David Hume, "Of Suicide," in T. H. Green and T. H. Grose (eds.), *Essays Moral, Political, and Literary* (London: Scientia Verlag Aalen, 1964), p. 414.

142. Sanders v. State, 54 Tex. Crim. 101, 105, 112 S.W. 68, 70 (1908).

143. The Texas Court of Criminal Appeals held that suicide had never been a crime in Texas and that aiding and abetting suicide also was not. The case involved a physician, Dr. Grace, who retired one evening, sleeping in one bed, his wife in the other, and his mistress on the floor between the two beds. The mistress, who was despondent, took her own life with a pistol that Dr. Grace had placed on a nightstand. Grace v. State, 44 Tex. Crim. 193, 69 S.W. 529 (1902). Dueling was first criminalized in Texas on Dec. 21, 1836. See Oliver C. Hartley, *A Digest of the Laws of Texas* (Philadelphia: Thomas, Cowperthwait, 1850), p. 288.

144. Common law did not generally excuse individuals from mayhem or murder on the basis of the defense of consent. See, for example, Matthew v. Ollerton (1693), Comberbach 218, where the court held that "if I licence a Man to beat me, such Licence is void . . . because 'tis against the Peace."

145. Immanuel Kant, *The Metaphysical Principles of Virtue: Part II of The Metaphysics of Morals,* trans. James Ellington (Indianapolis: Bobbs-Merrill, 1964), pp. 83–84; AK VI, 423-24.

146. "He who contemplates suicide will ask himself whether his action can be consistent with the idea of humanity as an end in itself. If, in order to escape from burdensome circumstances, he destroys himself, he uses a person merely as a means to maintain a tolerable condition up to the end of life." Kant, *Foundations of the Metaphysics of Morals,* trans. L. W. Beck, 6th ed. (Indianapolis: Bobbs-Merrill, 1976), p. 47; AK IV 429.

147. Kant in fact argues that masturbation is a violation of one's duty to oneself, which is more heinous than suicide. *The Metaphysical Principles of Virtue,* AK VI 425.

148. Kant, *Metaphysical Principles of Virtue*, AK VI 423.
149. Hume, "Of Suicide," p. 413.
150. Engelhardt and Malloy, "Suicide and Assisting Suicide: A Critique of Legal Sanctions," especially pp. 1022–27.
151. Norman Cantor, "A Patient's Decision to Decline Life-Saving Medical Treatment: Bodily Integrity Versus the Preservation of Life," *Rutgers Law Review* 26 (1973): 228–64.
152. Ludwig Edelstein, *The Hippocratic Oath: Text, Translation and Interpretation*, supp. no. 1 to *Bulletin of the History of Medicine* (Baltimore: Johns Hopkins University Press, 1943), pp. 10–15.
153. Paul Carrick, *Medical Ethics in Antiquity* (Dordrecht: D. Reidel, 1985).
154. Tex. Penal Code Ann. § 22.08 (Vernon 1974).
155. For an article that would seem to forward an obligation to refer those seeking assisted suicide to alternative providers if one is morally opposed, see Timothy Quill, Christine Cassel, and Diane Meier, "Care of the Hopelessly Ill: Proposed Clinical Criteria for Physician-Assisted Suicide," *New England Journal of Medicine* 327 (Nov. 5, 1992): 1380–83.
156. The phrase *captain of the ship* was introduced in the context of medical malpractice in the case of McConnell v. Williams, 361 Pa. 355, 65 A. 2d 243 (1959). This doctrine made nurses and others the borrowed servants of the physician performing surgery. As such, these other individuals were not regarded as independent agents or as employees of the hospital. The history of this doctrine, which is varied, does raise the question of the lines of responsibility and authority in health care generally.
157. S. J. Eisendrath and Albert R. Jonsen, "The Living Will: Help or Hindrance?" *Journal of the American Medical Association* 249 (Apr. 15, 1983): 2054–58.
158. A. M. Sadler, B. L. Sadler, and A. A. Bliss, *The Physician's Assistant—Today and Tomorrow* (New Haven, Conn.: Yale University Press, 1972).
159. For a comprehensive review of the lines of responsibility in health care, including the position of nurses, see Agich, *Responsibility in Health Care*.
160. For a study of the conflicts involved in maintaining institutional moral integrity, see Kevin Wm. Wildes, S.J., "Institutional Integrity: Approval, Toleration, and Holy War or 'Always True to You in my Fashion,'" *Journal of Medicine and Philosophy* 16 (Apr. 1991): 211–20.
161. From a moral perspective, one would need to bundle together a number of issues into an initial consent to participate in a particular health care association with its particular moral, financial, and medical advantages and disadvantages. In many countries, this would require rethinking malpractice law and reshaping it to allow individuals to consent to cheaper but somewhat more risky health care. See, for example, Mark A. Hall, "Informed Consent to Rationing Decisions," *Milbank Quarterly* 71 (1993): 645–68, and Paul S. Appelbaum, "Must We Forgo Informed Consent to Control Health Care Costs? A Response to Mark A. Hall," *Milbank Quarterly* 71 (1993): 669–76. See, also, Jonathan Frankel, "Medical Malpractice Law and Health Care Cost Containment: Lessons for Reformers from the Clash of Cultures," *Yale Law Journal* 103 (1994): 1297–1331.

# 8

---

## Rights to Health Care, Social Justice, and Fairness in Health Care Allocations: Frustrations in the Face of Finitude

The imposition of a single-tier, all-encompassing health care system is morally unjustifiable. It is a coercive act of totalitarian ideological zeal, which fails to recognize the diversity of moral visions that frame interests in health care, the secular moral limits of state authority, and the authority of individuals over themselves and their own property. It is an act of secular immorality.

A basic human secular moral right to health care does not exist—not even to a "decent minimum of health care." Such rights must be created.

The difficulty with supposed rights to health care, as well as with many claims regarding justice or fairness in access to health care, should be apparent. Since the secular moral authority for common action is derived from permission or consent, it is difficult (indeed, for a large–scale society, materially impossible) to gain moral legitimacy for the thoroughgoing imposition on health care of one among the many views of beneficence and justice. There are, after all, as many accounts of beneficence, justice, and fairness as there are major religions.[1]

Most significantly, there is a tension between the foundations of general secular morality and the various particular positive claims founded in particular visions of beneficence and justice. It is materially impossible both to respect the freedom of all and to achieve their long-range best interests. Loose talk about justice and fairness in health care is therefore morally misleading, because it suggests that there is a particular canonical vision of justice or fairness that all have grounds to endorse. Since this is not the case, as we have seen in chapters 2 and 3, "social justice" deserves the characterization Hayek gave it:

"Social justice" is not, as most people probably feel, an innocent expression of good will towards the less fortunate, but . . . it has become a dishonest insinuation that one ought to agree to a demand of some special interest which can give no real reason for it. If political discussion is to become honest it is necessary that people should recognize that the term is intellectually disreputable, the mark of demagogy or cheap journalism which responsible thinkers ought to be ashamed to use because, once its vacuity is recognized, its use is dishonest.[2]

Appeals to ideas of social justice in framing health care policy can be dishonest in suggesting a canonical agreement in secular moral reflection. Such agreement does not exist. They can be demagogic in inciting the coercive use of unjustified state force.

Rights to health care constitute claims on services and goods. Unlike rights to forbearance, which require others to refrain from interfering, which show the unity of the authority to use others, rights to beneficence are rights grounded in particular theories or accounts of the good. For general authority, they require others to participate actively in a particular understanding of the good life or justice. Without an appeal to the principle of permission, to advance such rights is to claim that one may press others into labor or confiscate their property. Rights to health care, unless they are derived from special contractual agreements, depend on particular understandings of beneficence rather than on authorizing permission. They may therefore conflict with the decisions of individuals who may not wish to participate in, and may indeed be morally opposed to, realizing a particular system of health care. Individuals always have the secular moral authority to use their own resources in ways that collide with fashionable understandings of justice or the prevailing consensus regarding fairness.

## Health care policy: the ideology of equal, optimal care

It is fashionable to affirm an impossible commitment in health care delivery, as, for example, in the following four widely embraced health care policy goals, which are at loggerheads:

1. The best possible care is to be provided for all.
2. Equal care should be guaranteed.
3. Freedom of choice on the part of health care provider and consumer should be maintained.
4. Health care costs are to be contained.

One cannot provide the best possible health care for all and contain health care costs. One cannot provide equal health care for all and respect the freedom of individuals peaceably to pursue with others their own visions of health care or to use their own resources and energies as they decide. For that matter, one cannot maintain freedom in the choice of health care services while containing the costs of health care. One may also not be able to provide all with equal health care that is at the same time the very best care because of limits on the resources themselves. That few openly address these foundational moral tensions at the roots of contemporary health care policy suggests that the problems are shrouded in a collective illusion, a false consciousness, an established ideology within which certain facts are politically unacceptable.

These difficulties spring not only from a conflict between freedom and beneficence, but from a tension among competing views of what it means to pursue and achieve the good in health care (e.g., is it more important to provide equal care to all or the best possible health care to the least-well-off class?). The pursuit of incompatible or incoherent health care is rooted in the failure to face the finitude of secular moral authority, the finitude of secular moral vision, the finitude of human powers in the face of death and suffering, the finitude of human life, and the finitude of human financial resources. A health care system that acknowledges the moral and financial limitations on the provision of health care would need to

1. endorse inequality in access to health care as morally unavoidable because of private resources and human freedom;
2. endorse setting a price on saving human life as a part of establishing a cost-effective health care system established through communal resources.

Even though all health care systems de facto enjoy inequalities and must to some extent ration the health care they provide through communal resources, this is not usually forthrightly acknowledged. There is an ideological bar to recognizing and coming to terms with the obvious.

Only a prevailing collective illusion can account for the assumption in U.S. policy that health care may be provided (1) while containing costs (2) without setting a price on saving lives and preventing suffering when using communal funds and at the same time (3) ignoring the morally unavoidable inequalities due to private resources and human freedom. This false consciousness shaped the deceptions central to the Clinton health care proposal, as it was introduced in 1994. It was advanced to support a health care system purportedly able to provide all with (1) the best of care and (2) equal care, while achieving (3) cost containment, and still (4) allowing those who wish the liberty to purchase fee-for-service health care.[3] While not acknowledging the presence of rationing, the proposal required silent rationing in order to contain costs by limiting access to high-cost, low-yield treatments that a National Health Board would exclude from the "guaranteed benefit package."[4] In addition, it advanced mechanisms to slow technological innovation so as further to reduce the visibility of rationing choices.[5] One does not have to ration that which is not available. There has been a failure to acknowledge the moral inevitability of inequalities in health care due to the limits of secular governmental authority, human freedom, and the existence of private property, however little that may be. There was also the failure to acknowledge the need to ration health care within communal programs if costs are to be contained. It has been ideologically unacceptable to recognize these circumstances.

Indeed, the Clinton proposal strengthens some of the worst misconceptions of the importance of high-cost, low-yield medicine by giving such a central importance to equality in access to health care. This is done despite the remarkably longer life expectancy of women versus men, the rich versus the poor, and high-status versus low-status individuals, which may in great measure be independent of access to health care.[6] This accent on personal health care is maintained despite long-standing evidence of the greater contribution of public health and other social changes to decreasing morbidity and mortality.[7] It is difficult to know why such a unique place should be given to health care versus other undertakings such as education, housing, and personal security, where individuals are allowed to secure better private basic education and housing, as well as private security services. The answers must lie in the ways in which personal health care appears to be central to the human struggle with finitude and death.

Reflections concerning the difficulties in limiting the use of health care resources have an ancient lineage and reveal a tight bond with the obsession to postpone death at all costs. Plato in Book 3 of the *Republic* recognizes the quandary of infinite expectations and finite resources that characterizes the challenge of health care choices. He is aware that private property may undermine societal efficiency as individuals attempt to extend their lives in a protracted struggle with death, as in the case of Herodicus, of whom Plato speaks with disapproval.[8] He concludes that the protracted treatment of chronic illnesses is boonless when medicine cannot restore citizens to their occupations and duties. Such individuals should instead accept death.[9] The *Republic* endorses acute health care, if it promises to restore individuals to a useful life, but very little, if any, chronic health care. Preventive health care would be provided in the form of gymnastics. Plato's reflections suggest the following general points: (1) humans have a difficulty in accepting their own limits; (2) limits should be acknowledged regarding the proper amount of resources to be invested in health care; (3) resources invested in health care often do not secure a high quality of life for those treated; and (4) such investments frequently constitute a major drain on common resources. For Plato, concerns regarding health care were expressed in terms of the goal of maintaining the polis, not in terms of isolated individual rights to health services.[10]

But individuals are the source of secular moral authority. This chapter explores the prospects for surmounting difficulties in framing a health care system, while recognizing the limits to achieving the most beneficent pattern for the distribution of health care resources:

1. It is impossible to discover a particular allocation of resources as generally obligatory because of the limits of secular reason (e.g., is it more important to invest communal resources in treating pediatric leukemia, or in treating the pains of the elderly suffering from degenerative osteoarthritis?);[11]
2. The authority of societies and states to appropriate the services of persons, forbid particular forms of health care provider–patient relationships, or draft health care workers to provide services is limited because the permission of individuals is the source of secular moral authority (e.g., the authority of the state, being drawn from its citizens, is circumscribed by the limited consent of its participants);
3. The authority of societies and states to appropriate and redistribute resources is limited by private property (e.g., there will be limits to the authority of the state to tax away private resources in order to provide medical care to preserve the health and save the life of indigents; a society must have legitimately acquired resources in order to establish a communal health system);
4. The opportunity for both individuals and groups to pursue health care is limited by the finitude of resources (e.g., one cannot invest all available resources in the maximum extension of life for all at all costs without radically draining resources from other major societal endeavors).

As a consequence, the secular moral legitimacy of attempts thoroughgoingly to achieve ideal systems for allocating resources to health care is severely limited.

## Justice, freedom, and inequality

Interests in justice as beneficence are motivated in part by inequalities and in part by needs. That some have so little while others have so much properly evokes moral concerns of beneficence. Still, as chapters 3 and 4 show, the moral authority to use force to set such inequalities aside is limited. These limitations are in part due to the circumstance that the resources one could use to aid those in need are already owned by other people. One must establish whether and when inequalities and needs generate rights or claims against others.

### The natural and social lotteries

"Natural lottery" is used to identify changes in fortune that result from natural forces, not directly from the actions of persons. The natural lottery shapes the distribution of both naturally and socially conditioned assets. The natural lottery contrasts with the social lottery, which is used to identify changes in fortune that are not the result of natural forces but the actions of persons. The social lottery shapes the distribution of social and natural assets. The natural and social lotteries, along with one's own free decisions, determine the distribution of natural and social assets. The social lottery is termed a lottery, though it is the outcome of personal actions, because of the complex and unpredictable interplay of personal choices and because of the unpredictable character of the outcomes, which do not conform to an ideal pattern, and because the outcomes are the results of social forces, not the immediate choices of those subject to them.

All individuals are exposed to the vicissitudes of nature. Some are born healthy and by luck remain so for a long life, free of disease and major suffering. Others are born with serious congenital or genetic diseases, others contract serious crippling fatal illnesses early in life, and yet others are injured and maimed. Those who win the natural lottery will for most of their lives not be in need of medical care. They will live full lives and die painless and peaceful deaths. Those who lose the natural lottery will be in need of health care to blunt their sufferings and, where possible, to cure their diseases and to restore function. There will be a spectrum of losses, ranging from minor problems such as having teeth with cavities to major tragedies such as developing childhood leukemia, inheriting Huntington's chorea, or developing amyelotrophic lateral sclerosis.

These tragic outcomes are the deliverances of nature, for which no one, without some special view of accountability or responsibility, is responsible (unless, that is, one recognizes them as the results of the Fall or as divine chastisements). The circumstance that individuals are injured by hurricanes, storms, and earthquakes is often simply no one's fault. When no one is to blame, no one may be charged with the responsibility of making whole those who lose the natural lottery on the ground of accountability for the harm. One will need an argument dependent on a particular sense of fairness to show that the readers of this volume should submit to the forcible redistribution of their resources to provide health care for those injured by nature. It may very well be unfeeling, unsympathetic, or uncharitable not to provide such help. One may face eternal hellfires for failing to provide aid.[12] But it is another thing to show in general secular moral terms that individuals owe others such help in a way that would morally authorize state force to redistribute their private resources and energies or to constrain their free choices with others. To be in dire need does not by itself create a secular moral right to be rescued from that need. The natural lottery creates inequalities and places individuals at disadvantage without creating a straightforward secular moral obligation on the part of others to aid those in need.

Individuals differ in their resources not simply because of outcomes of the natural lottery, but also due to the actions of others. Some deny themselves immediate pleasures in order to accumulate wealth or to leave inheritances; through a complex web of love, affection, and mutual interest, individuals convey resources, one to another, so that those who are favored prosper, and those who are ignored languish. Some as a consequence grow wealthy and others grow poor, not through anyone's malevolent actions or omissions, but simply because they were not favored by the love, friendship, collegiality, and associations through which fortunes develop and individuals prosper. In such cases there will be neither fairness nor unfairness, but simply good and bad fortune.

In addition, some will be advantaged or disadvantaged, made rich, poor, ill, diseased, deformed, or disabled because of the malevolent and blameworthy actions and omissions of others. Such will be unfair circumstances, which just and beneficent states should try to prevent and to rectify through legitimate police protection, forced restitution, and charitable programs. Insofar as an injured party has a claim against an injurer to be made whole, not against society, the outcome is unfortunate from the perspective of society's obligations and the obligations of innocent citizens to make restitution. Restitution is owed by the injurer, not society or others. There will be outcomes of the social lottery that are on the one hand blameworthy in the sense of resulting from the culpable actions of others, though on the other hand a society has no obligation to rectify them. The social lottery includes the exposure to the immoral and unjust actions of others. Again, one will need an argument dependent on a particular sense of fairness to show that the readers of this volume should submit to the forcible redistribution of their resources to provide health care to those injured by others.

When individuals come to purchase health care, some who lose the natural lottery will be able at least in part to compensate for those losses through their winnings at the social lottery. They will be able to afford expensive health care needed to restore health and to regain function. On the other hand, those who lose in both the natural and the social lottery will be in need of health care, but without the resources to acquire it.

## The rich and the poor: differences in entitlements

If one owns property by virtue of just acquisition or just transfer, then one's title to that property will not be undercut by the tragedies and needs of others. One will simply own one's property. On the other hand, if one owns property because such ownership is justified within a system that ensures a beneficent distribution of goods (e.g., the achievement of the greatest balance of benefits over harms for the greatest number or the greatest advantage for the least-well-off class), one's ownership will be affected by the needs of others. In chapter 4, we saw why property is in part privately owned in a strong sense that cannot be undercut by the needs of others. In addition, all have a general right to the fruits of the earth, which constitutes the basis for a form of taxation as rent to provide fungible payments to individuals, whether or not they are in need. Finally, there are likely to be resources held in common by groups that may establish bases for their distribution to meet health care concerns. The first two forms of entitlement or ownership exist unconstrained by medical or other needs. The last form of entitlement or ownership, through the decision of a community, may be conditioned by need.

The existence of any amount of private resources can be the basis for inequalities that secular moral authority may not set aside. Insofar as people own things, they will have a right to them, even if others need them. Because the presence of permission is cardinal, the test of whether one must transfer one's goods to others will not be whether such a redistribution will not prove onerous or excessive for the person subjected to the distribution, but whether the resources belong to that individual. Consider that you may be reading this book next to a person in great need. The test of whether a third person may take resources from you to help that individual in need will not be whether you will suffer from the transfer, but rather whether you have consented—at least this is the case if the principle of permission functions in general secular morality as this book has shown. The principle of permission is the source of authority when moral strangers collaborate, because they do not share a common understanding of fairness or of the good. As a consequence, goal-oriented approaches to the just distribution of resources must be restricted to commonly owned goods, where there is authority to create programs for their use.

Therefore, one must qualify the conclusions of the 1983 American President's Commission for the Study of Ethical Problems that suggest that excessive burdens should determine the amount of tax persons should pay to sustain an adequate level of health care for those in need.[13] Further, one will have strong grounds for morally condemning systems that attempt to impose an all-encompassing health care plan that would require "equality of care [in the sense of avoiding] the creation of a tiered system [by] providing care based only on differences of need, not individual or group characteristics."[14] Those who are rich are always at secular moral liberty to purchase more and better health care.

*Drawing the line between the unfortunate and the unfair*

How one regards the moral significance of the natural and social lotteries and the moral force of private ownership will determine how one draws the line between circumstances that are simply unfortunate and those that are unfortunate and in addition unfair in the sense of constituting a claim on the resources of others.

Life in general, and health care in particular, reveal circumstances of enormous tragedy, suffering, and deprivation. The pains and sufferings of illness, disability, and disease, as well as the limitations of deformity, call on the sympathy of all to provide aid and give comfort. Injuries, disabilities, and diseases due to the forces of nature are unfortunate. Injuries, disabilities, and diseases due to the unconsented-to actions of others are unfair. Still, outcomes of the unfair actions of others are not necessarily society's fault and are in this sense unfortunate. The horrible injuries that come every night to the emergency rooms of major hospitals may be someone's fault, even if they are not the fault of society, much less that of uninvolved citizens. Such outcomes, though unfair with regard to the relationship

RIGHTS TO HEALTH CARE, SOCIAL JUSTICE, AND FAIRNESS 383

of the injured with the injurer, may be simply unfortunate with respect to society
and other citizens (and may licitly be financially exploited). One is thus faced
with distinguishing the difficult line between acts of God, as well as immoral acts
of individuals that do not constitute a basis for societal retribution on the one
hand, and injuries that provide such a basis on the other.

A line must be created between those losses that will be made whole through
public funds and those that will not. Such a line was drawn in 1980 by Patricia
Harris, the then secretary of the Department of Health, Education, and Welfare,
when she ruled that heart transplantations should be considered experimental and
therefore not reimbursable through Medicare.[15] To be in need of a heart transplant and not have the funds available would be an unfortunate circumstance but
not unfair. One was not eligible for a heart transplant even if another person had
intentionally damaged one's heart. From a moral point of view, things would
have been different if the federal government had in some culpable fashion
injured one's heart. So, too, if promises of treatment had been made. For example, to suffer from appendicitis or pneumonia and not as a qualifying patient
receive treatment guaranteed through a particular governmental or private insurance system would be unfair, not simply unfortunate.

Drawing the line between the unfair and the unfortunate is unavoidable because it is impossible in general secular moral terms to translate all needs into
rights, into claims against the resources of others. One must with care decide
where the line is to be drawn. To distinguish needs from mere desires, one must
endorse one among the many competing visions of morality and human flourishing. One is forced to draw a line between those needs (or desires) that constitute
claims on the aid of others and those that do not. The line distinguishing unfortunate from unfair circumstances justifies by default certain social and economic
inequalities in the sense of determining who, if any one, is obliged in general
secular morality to remedy such circumstances or achieve equality. Is the request
of an individual to have life extended through a heart transplant at great cost, and
perhaps only for a few years, a desire for an inordinate extension of life? Or is it a
need to be secure against a premature death? So, too, for treatment in an intensive
care unit when this will only postpone death a few months or convey only a small
(e.g., 3 percent) chance of surviving but at great cost (e.g., the treatment will cost
over $200,000 dollars, thus saving lives at over $6 million per life saved!). The
difficulty of discovering answers to such questions has already been explored in
chapters 2 and 3. Taking a particular position in these matters requires endorsing
a particular moral vision. Outside a particular view of the good life, needs do not
create rights to the services or goods of others.[16] Indeed, outside of a particular
moral vision there is no canonical means for distinguishing desires from needs.

There is a practical difficulty in regarding major losses at the natural and social
lotteries as generating claims to health care: attempts to restore health indefinitely
can deplete societal resources in the pursuit of ever-more incremental extensions

of life of marginal quality. A relatively limited amount of food and shelter is required to preserve the lives of individuals. But an indefinite amount of resources can in medicine be committed to the further preservation of human life, the marginal postponement of death, and the marginal alleviation of human suffering and disability. Losses at the natural lottery with regard to health can consume major resources with little return. Often one can only purchase a little relief, and that only at great costs. Still, more decisive than the problem of avoiding the possibly overwhelming costs involved in satisfying certain health care desires (e.g., postponing death for a while through the use of critical care) is the problem of selecting the correct content-full account of justice in order canonically to distinguish between needs and desires and to translate needs into rights.

*Beyond equality: an egalitarianism of altruism versus*
*an egalitarianism of envy*

The equal distribution of health care is itself problematic, a circumstance recognized in *Securing Access to Health Care,* the 1983 report of the President's Commission.[17] The difficulties are multiple:

1. Although in theory, at least, one can envisage providing all with equal levels of decent shelter, one cannot restore all to or preserve all in an equal state of health. Many health needs cannot be satisfied in the same way one can address most needs for food and shelter.
2. If one provided all with the same amount of funds to purchase health care or the same amount of services, the amount provided would be far too much for some and much too little for others who could have benefited from more investment in treatment and research.
3. If one attempts to provide equal health care in the sense of allowing individuals to select health care only from a predetermined list of available therapies, or through some managed health care plan such as accountable (to the government) health care plans or regional health alliances, which would be provided to all so as to prevent the rich from having access to better health care than the poor, one would have immorally confiscated private property and have restricted the freedom of individuals to join in voluntary relationships and associations.

That some are fortunate in having more resources is neither more nor less arbitrary or unfair than some having better health, better looks, or more talents. In any event, the translation of unfortunate circumstances into unfair circumstances, other than with regard to violations of the principle of permission, requires the imposition of a particular vision of beneficence or justice.[18]

The pursuit of equality faces both moral and practical difficulties. If significant restrictions were placed on the ability to purchase special treatment with one's resources, one would need not only to anticipate that a black market would inevitably develop in health care services, but also acknowledge that such a black market would be a special bastion of liberty and freedom of association justified in general secular moral terms. As chapters 2, 3, and 4 have shown, there would be no secular moral authority to interfere in that market. In general secular moral terms, providing bribes or gratuities to acquire better health care, even in violation of the law, could be understood as the acts of freedom fighters or resisters against unjust and unfair state oppression, statements of the Clinton health care proposal to the contrary notwithstanding.[19] In any event, those with political power and privilege will tend to be able directly or indirectly to acquire better health care for themselves and their families. When the law prohibits the satisfaction of any strong, important set of human concerns and desires, a black market inevitably develops. For this reason, it is difficult to identify truly egalitarian systems anywhere in the world.

Health care policy is a challenge for egalitarianism because of the dramatic character of the inequalities it faces (e.g., some die young, others live long and full lives; some suffer from lifelong debilitating diseases, others live long and relatively pain-free lives). If this life is all there is, and if here in this world all meaning is to be found, many will wonder whether any inequalities in this ultimate area may be tolerated. Inequalities in health care appear as ultimate inequalities, although differences in life expectancy due to income, gender, and social status are much more significant. Women, for example, in most developed countries live over five years longer than men and the difference in life expectancy between countries that invest modestly and those that invest substantially is relatively minor.[20] Still, the focus of egalitarian concerns is often disproportionately on health care rather than on inequalities in wealth, housing, education, and even security, which are omnipresent (e.g., the rich can hire armed guards while the poor must rely on ordering police protection, such as it is). For example, Robert Evans, in examining the Canadian government's monopolization of health care insurance so as to impose one encompassing health care system on all, recognizes that many conflate the freedom to use one's own resources to buy better health care with "the idea that one person's life and limb is more valuable than another's, more worth saving on the basis of his/her ability to pay, [which] comes rather close to denying a fundamental 'cherished illusion' of equality which underlies our political and judicial system."[21] If one regards this abhorrence, and the illusion that sustains it, as having the moral significance of creating (or allowing the acknowledgment of) an obligation to use force to avoid such conditions, one will have committed oneself to a health system that aims at equal care for all, even if this requires coercively restricting peaceable private choice. For example, to defend this illusion, Canada acts immorally, and the Clinton plan suggested interventions that would have been immoral in general secular terms.

In order to avoid such immorality, health care systems must acknowledge the secular moral limitations on state power and eschew such excesses.

The health care arts and sciences are projects of finite men and women with finite resources, living and practicing their professions in the face of often horrible human tragedy and within moral limitations that forbid them from attempting all they could in order to help others. These limits define where inequalities are not inequities, and where unfortunate outcomes are not unfair. There will still be the possibility of blunting many of the unfortunate outcomes of natural forces and social undertakings. Within the constraints of secular moral authority, it will be proper to attempt to set some inequalities aside by using commonly owned resources to aid those in need. But this requires distinguishing between two forms of egalitarianism: an egalitarianism of envy and an egalitarianism of altruism.

An egalitarianism of envy holds that a second world is worse than a first if, all else being equal, the second world differs from the first in some person's being better off in the second world without anyone being worse off. From this perspective the good fortune of someone can be regarded as unfair in itself or to all others. First, the good fortune of having more than others may be held to be unfair if the fortune is unprincipled, if it simply happens and is thus not deserved. For Rawls's account to which we will shortly turn, good fortune is fair if it redounds to the benefit of the least-well-off class. Otherwise, good fortune exists without justification, without a warrant of fairness, and is in that sense unfair. The good fortune of some can be tolerated only if it advantages the least well off (i.e., "you may have more only if that helps me [a member of the least-well-off class]"); otherwise, the contractors of the original position would not allow it. Second, good fortune may be seen simply as robustly unfair in disturbing equality. By giving a prior morally canonical status to all being equal, this form of egalitarianism legitimates taking from those who have by good fortune received more. In its strongest form it legitimates making all worse off if this will realize equality. This egalitarian attitude trades on an envy that would justify "a moral feeling of displeasure or ill-will at the superiority of [another person] in happiness, success, reputation or the possession of anything desirable."[22] Such an endorsement of equality is immoral in general secular terms because it affirms ill will in the sense of an approval of coercive force to take from those who have more so that they are leveled to the position of those who have less.[23] In its perspective, good fortune cannot be recognized as a morally nonprincipled given, as neither fair nor unfair. The fortune of some and the consequent (i.e., comparative) relative misfortune of others are not recognized as simply happening, but as creating a claim in fairness to have such circumstances rectified.

With respect to health care, an egalitarianism of envy endorses a world in which no one had access to lung transplants (or other high-cost interventions) over a world in which only the rich would have access. This understanding can lead to the illegitimate use of state force: (1) in forbidding the rich from purchasing better care or (2) in slowing technological development to ensure that it would be available only when it can be provided for all. Such strategies limiting access and/or medical progress would be endorsed, even if this led to death and suffering, as long as equality was achieved.

Whether the relative fortune of some is to be understood in terms of the satisfaction or goods realized in the achievement of a human perfection (e.g., the nobility of human character realized in those of good breeding, ample resources, and cultivated manners—those who live *humaniter*) or in terms of the dissatisfaction it engenders due to the comparatively inferior fortune of others depends on the vision of the good or of justice invoked. To justify coercive egalitarianism in general secular moral terms, one must secure the canonical normativity of a particular moral understanding or ranking of values and the authorization of force on its behalf, which we have seen in chapters 2 and 4 is not possible.

In contrast, an egalitarianism of altruism appeals to the sympathy of others to help those suffering. An egalitarianism of altruism holds that a second world is worse than the first if one of the inhabitants of the second world experiences pain, deformity, disability, or an unwelcome earlier death that is not experienced in the first world. Egalitarianism of this genre is not concerned whether some have more, only whether some suffer. Inequalities are not in themselves disvalued. What is disvalued is suffering or that some lack an important good. Equality in goods, abilities, possessions, and experiences is not valued for its own sake. Rather, what is valued is the good to be achieved through a particular intervention. In terms of an egalitarianism of altruism, one is concerned to provide an expensive treatment to those who need it, not to withhold from the rich who might be able to purchase it. Such an egalitarianism can legitimately, within the constraints set by the principle of permission, motivate choices regarding the use of commonly owned resources.

## From macroallocations to microallocations

One must decide how much should be invested in health care as well as who should receive costly medical interventions. Different levels of health care choices interact. Each level brings its own moral interests and problems, while each level influences the other and shapes the character of its quandaries. Somewhat procrusteanly, these can be viewed as four levels of concerns.[24]

### Higher-level macroallocational choices

There is an interest in determining what level of resources should be devoted to health care. Yet no secular government or any individual may determine what portion of total available resources should be given to health care. The common funds in the hands of societies and states may be subject to explicit allocational choices. A society may need to decide, for example, what portion of its common resources should be invested in defense, education, the construction of museums, health care, and so on. Here the question will arise whether one may in general hold that health care expenditures have a more pressing claim on a society's attention and resources than, for example, laying out formal gardens or protecting endangered species. The difficulty is, as we have already seen, that there is no canonical ranking of "needs," such as the needs that justify feeding the starving, providing housing for the homeless, supporting the fine arts, or saving endangered species. Such rankings must be established by particular agreement for particular communal undertakings.

*Lower-level macroallocational choices*

In order adequately to appreciate the difficulty of discovering the proper pattern for health care allocations, one must examine what is encompassed. Health care, after all, includes not only the treatment of coronary artery disease, cancer, pneumonia, and tuberculosis, but arthritis, headaches, athlete's foot, and acne. Health care includes as well the psychiatric treatment of neuroses and the general support given by physicians to the worried well and vexed ill. It encompasses genetic counseling and the provision of contraceptives. Cosmetic surgery to raise sagging breasts and buttocks and to make noses better conform to prevailing cultural and aesthetic norms also falls within its purview. To decide which of these health care undertakings is more or less worthy of urgent support, one must decide which count as true needs, and which are mere desires. One must fashion a hierarchy of needs and desires to rank the claims made by different areas of health care for support. We have already seen in chapter 2 why it will be impossible to discover in general secular terms a single and univocal normative hierarchy that will determine how much of a communal budget should be allocated to the cure and treatment of pediatric leukemia versus the cataracts of the elderly. If such a hierarchy cannot be discovered, one will need to determine how one is fairly to create such hierarchies for the allocation of communal resources.

*Higher-level microallocational choices*

In deciding which patients should receive what forms of treatment, one makes choices against background assumptions about the ways in which resources ought to be allocated to particular kinds of patients. Although the focus is on particular sorts of patients (e.g., patients with particular likelihoods of surviving with particular investments of resources), they are seen through presumptions regarding the proper patterns within which such choices should be made. If the question is the provision of kidney transplants to patients with end-stage renal disease, one must decide how one ought in general to select recipients if there is an insufficient number of organs available for transplantation or insufficient funds to provide for the care of all. One must determine whether such health care should be provided (1) equally to all in need (and, if resources are not sufficient, to those chosen by a lottery), (2) to all who can pay or who have family, friends, acquaintances, or sympathetic third parties who will pay for the treatment, (3) to those individuals who are most likely to return to a productive life and thus maximally benefit society, or (4) in terms of some other set of considerations, such as providing treatment to those who merit it through special services to society. The choice of a vision for proper microallocational decisions, as well as the recognition of the limits of one's moral authority coercively to impose particular allocatory patterns, sets the stage for, but does not absolutely determine, those decisions. One may still argue that in particular cases particular forms of exceptions should be allowed. Moreover, because there will not be sufficient secular moral authority to forbid private individuals or hospital systems from departing from generally endorsed allocatory patterns, there will be the secular moral right to fashion numerous parallel approaches to the microallocation of organs, including their purchase and sale on the open market.

*Lower-level microallocational choices*

Charles Fried has argued that physicians and other health care providers should not make allocational decisions.[25] Those in charge of communal funds (e.g., officials appointed for this purpose by governments or through insurance contracts) may properly establish patterns for the availability of communal resources. Hospital administrators may also determine the portion of the hospital budget that will be allocated to particular hospital services. In addition, they may establish allocatory procedures and patterns for particular services to particular kinds of patients. They may set the pattern for microallocations.

In contrast, individual physicians and other health care professionals may properly seek to secure the best care for their patients, even if the pursuit of such care conflicts with the ideal pattern for microallocations. Fried can be understood as holding that the tension between physicians and bureaucrats is wholesome, somewhat on the model of the tension between defense and prosecuting attorneys. The counsel for the defense attempts to establish the defendant's innocence with all available energies, even if that attorney believes the defendant is in fact guilty, while the prosecutor attempts to establish the guilt of the defendant, even in the face of doubts regarding the guilt of the defendant. The Anglo-American adversary system of law presumes that this conflict will optimally disclose truth in the service of justice. So, too, one might hold that from the conflict between the hospital administration seeking to impose a particular efficient or mandated system of health care and the physician seeking to acquire for a patient the very best health care regardless of the system, there will develop the best balancing of forces needed to secure a health care system attentive both to general goals of efficiency and cost consciousness, as well as the individual needs and desires of patients.

There are moral limits on the extent to which health care professionals may secure resources for their patients, even in order to save their lives. Health care professionals may energetically explore all avenues for support and may be as strong advocates as possible. But they may not "game the system" by lies or through fraud. After all, if they believe lifesaving treatment is owed their patients, and such is not forthcoming from the government, private insurance, or the charity of others, then such health care professionals may sell their own assets to raise funds. Physicians are wrong if they believe they are obliged to provide patients all the treatment they need, even when they must take the needed resources by fraud, for this violates the principle of permission.

The more the pattern or principle for microallocational choices functions as a rule of thumb, the more there will be a distance between higher-level microallocational choices regarding what pattern of choosing particular levels of treatment is proper for particular kinds of patients, and lower-level microallocational decisions about the proper level of treatment for particular patients. As this distance increases, the lower-level microallocational choices will put pressures on the system as a whole, which may lead to recasting the rules of thumb, and consequently reshaping lower-level macroallocational choices, and then in the end revising the higher-level macroallocational pattern. If, out of consideration for particular patients, physicians continually secure funds for expensive lifesaving treatments, this will force a reconsideration of the policies for macroallocational choices. There is a dialectic among these four levels.

*Gambling with human life, and setting a price on health and survival*

Health care systems must take account of the probabilistic character of empirical knowledge in determining what resources are to be invested in diminishing particular risks of death, disability, suffering, dysfunction, and disfigurement. The many uncertainties of medical knowledge and the high costs of medical interventions invite one to gamble with human life and human suffering. Such gambles are a part of human life. One builds bridges, cars, and factories that are safe up to a point but not perfectly safe. One accepts less than the safety one would achieve if one attempted to protect lives at any cost. One thus sets a price on saving life and gambles with the lives and suffering of individuals. In general, people seem adverse to acknowledging this circumstance. Many find this circumstance particularly troublesome in health care. But health is where such choices must repeatedly be made. Again, if a patient has at most a 3 percent chance of survival, and the cost of treatment will be over $200,000, then one will be saving life at the cost of over $6 million. Does it matter whether a person has a life expectancy of one, ten, or sixty years? How is one to take account of data indicating that almost half a million dollars is invested in critical care treatment of patients with hematological cancers for every year of life secured at home?[26] There are no content-full secular moral answers to such questions. From a permission-based account of health care allocations, it will be acceptable to create policies regarding when it is worth trying to save lives. A secular health care system will need to shoulder the task of fashioning choices about how to invest communal resources in gambling with human suffering and death.

In all of this, people will seek moral guidance. They will want concrete moral advice in matters bearing on life, death, suffering, and disability. One is thus returned to the fundamental issue of whether and how just patterns for the distribution of resources to and in health care can be discovered, or whether and how they must be created through some form of common and fair negotiation or agreement. The issue of whether one can know truly what a just pattern of health care distribution should be, or whether one must instead in some procedurally fair, and in that sense just, fashion create a pattern of health care distribution, lies at the very heart of the question of justice in heath care. One must decide to what extent the pattern for justice in health care distributions at the macro- and micro-levels can be discovered and the extent to which such a pattern is properly the product of a fair procedure of negotiation and agreement among the individuals involved.

### Conflicting models of justice: from content to procedure

John Rawls's *A Theory of Justice* and Robert Nozick's *Anarchy, State, and Utopia* offer contrasting understandings of what should count as justice or fairness. They sustain differing suggestions regarding the nature of justice in health care. They provide a contrast between justice as primarily structural, a pattern of distributions that is amenable to rational disclosure, versus justice as primarily procedural, a matter of fair negotiation.[27] In *A Theory of Justice* Rawls forwards an expository device of an ahistorical perspective[28] from which to discover the proper pattern for the distribution of resources, and therefore presumably for the distribution of health care resources. In this understanding, it is assumed that societally based entitlements have moral priority. Nozick, in contrast, advances a historical account of just distributions within which justice depends on what individuals have agreed to do with and for each other. Nozick holds that individually based entitlements are morally prior to societally based entitlements. In contrast with Rawls, who argues that one can discover a proper pattern for the allocation of resources, Nozick argues that such a pattern cannot be discovered and that instead one can only identify the characteristics of a just process for fashioning rights to health care.

Rawls's argument is of interest because of his claim to be able to discover the proper principles to be followed in distributing primary social goods. Although he avoids the issue of allocating health care resources, and though he has significantly limited the claims for his account,[29] his theory is often invoked in the discussion of the distribution of health care resources.[30] To appreciate Rawls, one might approach the problem of distributive justice through considering how one might divide plots of land on an unowned island.[31] Let us imagine that some readers of this book are adrift in a powerless boat approaching an uninhabited and unowned island. Let us also imagine that all have an equal interest in owning land on the island. We might all assign by agreement to one individual the task of managing the distribution. That individual would need to survey the island and divide it equally. To ensure fairness, we might give to that individual the destiny of taking that parcel of land that no one else wanted, the last parcel left after all others had selected a tract. The distributor would wish to lay out tracts with great care, to ensure that each tract would be equal. Or if the tracts were unequal, the inequality would produce an advantage for the person receiving the smaller tract, so that it would be as desirable as the rest. In this way we could establish a procedure for the just distribution of the land, in that no one would have a basis for protesting the share received. The procedure would be so structured as to protect the interests of all. All of this presumes the island is unowned and that we all have a similar understanding of the value of the tracts of land and the risks at stake.

Rawls has developed this procedure on a grand scale in terms of an ahistorical contractual position that serves as an expository device to disclose the implications of one liberal democratic version of justice or fairness. He introduces his intellectual standpoint by asking us to imagine what would count as a just distribution of the primary social goods to which representative original contractors would agree. In so doing, he presumes that things in the world are not already owned. He presumes as well that all would want an equal distribution of income and wealth unless an unequal distribution would be to the advantage of the person receiving the smallest allocation. Rawls develops the conceptual machinery for this procedure around six key assumptions: (1) that there is a single, "thin," normative view of what should characterize a rational contractor (i.e., that such rational contractors have certain interests expressed in a minimal or thin theory of the good that supports a particular lexical ordering of the primary social goods, one that ranks liberty higher than the other primary social goods);[32] (2) that such contractors are risk-aversive and therefore unwilling to take the risk of being a member of an exploited class (e.g., as might occur in a utilitarian scheme, which would distribute the primary social goods so as to create the greatest good for the greatest number, with the possibility of some harm to a small minority);[33] and that (3) such contractors lack envy and are therefore willing to accept unequal distributions if they redound to the benefit of the least-advantaged class in that society[34] (i.e., thereby ensuring all who risk an unequal distribution against receiving less than they would have through an equal distribution); (4) that a reference state of equality can be specified (such a reference state could not be specified if there were not a fundamental agreement regarding values so that equality could be calculated); (5) that the contractors act as if they were heads of families; and (6) that these rational contractors can be envisioned as deciding on their circumstances from the perspective of an original contracting position within which they are ignorant of circumstances that would otherwise bring them to be "biased" contractors, such as (a) their position in society, (b) their natural assets and abilities, (c) their conception of the good, including their rational plan of life, (d) special features of their psychology, (e) the particular circumstances of their society, and (f) the generation to which they belong.[35]

By placing the distribution of natural assets and abilities behind the veil of ignorance, as well as one's position in society, Rawls erases many of the usual lines between what is unfair and what is simply unfortunate. His hypothetical contractors will want to structure society so as to compensate for receiving fewer assets and abilities, thus rendering uncorrected advantages from such assets and abilities unfair. In this way Rawls seeks to secure a moral obligation to compensate others for the unfortunate results of the natural lottery (i.e., the outcomes of natural forces) and the social lottery (i.e., the outcomes of the choices of individuals and society). If one does not yet know whether one will be favored by the natural or social lottery, and if all things are still unowned, one will wish to distribute resources so as to ensure against possible losses in either of these lotteries. Indeed, even if persons already have entitlements, one will be tempted to impeach their claims for one's own advantage. One will not be inclined to find a social arrangement acceptable unless it secures one's advantage. Unfortunate outcomes therefore become unfair outcomes, outcomes that individuals in the original position would have seen as requiring compensation as an element of an acceptable social structure. In this fashion, one can presumably argue for health care insurance as a basic right.

In these terms John Rawls advances his two principles of justice, as those that would be endorsed by individuals in his account of the original position.

First Principle

Each person is to have an equal right to the most extensive total system of equal basic liberties compatible with a similar system of liberty for all.

Second Principle

Social and economic inequalities are to be arranged so that they are both:
(a) to the greatest benefit of the least advantaged, consistent with the just savings principle, and
(b) attached to offices and positions open to all under conditions of fair equality of opportunity.[36]

With respect to issues of health care, one will have to decide whether health care is governed under the first principle (i.e., is a condition of liberty), or the first or second half (i.e., is a condition of fair equality) of the second principle.

If the allocation of health care resources is like Rawls's allocation of income and wealth, differences in allocation will be justifiable as long as these differences redound to the benefit of the least-well-off class. There will then be a problem of defining the least-well-off class with regard to either economic characteristics or economic plus health status characteristics.[37] At the very least, it is difficult to understand why contractors, given Rawls's account of their risk-aversiveness, would not require distributions of resources to the benefit of the medically worst-off up to the point at which such redistributions would decrease the welfare status of the least-well-off. Since dying young is a great disadvantage, the claims for high-cost, low-yield treatment for those who would die young or for the young disabled would likely be quite significant. If the allocation of health care resources is integral to fair equality of opportunity (e.g., equality of life-span), one will need to allocate funds for health care prior to allocations for other primary social goods such as income support or the achievement of an attractive standard of living. Improving health and compensating for disability would take precedence over improving the welfare status, otherwise considered, of the least-well-off. If this is the case, one will face very strong claims for resources on the part of the incapacitated and those who die young, which would lead to expending significant resources in the pursuit of only modest gains in health status so as to achieve a modicum of greater equality of opportunity. Since equality of opportunity would seem in issues of health to include at least living in good health into middle age, if not having at least a life expectancy equal to most, resources would be drained from the old to the young to postpone death and remedy disabilities. The claims would even be yet more robust if health care were understood as a condition for maintaining the ability to exercise basic liberties—that is, they would trump even considerations of equality of opportunity.

Rawls's ahistorical foundation for the allocation of resources is, to borrow from Nozick, an end-state view of distributive justice. It provides principles that individuals should find acceptable as a basis for the distribution of commonly owned resources, if they consider themselves outside of any already established system of property rights, as if all were owned in common. Nozick, in contrast, gives a historical account. He assumes (1) that the condition for morality is mutual respect, and (2) that people actually already own things prior to any particular society. Therefore, the principles of justice are those of just acquisition, just transfer, and retribution for past injustices in acquisition or transfer under the general formal principle of justice, *"From each as they choose, to each as they are chosen."*[38] As a result, for Nozick in *Anarchy, State, and Utopia,* the results of the natural and social lotteries are unfortunate, though not unfair, insofar as they have not been influenced by unjustified force, coercion, or over-reaching. Unfortunate (or, for that matter, fortunate) outcomes do not of themselves create obligations in justice. For Nozick, moral agents are not obliged out of considerations of fairness to attempt to blunt the consequences of the natural lottery through which some are born healthy and others with serious diseases. In addition, for Nozick the adverse outcomes of the social lottery, through which some are wealthy through gifts, inheritances, or the cooperation of others, and others impoverished, are also simply unfortunate if unjustified societal force, coercion, or overreaching has not been involved. Although individuals may have acted unfairly, for which compensation will be due from the accountable individuals, when this is not possible, matters will simply be unfortunate from the perspective of others in that they will not be obliged to make the injured whole. That some do not have funds to pay for health care does not of itself create a societal obligation of redress. Nor is it a moral affront that some have funds to purchase health care that others need but cannot afford.

The differences between Nozick of *Anarchy, State, and Utopia* and Rawls of *A Theory of Justice* express themselves in different accounts of entitlements and ownership, and in different understandings of nonprincipled fortune and misfortune. For Rawls, one has justifiable title to goods if such a title is part of a system that ensures the greatest benefit to the least advantaged, consistent with a just-savings principle, and with offices and positions open to all under conditions of fair equality and opportunity, and where each person has an equal right to the most extensive total system of equal basic liberties compatible with a similar system of liberty for all. In contrast, for Nozick, one simply owns things: "Things come into the world already attached to people having entitlements over them."[39] If one really owns things, there will be freedom-based limitations on principles of distributive justice. One may not use people or the property without their permission or authorization. The needs of others will not erase one's property rights. The readers of this book should consider that they may be wearing wedding rings or other jewelry not essential to their lives, which could be sold to buy antibiotics to save identifiable lives in the third world. Those who keep such baubles may in part be acting in agreement with Nozick's account and claiming that "it is my right to keep my wedding ring for myself, even though the proceeds from its sale could save the lives of individuals in dire need."

Nozick's account requires a distinction between someone's secular moral rights and what is right, good, or proper to do. At times, selling some (perhaps all) of one's property to support the health care of those in need will be the right thing to do, even though one has a secular moral right to refuse to sell. This contrast derives from the distinction Nozick makes between *freedom as a side constraint,* as the very condition for the possibility of a secular moral community, and *freedom as one value among others.* This contrast can be understood as a distinction between those claims of justice based on the very possibility of a moral community, versus those claims of justice that turn on interests in particular goods and values, albeit interests recognized in the original position. For Nozick, one may not use innocent free persons without their consent, even if that use will save lives by providing needed health care or securing equality of opportunity. Even if such would be a good thing to do (e.g., in this sense of saving lives), no one has a right to do it. Because for Nozick one needs the *actual* consent of *actual* persons in order to respect them as free persons, their rights can morally foreclose the pursuit of many morally worthy goals. In contrast, Rawls treats freedom or liberty as a value. As a consequence, in developing just institutions, Rawls does not require actual consent of those involved. As a result, Rawls would allow rights to self-determination to be limited in order to achieve important social goals.

The difference between Rawls's and Nozick's accounts in great measure derives from the circumstance that Rawls's theory of justice turns on an invitation to imagine what it would be like to sketch the principles of justice as fairness, so that no matter into what class one is born, one would not have grounds for claiming that membership in that class is rationally unacceptable. From this perspective unjustified good fortune or misfortune must be corrected. All distributions of fortune must be addressed from the perspective of the original position. Yet this perspective does not appear to give us useful guidance for the hard decisions in health care policy (e.g., how ought one to balance the importance of avoiding early death with the importance of avoiding suffering). Moreover, insofar as guidance is forthcoming, this perspective may generate unmanageable claims (e.g., to do everything to equalize life expectancies or compensate for disabilities). Nozick challenges why one should assume such an ahistorical viewpoint, if indeed people actually own things. His retort in *Anarchy, State, and Utopia* is that a position such as Rawls's would deliver principles of distributive justice that rational individuals should take to be normative, only if people do not already (in the order of justification) own themselves and things privately and in addition embrace certain particular views of rationality and justice. However, people do already own themselves as well as things privately, as Nozick and this book in chapter 4 have argued. Freedom is not simply one value among others, but the source of moral authority expressed in choice or permission. It is the source of moral authority when moral strangers collaborate.

In this fashion, one can offer a foundation for Nozick's otherwise unsecured points of departure.[40] One can place Nozick's contentions in chapters 2 and 3 by construing them as laying out the necessary conditions for the possibility of a moral structure that can bind moral strangers. The limited state is the morally authoritative structure that members of morally diverse communities can, as moral strangers, recognize as mutually binding. As a consequence of this justification, even if a fair distribution could be effected in Rawls's terms, it would represent only one ideological viewpoint. It would have no generally binding authority. Moreover, if a state of affairs came into existence that conformed to Rawlsian requirements, free individuals would be in secular moral authority through their own free transactions to erase that state of affairs. Since authority is derived from individuals, it is they who give communal structures their moral standing. Somewhat oversimplistically put, authority comes from the governed, not from a rationally authoritative vision of justice or fairness. From this perspective, the proper amount of resources to be given to health care is to be created by agreement, not discovered in an original position. One does not have to attempt the impossible, namely, to derive normative content-full principles like rabbits out of a philosophical hat. Instead, one derives authority from the consent of actual individuals.

This contrast between Rawls and Nozick can be appreciated more generally as a contrast between two quite different principles of justice, each of which has strikingly different implications for the allocation of health care resources.

1.  Freedom- or permission-based justice is concerned with distributions of goods made in accord with the notion of the secular moral community as a peaceable social structure binding moral strangers, members of diverse concrete moral communities. Such justice will therefore require the consent of the individuals involved in a historical nexus of justice-regarding institutions understood in conformity with the principle of permission. The principle of beneficence may be pursued only within constraints set by the principle of permission.
2.  Goals-based justice is concerned with the achievement of the good of individuals in society, where the pursuit of beneficence is not constrained by a strong principle of permission, but driven by some particular understanding of morality, justice, or fairness. Such justice will vary in substance as one attempts, for example, to (a) give each person an equal share; (b) give each person what that person needs; (c) give each person a distribution as a part of a system designed to achieve the greatest balance of benefits over harms for the greatest number of persons; (d) give each person a distribution as a part of a system designed to maximize the advantage of the least-well-off class within conditions of equal liberty for all and of fair opportunity.

Allocations of health care in accord with freedom- or permission-based justice must occur within the constraint to respect the free choices of persons, including their exercise of their property rights. Allocations of health care in accord with goals-based justice will need to establish what it means to provide a just pattern of health care, and what constitutes true needs, not mere desires, and how to rank the various health goals among themselves and in comparison with nonhealth goals. Such approaches to justice in health care will require a way of ahistorically discovering the proper pattern for the distribution of resources.

Permission-based and goals-based approaches to justice in health care contrast because they offer competing interpretations of the maxim, "Justitia est constans et perpetua voluntas jus suum cuique tribuens" (Justice is the constant and perpetual will to render everyone his due).[41] A permission-based approach holds that justice is first and foremost giving to each the right to be respected as a free individual as the source of secular moral authority, in the disposition of personal services and private goods: that which is due (*ius*) to individuals is respect of their authority over themselves and their possessions. In contrast, a goals-based approach holds that justice is receiving a share of the goods, which is fair by an appeal to a set of ahistorical criteria[42] specifying what a fair share should be, that is, what share is due to each individual. Since there are various senses of a fair share (e.g., an equal share, a share in accordance with the system that maximizes the balance of benefits over harms, etc.), there will be various competing senses of justice in health care under the rubric of goals-based justice.

We are returned here to the foundational issues addressed in chapters 2, 3, and 4. There is no canonical moral vision or understanding of basic claims on resources in terms of which equality or fairness can be required. There is no way to establish the ranking of economic liberties versus political liberty or liberty from the threat of arbitrary violence without begging the cardinal question of which is more important. As has been noted, if one reconstructs the settled moral intuitions in these matters of liberals from Cambridge, Massachusetts, they will be quite different from those who find the government of Singapore congenial. The selection of a thin theory of the good to motivate the contractors in the original position depends on a choice that cannot be justified in general secular terms. Nor is there a canonical understanding of acceptable risks. There is no canonical content-full vision of justice to shape secular health care policy. As a result, a justification for allocation choices regarding resources must be restricted to communal resources. Such choices can derive their authority only from the permission of those involved.

In this light, Nozick's account can be recast, given a foundation, and up to a point used to illustrate the dilemma of secular health care policy in large-scale states. Because there is no canonical content-full vision of the good, fairness, or justice, the authority for the distribution of goods must be derived from common agreement. If states legitimately possess communal property, these can legitimately be the object of allocatory decisions pursuant to the constitutions of those states. But careful distinctions will need to be drawn between communal and private properties. Moreover, persons as well as their property and services may not be used without their permission.

## The moral inevitability of a multitier health care system

Public health care systems are communal attempts to ensure against losses at the natural and social lotteries through planned human beneficence. They function to blunt the tragedies of nature as well as the uncaring and evil choices of persons, including those who will not respond with sympathy to those in need. They are social constructs established to relieve individuals of some of the anxieties associated with the fear of disability, suffering, disease, and death.[43] They are one of many human attempts to render nature congenial to persons.

This volume's analyses of the principles of permission and beneficence and of entitlements to property support a multitier system of health care. On the one hand, not all property is privately owned. Nations and other social organizations may invest their common resources in ensuring their members against losses in the natural and social lotteries. On the other hand, as we have seen in chapter 5, not all property is communal. There are private entitlements, which individuals may freely exchange for the services of others. The existence of a multitier system (whether officially or unofficially) in nearly all nations and societies reflects the existence of both communal and private entitlements, of social choice and individual aspiration. A two-tiered system with inequality in health care distribution is both morally and materially inevitable.

In the face of unavoidable tragedies and contrary moral intuitions, a multitiered system of health care is in many respects a compromise. On the one hand, it provides some amount of health care for all, while on the other hand allowing those with resources to purchase additional or better services. It can endorse the use of communal resources for the provision of a decent minimal or basic amount of health care for all, while acknowledging the existence of private resources at the disposal of some individuals to purchase better basic as well as luxury care. While the propensity to seek more than equal treatment for oneself or loved ones is made into a vicious disposition in an egalitarian system, a multitier system allows for the expression of individual love and the pursuit of private advantage, though still supporting a general social sympathy for those in need. Whereas an egalitarian system must suppress the widespread human inclination to devote private resources to the purchase of the best care for those whom one loves, a multitier system can recognize a legitimate place for the expression of such inclinations. A multitier system (1) should support individual providers and consumers against attempts to interfere in their free association and their use of their own resources, though (2) it may allow positive rights to health care to be created for individuals who have not been advantaged by the social lottery.

The serious task is to decide how to define and provide a decent minimum or basic level of care as a floor of support for all members of a society, while allowing money and free choice to fashion special tiers of services for the affluent. In addressing this general issue of defining what is to be meant by a decent minimum basic level or a minimum adequate amount of health care, the American President's Commission in 1983 suggested that in great measure content is to be created rather than discovered by democratic processes, as well as by the forces of the market. "In a democracy, the appropriate values to be assigned to the consequences of policies must ultimately be determined by people expressing their values through social and political processes as well as in the marketplace."[44] The Commission, however, also suggested that the concept of adequacy could in part be discovered by an appeal to that amount of care that would meet the standards of sound medical practice. "Adequacy does require that everyone receive care that meets standards of sound medical practice."[45] But what one means by "sound medical practice" is itself dependent on particular understandings within particular cultures. Criteria for sound medical practice are as much created as discovered. The moral inevitability of multiple tiers of care brings with it multiple standards of proper or sound medical practice and undermines the moral plausibility of various obiter dicta concerning the centralized allocation of medical resources.[46]

Indeed, the arguments in chapters 2, 3, 4, and 5 lead to the conclusion that concepts of adequate care are not discoverable outside of particular views of the good life and of proper medical practice. In nations encompassing diverse moral communities, an understanding of what one will mean by an adequate level or a decent minimum of health care will need to be fashioned, if it can indeed be agreed to, through open discussion and by fair negotiation. In some small-scale communities such as the BaMbuti, there may be little commitment of common resources to the endeavors of modern health care. For such communities, a decent level of such care may be little or no care. In nations such as the United Kingdom, the decent minimum of care may not include hemodialysis for individuals over a particular age or coronary bypass surgery for any but the most promising candidates (or at least there will be informal ways of discouraging such treatment).[47] For many elsewhere, such a minimal level of investment will not count as a decent level. For Roman Catholics and others in the United Kingdom, the provision of abortions through the National Health Service will be unacceptable, making the United Kingdom's basic package morally problematic.

One creates through negotiation an amount of health care that becomes de facto the decent minimal amount for a polity, though it always remains open to further critique, discussion, and alteration. In smaller social groups that share a common view of the good life, one may be able to appeal to a common vision to discover what should count as a decent minimum of health care. But across communities there will be different moral visions along with different understandings of what should count as a decent minimum of health care or a standard of services that comports with sound medical practice. This diversity will provide a motivation for particular groups to provide particular packages of health care that reflect moral concerns regarding the character of proper health care delivery, rather than concerns to have access to better basic or to luxury health care. For example, out of concerns to avoid supporting morally inappropriate care (e.g., abortion and euthanasia), and in order to establish a worldwide basic package for all its members, one might imagine the Roman Catholic church requiring all of its members to devote 40 percent of their tithe to the church for health care. In this way, all Roman Catholics could carry with them through the world a basic guaranteed package of services, which would be in accord with their moral commitments. Those who wish more could purchase it. One would receive care *secundum status.*

Or one could envisage various groups creating their own special health care packages integrated with the basic package for a polity. Just as in Germany, citizens who are Roman Catholic or members of the Evangelical Reformed church are visited with a tax surcharge for spiritual services, different groups could pay different amounts (or receive refunds) for their special moral commitments with respect to abortion, sterilization, third-party-assisted suicide, euthanasia, and the like, insofar as these are made part of health care agreements. There might be special discounts for signing agreements to limit treatment or be euthanatized. Among the moral advantages of this approach would be that one would not need to be involved in the provision of health care one knew to be immoral. In particular, one would not be taxed to support what one recognizes to be immoral endeavors. Moreover, one could clearly distance oneself from their provision.

These diverse health care packages could in some circumstances be provided in the same building, just as hospitals now have private and semiprivate rooms. In other cases, such moral diversity could be realized in separate facilities. In either case, there could be special criminal and civil law that would protect against health care being provided to patients or in areas where it had by agreement been held to be morally offensive. Thus, for example, those who opposed euthanasia and joined a noneuthanasia health insurance system or sickness fund could be assured against being euthanatized. Those who performed abortions in a nonabortion hospital could be held criminally and civilly liable.

Outside of communities that share a moral vision, one will need to create policy for the use of common resources. Often this will proceed best through a dialogue among citizens, politicians, and health care experts. In this way, one may be able to fashion a basic package of health care for all citizens. But there will inevitably be different levels of care and different standards. Those who have the resources will demand first-class basic along with supplementary care. To borrow a metaphor from Gilbert Welch, though one may provide all with coach health care, so that none need be treated "stand-by," some will always upgrade to business and first-class care.[48]

The best example of an open democratic dialogue creating a basic package of health care is what was forwarded as the so-called Oregon Plan.[49] The plan was developed in order to cover all Oregonians below the poverty line. The idea was to decrease the use of high-cost, low-yield interventions in order to provide all indigents with a level of care likely to secure morbidity and mortality relief on a par with that achieved by the basic health care guaranteed in many countries.[50] The hope was to require all employers to provide this minimal package to all their employees. A poll was taken to determine how citizens ranked the various health care services that could be provided. Public meetings were held in forty-seven of the forty-nine counties of Oregon to explore the balancing of interest in different treatments. After all, one must decide whether a basic package of care will cover root-canal work as well as critical care for neonates with birth weights under 500 grams. The plan was clearly committed to multitier health care provision. Providers would not be held criminally or civilly liable for the nonprovision of treatment, if when the treatment was not covered under the basic Oregon Plan they indicated its merit and the need to purchase it privately. Nor would individuals or companies be coercively prevented by state force from buying or selling private basic or luxury health care or health care insurance.

Because federal law and limited effective states' rights constrained the Oregon Plan to address only issues of Medicaid and basic mandated insurance for employees, and because of the intrusions of the Americans with Disabilities Act (the plan would not have provided neonatal intensive care for newborns with birthweights under 500 grams, or liver transplants for alcoholics, which omissions were held to be invidiously discriminatory), the Oregon Plan was not allowed to proceed as first envisioned. Still, the plan showed that it was possible for citizens, politicians, and health care experts to enter into a dialogue aimed at creating a basic package of health care without interfering in the rights of individuals to purchase better basic or supplementary care. It laid the basis for an important cultural achievement: recognizing and working within the constraints set by the probabilistic character of health care reality and the limits of moral authority, human life, and human resources.

The Oregon Plan represented a first hesitant and difficult break with the American health care ideology and its regnant deceptions. Understood in this light, the original Oregon Plan had the special virtue of recognizing: (1) the moral inevitability of inequality in health care; (2) the moral necessity of creating the proper character of basic health care packages, rather than discovering their appropriate content; (3) the moral necessity of recognizing the finitude of life and resources and then setting a price on saving life and treating suffering, disability, and deformity; (4) the moral allowability of responding with sympathy and altruism as expressed in the fashioning of a basic health care package from communal resources; (5) the moral challenge of sustaining a secular culture able to gamble with human life and suffering in the face of limited moral authority and vision; and (6) the moral necessity of the limited character of all secular projects, including that of treating disease, disability, and deformity.

Understood most generally, these reflections can be seen as indicating the moral inevitability of the following principle in fashioning health care allocations:

---

### PRINCIPLE OF HEALTH CARE ALLOCATION

People are free to purchase the health care they can buy and to provide the health care others wish to give or to sell.

A. The principle of permission allows persons with common resources to act beneficently by creating a package of health care that can be guaranteed to others, thus creating basic expectations for care and treatment. The principle recognizes the following secular moral constraints:

1. A private tier of health care is morally unavoidable.
2. A public or communal tier of health care may, but need not, be created out of communal funds.
3. There is no canonical, secularly discoverable normative comparison or ranking of health care needs and desires with other needs and desires, or among health care needs and desires; all such orderings or rankings must be created. There is no secularly obligatory rule of rescue that is independent of particular agreement.
4. Health care in almost all morally defensible circumstances will be multitier so that when a basic package is provided for the indigent, more ample or better quality basic as well as luxury care may be purchased by the affluent.
5. An all-encompassing, single-payer plan, as has existed in Canada, is morally impermissible because it violates fundamental principles of secular morality. It is in this sense immoral.[51]
6. Inequalities in health care are morally inescapable because individuals are free and differ in the scope of their needs and resources.
7. Whether or not they are geographically located, given the limited secular moral authority of large-scale governments spanning pluralist societies, communities (e.g., the Roman Catholic) may develop their autonomous health care systems so that they need not be involved in morally objectionable health care services (e.g., be involved in abortion and euthanasia) and so that such services may be forbidden in their own facilities.

B. Maxim: Give to those who need or desire health care that which they, you, or others are willing to pay for or provide gratis.

---

This principle, like all the principles in this volume, summarizes a cluster of moral issues salient in the peaceable collaboration of moral strangers. It also underscores. that the foundation of the secular moral authority binding moral strangers is derived from the permission of individuals. The principle of health care allocation does not disclose what concretely is good, proper, praiseworthy, or morally appropriate for individuals to provide to others in need of health care. That can only be discovered within the right community of moral friends.

### Conclusions: creating rights to health care in the face of moral diversity

Particular health care systems with particular guaranteed basic minimums of health care services reflect explicit as well as implicit choices of particular goals and values, rather than others. They involve ranking some goals and values higher, and others lower. In general secular moral terms, the circumstance that patients in one system or tier will be guaranteed care not provided in another, that patients who are salvageable in one system or tier will die in another tier for lack of the same care, is not a testimony to secular moral malfeasance, but to the different powers, fortune, choices, and visions of free men and women. There are limits to our capacity secularly to discover what we ought to do together. There are limits to our secular moral authority to require others to conform to one moral vision or one content-full understanding of justice or fairness.

Our secular moral limitations argue against uniformity in health care packages and in favor of the affirmative acceptance of a diversity of approaches to providing health care. One of the strongest arguments in favor of recognizing this diversity is rooted in the obligation not to interfere with the peaceable religious appreciation of the immorality of many of the health care services that will be seen as unproblematic by those without the benefit of grace (e.g., abortion). In addition, varying concerns with amenities and superior quality of care will make augmented basic and supplementary packages highly attractive to those with the resources to purchase them. If one takes moral diversity seriously, whether expressed in religious understandings or in desires for augmented or superior care, one will need to tolerate the fashioning of parallel health care systems with diverse basic packages of care. Concerns raised in chapters 6 and 7 regarding the moral impropriety of many of the interventions that secular moral institutions must tolerate further strengthen the obligation to acknowledge in health care the moral diversity that characterizes the human condition. When we meet as moral strangers, we must settle for deciding fairly what we will do together. When we cannot together discover what we ought to do, then we must often agree peaceably to go our own ways. Partially parallel health care systems can allow the segmentation of health care delivery in areas of significant moral disagreement. Our moral differences need not lead us to total separation, but only to parting company in certain areas of health care delivery.

## Notes

1. Discussions regarding the allocation of health care resources have spawned a wide range of conflicting visions. See, for example, Thomas J. Bole and William Bondeson (eds.), *Rights to Health Care* (Dordrecht: Kluwer, 1991); Daniel Callahan, *What Kind of Life: The Limits of Medical Progress* (New York: Simon & Schuster, 1990); Larry Churchill, *Rationing Health Care in America* (Notre Dame, Ind.: University of Notre Dame Press, 1987); Paul Menzel, *Strong Medicine: The Ethical Rationing of Health Care* (New York: Oxford University Press, 1990). See, also, Dan Brock, *Life and Death: Philosophical Essays in Biomedical Ethics* (New York: Cambridge University Press, 1993), especially pp. 235–416.
2. Friedrich A. Hayek, *Law, Legislation, and Liberty* (Chicago: University of Chicago Press, 1976), p. 97.

3. The White House Domestic Policy Council, *The President's Health Security Plan* (New York: Times Books, 1993). For reflections on this proposal, see "The Clinton Plan: Pro and Con," *Health Affairs* 13 (Spring 1994): 1–273, and "Mandates: The Road to Reform?" *Health Affairs* 13 (Spring 1994): 1–302. For an attempt to provide moral underpinnings to the Clinton proposal, see Dan W. Brock and Norman Daniels, "Ethical Foundations of the Clinton Administration's Proposed Health Care System," *Journal of the American Medical Association* 271 (Apr. 20, 1994), 1189–96. For a critical moral assessment of the Clinton proposal, see Norman Daniels, "The Articulation of Values and Principles Involved in Health Care Reform," *Journal of Medicine and Philosophy 19* (Oct. 1994): 425–33; H. Tristram Engelhardt, Jr., "Health Care Reform: A Study in Moral Malfeasance," *Journal of Medicine and Philosophy* 19 (Oct. 1994), 501–16; George Khushf, "Ethics, Policies, and Health Care Reform," *Journal of Medicine and Philosophy* 19 (Oct. 1994): 397–405; Richard D. Lamm, "Rationing and the Clinton Health Plan," *Journal of Medicine and Philosophy 19* (Oct. 1994): 445–54; Laurence B. McCullough, "Should We Create a Health Care System in the United States?" *Journal of Medicine and Philosophy* 19 (Oct. 1994): 483–90. For an overview of the process by which the original Clinton plan was framed, see Laurence J. O'Connell, "Ethicists and Health Care Reform: An Indecent Proposal?" *Journal of Medicine and Philosophy* 19 (Oct. 1994): 419–24, and Marian Gray Secundy, "Strategic Compromise: Real World Ethics," *Journal of Medicine and Philosophy* 19 (Oct. 1994): 407–17. Finally, for a presentation of the conflicts between the moral integrity of one religious community and the Clinton health care proposals, see James T. McHugh, "Health Care Reform and Abortion: A Catholic Moral Perspective," *Journal of Medicine and Philosophy* 19 (Oct. 1994): 491–500.

4. The White House Domestic Policy Council, *The President's Health Security Plan*, p. 43.

5. Innovation would be discouraged as drug prices are subject to review as reasonable. The White House Domestic Policy Council, *The President's Health Security Plan*, p. 45. If one cannot make a good profit by developing new drugs, it will be more attractive to develop video games, where there is less likely to be a public concern about unreasonable profits. In such circumstances, one will have a society with widely enjoyed video games, but which will likely lack sufficient new drugs to respond to multidrug-resistant tuberculosis and other diseases.

6. J. K. Iglehart, "Canada's Health Care System Faces Its Problems," *New England Journal of Medicine* 322 (Feb. 22, 1990): 562–68; M. G. Marmot, George D. Smith, Stephen Stansfeld, et al., "Health Inequalities among British Civil Servants: The Whitehall II Study," *Lancet* 337 (June 8, 1991): 1387–93; G. J. Schieber, J.-P. Poullier, and L. M. Greenwald, "Health Spending, Delivery, and Outcomes in OECD Countries," *Health Affairs* 12 (Summer 1993): 120–29.

7. Rene Dubos, *Man Adapting* (New Haven Conn.: Yale University Press, 1969).

8. Plato, *Republic* 3.406a–b.

9. Plato, *Republic* 3.407–8.

10. Gregory Vlastos, "The Rights of Persons in Plato's Conception of the Foundations of Justice," in H. T. Engelhardt, Jr., and Daniel Callahan (eds.), *Morals, Science, and Sociality* (Hastings-on-Hudson, N.Y.: Hastings Center, 1978), pp. 172–201.

11. See, for example, the discussion in F. M. Kamm, *Morality, Mortality,* vol. 1, *Death and Whom to Save from It* (New York: Oxford University Press, 1993).

12. In considering how to respond to the plight of the impecunious, one might consider the story Jesus tells of the rich man who fails to give alms to "a certain beggar named Lazarus, full of sores, who was laid at his gate, desiring to be fed with the crumbs which fell from the rich man's table" (Luke 16:20–21). The rich man, who was not forthcoming with alms, was condemned eternally to a hell of excruciating torment.

13. President's Commission for the Study of Ethical Problems in Medicine and Biomedical and Behavioral Research, *Securing Access to Health Care* (Washington, D.C.: U.S. Government Printing Office, 1983), vol. 1, pp. 43–46.

14. The White House Domestic Policy Council, "Ethical Foundations of Health Reform," in *The President's Health Security Plan,* p. 11.

15. H. Newman, "Exclusion of Heart Transplantation Procedures from Medicare Coverage," *Federal Register* 45 (Aug. 6, 1980): 52296. See also H. Newman, "Medicare Program: Solicitation of Hospitals and Medical Centers to Participate in a Study of Heart Transplants," *Federal Register* 46 (Jan. 22, 1981): 7072–75.

16. The reader should understand that the author holds that almsgiving is one of the proper responses to human suffering (in addition to being an appropriate expression of repentance, an act of repentance to which surely the author is obligated). It is just that the author acknowledges the limited secular moral authority of the state to compel charity coercively. Jesus said, "If you want to be perfect, go, sell your possessions and give to the poor, and you will have treasure in heaven. Then come, follow me" (Matthew 19:21). There is no evidence that He said, "If you would be perfect, become a political activist on behalf of the poor, establish a progressive redistributive tax system, and use state force to be sure all support a welfare program." Being committed to aiding the poor is not equivalent to being committed to using state force to compel nonbelievers to be charitable. Moreover, the final emphasis is on following Jesus. An Orthodox interpretation of the meaning of this phrase is provided by St. Athanasius (296–373), who recounts that St. Anthony the Great of the Desert (250–356), when he heard this reading from the Gospels, sold what he had and then eventually became the great leader of Christian monasticism. See St. Athanasius, *The Life of St. Anthony.* The author's criticism of attempts by philosophers to provide a secular philosophical justification for governmentally imposed, coercive redistributive schemes does not imply that he holds that one should not follow the authentic injunction of the Gospels.

17. President's Commission, *Securing Access to Health Care,* vol. 1, pp. 18–19.

18. Since Rawls's theory of justice invites one in the original position to regard all responses to good fortune and misfortune from the perspective of how one would establish social institutions to respond so that one would regard arrangements as acceptable (i.e., as maximizing within certain constraints one's position, should one be in the least-well-off class), all fortunate and unfortunate outcomes must be regarded as either fair or unfair; there are no mere neutral happenings of fate or chance.

19. Matters appear differently within particular ideologies and religions. For example, just as Christianity has traditionally required slaves to remain subject to their masters,

Christianity has set as the ideal for its members—that of submitting to laws insofar as this does not violate the canons of the Church or the teaching received from the Apostles. Thus, in submission one is a martyr for the Faith.

20. See, for example, Marmot, Smith, Stansfeld, et al., "Health Inequalities among British Civil Servants: The Whitehall II Study," for a study of the impact of status on life expectancy. Iglehart notes that after fifteen years of an all-encompassing health care system, there was a 5.6 year difference in life expectancy between highest-earning males and lowest-earning males in Canada. Iglehart, "Canada's Health Care System Faces Its Problems."

21. Robert G. Evans, "Health Care in Canada: Patterns of Funding and Regulation," *Journal of Health Politics, Policy and Law* 8 (Spring 1983): 30. See also *Strained Mercy: The Economics of Canadian Health Care* (Toronto: Butterworths, 1984).

22. *Oxford English Dictionary* (1993), vol. 3, p. 232.

23. Those who hold that an egalitarianism of envy is justified will affirm moral intuitions such that they will prefer a world in which, all else being equal, individuals are equal rather than some individuals having greater happiness, power, satisfaction, and so forth. Thus, if they are asked to judge which is better, world A with ten individuals who are fully equal, and world B in which one individual by mutation develops the ability to "see" radiation and therefore avoid certain risks but only for that individual, world A will be regarded as preferable to world B.

24. I use the term *macroallocation* to identify allocations among general categories of expenditures. I use the term *microallocation* to indicate choices among particular individuals as to who will receive resources and in what amount.

25. Charles Fried, "Rights and Health Care—Beyond Equity and Efficiency," *New England Journal of Medicine* 293 (July 31, 1975): 241–45.

26. David Schapira, James Studnicki, et al., "Intensive Care, Survival, and Expenses of Treating Critically Ill Cancer Patients," *Journal of American Medical Association* 269 (Feb. 10, 1993): 783–88.

27. John Rawls, *A Theory of Justice* (Cambridge, Mass.: Harvard University Press, 1971), and Robert Nozick, *Anarchy, State, and Utopia* (New York: Basic Books, 1974).

28. "Ahistorical" is used not to identify not just accounts that abstract from particular social, cultural, and historical circumstances, but also accounts that do not attend to the actual history of actual agreements that convey actual permission or authority. They rely instead on a conceptual standpoint in which consent, permission, or agreement is seen to be rationally justified, even if it is not actually forthcoming in the real history of human agreements.

29. In his *A Theory of Justice*, Rawls gives indications that he has not forwarded a general philosophical foundation for the notion of fairness he endorses. When reading his remark that "I shall be satisfied if it is possible to formulate a reasonable conception of justice for the basic structure of society conceived for the time being as a closed system isolated from other societies" (p. 8), one might conclude that Rawls is simply stepping back from an account of international justice. But in his article "Justice as Fairness: Political Not Metaphysical," it becomes clear that justice as fairness is a political conception, not a foundational moral conception. "Justice as fairness is

intended as a political conception of justice for a democratic society, it tries to draw solely upon basic intuitive ideas that are embedded in the political institutions of a constitutional democratic regime and the public traditions of their interpretation.'' *Philosophy and Public Affairs* 14 (Summer 1985): 225. By the time one comes to *Political Liberalism*, this is acknowledged quite openly. ''Political liberalism, then, aims for a political conception of justice as a freestanding view. It offers no specific metaphysical or epistemological doctrine beyond what is implied by the political conception itself.'' John Rawls, *Political Liberalism* (New York: Columbia University Press, 1993), p. 10. As a consequence, any application of Rawls's theory of justice in the allocation of health care resources will be useful only in a community in which there is general agreement regarding its foundational commitments.

30. See, for example, Norman Daniels, *Just Health Care* (Cambridge: Cambridge University Press, 1985); ''Health Care Needs and Distributive Justice,'' *Philosophy and Public Affairs* 10 (Spring 1981): 146–79; ''Rights to Health Care and Distributive Justice: Programmatic Worries,'' *Journal of Medicine and Philosophy* 4 (June 1979): 174–91; and *Just Health Care* (New York: Cambridge University Press, 1985). Also Ronald Green, ''Health Care Justice in Contract Theory Perspective,'' in R. Veatch and R. Branson (eds.), *Ethics and Health Policy* (Cambridge, Mass.: Ballinger, 1976), pp. 111–26. For a review of some of these issues, see John C. Moskop, ''Rawlsian Justice and a Human Right to Health Care,'' pp. 329–38, and Lawrence Stern, ''Opportunity and Health Care: Criticisms and Suggestions,'' pp. 339–61, both in *Journal of Medicine and Philosophy* 8 (Nov. 1983). A detailed review of issues in justice in health care is provided as well by Earl E. Shelp (ed.), *Justice and Health Care* (Dordrecht: Reidel, 1981).

31. Readers will recognize this island as one in the archipelago of philosophers' islands: fictive situations used to control for the usual variables of life. Here this island offers territory previously unowned and uninhabited, and therefore available for *original* possession. Using this example, one can ask how the process of distributing property in a just fashion should occur without addressing such special issues as making restitution for past injustices.

32. Rawls, *Theory of Justice,* pp. 395–99.

33. John Hersanyi, ''Can the Maximin Principle Serve as a Basis for Morality? A Critique of John Rawls's Theory,'' *American Political Science Review* 6 (1975); 594–606.

34. See Rawls, *Theory of Justice,* p. 143.

35. Ibid., p. 137.

36. Ibid., p. 302.

37. See, for example, Nozick's discussion of who should count as the worst-off class—representative depressives, alcoholics, or paraplegics? *Anarchy, State, and Utopia,* pp. 189–91.

38. Nozick, *Anarchy, State, and Utopia,* p. 160.

39. Ibid.

40. There are many similarities between Locke and Nozick. Both begin with the assumption of certain human rights. John Locke secures his in a particular background theology. In the absence of that theology, indeed, in a secular context, an underpinning must be given for Nozick's entire account. Fortunately for Nozick, the project of securing authority through permission when moral strangers meet can provide a basis

for securing the centrality of freedom as a side constraint and individuals as a source of secular moral authority.
41. Flavius Petrus Sabbatius Justinianus, *The Institutes of Justinian*, trans. Thomas C. Sandars (1922; repr. Westport, Conn,: Greenwood Press, 1970), 1.1, p. 5.
42. These criteria may take historical, empirical, and other data into consideration. They, however, exclude certain patterns from the free peaceable choice of actual individuals and thus impose an ahistorical constraining pattern on their choices, which pattern reflects some particular vision or understanding of the proper account of goods or of the good.
43. Fear of the blind forces of nature has been a theme throughout human history. With the development of preventive medicine, modern medical treatment, and health or sickness insurance schemes, the fear of disease, pestilence, and plague has been blunted. To appreciate the full force of this fear one must look to the past when there was less of a sense of control and more a sense of hopelessness in the face of fate. This is well expressed in the opening to the thirteenth-century collection of songs and poems Carl Orff set to music for the cantata *Carmina Burana: Cantiones Profanae* (Mainz: B. Schott's Söhne, 1953; my translation):

| | |
|---|---|
| O Fortuna, | O Fortune |
| velut Luna | always changing |
| statu variabilis, | like the moon, |
| semper crescis | forever you wax |
| aut decrescis; . . . | and wane; . . . |

This general appreciation of a lottery of fate in which one alternately wins and loses included a sense of the natural and social lotteries' bearing on health status. The second strophe begins:

| | |
|---|---|
| Sors immanis | Lottery monstrous |
| et inanis, | and blind, |
| rota tu volubilis, | your turning wheel |
| status malus, | forever dissolves |
| vana salus | both misfortune |
| semper dissolubilis, . . . | and fruitless health, . . . |

The third strophe begins:

| | |
|---|---|
| Sors salutis | O Lottery of health |
| et virtutis | and of strength |
| michi nunc contraria. | you are now against me. |

    The poem captures what we have often forgotten, namely, the terror that seized our ancestors as plagues recurringly passed through cities and when life generally was much less secure. The majority of individuals in modern developed industrialized societies have little appreciation of these past realities and of the present life of millions in many developing countries who still live in such circumstances.
44. President's Commission, *Securing Access to Health Care*, vol. 1, p. 37.
45. Ibid.
46. For an example of a series of obiter dicta regarding the appropriate allocation of scarce medical resources, see Council on Ethical and Judicial Affairs, American Medical Association. "Ethical Considerations in the Allocation of Organs and Other Scarce

Medical Resources Among Patients,'' *Archives of Internal Medicine* 155 (Jan. 9, 1995): 29–40. For a study that addresses the problem of coming to terms with different tiers of health care, see E. Haavi Morreim, *Balancing Act* (Dordrecht: Kluwer, 1991).

47. Thomas Halper, *The Misfortunes of Others: End-stage Renal Disease in the United Kingdom* (Cambridge: Cambridge University Press, 1989). For a recent critical examination of the National Health Service, see Baruch A. Brody and Reider K. Lie, ''Methodological and Conceptual Issues in Health Care System Comparisons: Canada, Norway, and the United States,'' 437–63; Jean–Pierre Poullier, ''Eppur si muove: Comment on Baruch Brody and Reider Lie,'' 465–73; Brody and Lie, ''Response to Poullier,'' 475–76, all in *Journal of Medicine and Philosophy* 18 (Oct 1993).

48. H. G. Welch, ''Health Care Tickets for the Uninsured,'' *New England Journal of Medicine* 321 (Nov. 2, 1989): 1261–64.

49. Martin A. Strosberg, Joshua M. Wiener, Robert Baker (eds.), *Rationing America's Medical Care: The Oregon Plan and Beyond* (Washington, D.C.: Brookings Institution, 1992). See also Congress of the United States Office of Technology Assessment, *Evaluation of the Oregon Medicaid Proposal* (Washington, D.C.: U.S. Government Printing Office, 1992), and John K. Iglehardt, ''Health Care Reform: The States,'' *New England Journal of Medicine* 330 (Jan. 6, 1994): 75–79. See, also, Paige R. Sipes-Metzler, ''Oregon Health Plan: Ration or Reason,'' *Journal of Medicine and Philosophy* 19 (Aug. 1994): 305–14.

50. When one compares the amount of resources invested in health care in the OECD countries with the life expectancies achieved at birth, at sixty years, and at eighty, one discovers that, though there are significant differences in absolute investments, as well as in the percentage of the gross domestic product deployed for health care (the United States investing about $2,868 per person in 1991 compared with Germany's $1,659, the United Kingdom's $1,043, and Greece's $404), there are very little differences in life expectancies. Schieber et al., ''Health Spending, Delivery, and Outcomes in OECD Countries,'' 120–29. For a discussion of the reliability of the OECD data, see David Seedhouse, *Fortress NHS: A Philosophical Review of the National Health Service* (Chichester: John Wiley, 1994). For a discussion of the reliability of these data, see Brody and Lie, ''Methodological and Conceptual Issues in Health Care System Comparisons: Canada, Norway, and the United States,'' 437–64, Poullier, ''Eppur si muove: Comment on Baruch Brody and Reider Lie,'' 465–74, and Brody and Lie, ''Response to Poullier,'' 475–76. Even if the data were up to a point unreliable, they would not change the general point that dramatic differences in expenditures do not realize dramatic differences in life expectancy.

51. The ill-fated Clinton proposal for health care change serves as a moral exemplar of how not to engage in health care reform. From initially suggesting that it was possible to fashion a useful health reform proposal for a quarter of a billion people in one hundred days without public meetings and without careful comparison of American versus foreign experiences, to framing an actual proposal within the deceptions of an ideology that forbade acknowledging rationing, the proposal was a study in disingenuity. It should be featured in bioethics casebooks in the future as an example of what not to do.

# 9

## Reshaping Human Nature:
## Virtue with Moral Strangers
## and Responsibility without Moral Content

### Cosmic disorientation

We find ourselves alone. We are left without ultimate purpose or orientation.[1] We
have retreated to our own devices. Deaf to grace, we are left to guide ourselves.
For a while Sisyphus may defiantly face the rock. For some, "the struggle itself
toward the heights is enough to fill a man's heart. [Some may] imagine Sisyphus
happy" rather than in hell.[2] In rebellion there can be a perverse but profound
joy.[3] But whatever the matter may be for gods, unlike Sisyphus, we do not roll
the rock forever. Our choices are in the face of death and with those with whom
we share no ultimate convictions. Contemporary thought is marked by a growing
distance from ultimate orientation and purpose. Blind to final purposes, we turn
to ourselves for meaning. As moral strangers, within the fabric of secular morality, we confront godlike choices with impoverished human vision, and without
ultimate guideposts.

In these circumstances, we must articulate a secular ethics and bioethics.
Secular bioethics is framed this side of a major moral change, a collapse of
traditional expectations, and an intellectual reorientation. Our dominant culture
can no longer find our special place in the cosmos. The commitments that shaped
our thought for over a millennium and a half have been abandoned, at least by the
dominant culture. These changes have been a long time coming. As the first
chapter recalled, Nicolaus Copernicus, an employee of the Frauenburg Cathedral
in East Prussia, with his *De revolutionibus orbium coelestium* (1543) contributed

unwittingly to a vision that obscured our cosmic uniqueness and strengthened a secular view of reality. The change in astronomical perspective became a byword for a radical alteration in the understanding of our condition. We no longer experience ourselves as in the center of things, but as living on an obscure planet, orbiting an insignificant star, which is a member of one of innumerable galaxies. There no longer seems to be anything special about who we are. As Nietzsche recognized, modern science invites nihilism.[4] So, too, with the publication on November 24, 1859, of Charles Darwin and A. R. Wallace's *On the Origin of Species by Means of Natural Selection, or the Preservation of Favoured Races in the Struggle for Life*, our special status as humans seems obscured as well. Our nature appears the result of chance. Instead of a descent of human nature from the creative act of God, ''Adam, the son of God'' (Luke 3:38), we have been offered a *Descent of Man, and Selection in Relation to Sex* (1871).

This book ends where it began, against the background of these vast cultural changes. We confront the challenge of collaborating as moral strangers in a secular world deprived of canonical, guiding moral content. We began with the implications this has for moral issues in health care, for establishing a secular bioethics. We explored what moral standards are available when ultimate secular moral standards cannot be discovered. As chapter 5 showed, these difficulties do not bear solely on moral values, but on values in general, and in particular on the values associated with judgments of disease and health. Since medicine and the biomedical sciences are becoming ever more a means for refashioning and re-shaping human nature, we are concerned not only with what men and women ought to do, but with what they ought to become, with how we may refashion ourselves. Such choices involve moral, aesthetic, and other values that affirm what is good, beautiful, and proper human form and structure. Such judgments also incorporate views about what is natural or unnatural.

The appeal to human nature as a guide for moral action has been taken from us, or is at least profoundly restricted, when we can no longer acknowledge a design, but only the results of the blind forces of mutation, genetic drift, and natural selection. As chapter 5 has shown, this leads us in general secular contexts to specifying diseases in terms of the values of particular individuals, communities, and cultures. Because the composition of the values that structure the language of disease and health are more created than discovered, we are again thrown back upon ourselves. The result is not only disorientation in the sense of a loss of transcendent moorings, but also a reorientation in terms of what one might call a new transcendental mooring: persons as the center and source of general secular meaning. Even if we do not recognize our special place in nature, and even if our very nature as humans seems the arbitrary outcome of blind causal forces, we can make judgments about ourselves, our nature, and our projects.

There is a distance between us as persons and us as humans. The distance is the gulf between a reflective, manipulative being and the object of its reflection and manipulation. From our perspective as persons with particular understandings, views, and hopes, we can decide whether this is the best of places in the cosmos. If we find it unsatisfactory, we can even plot ways of changing our location. We can decide whether this is the best of natures and seek ways to refashion it if we find it wanting. As persons we can make our bodies objects of our judgment and manipulation. We can find ways in which we could have been better fashioned and redesign our genetic reconstruction accordingly.[5]

So far, our interventions have been humble. Through both passive and active immunization we have provided immunity to diseases without actually suffering those diseases. We have developed prosthetic lenses, valves, and joints. We have learned to control the usual mechanisms for rejecting foreign tissues so as to transplant organs. We have come to understand hormonal mechanisms so that we can break the natural bond between sexual intercourse and reproduction.

In the future our ability to constrain and manipulate human nature to follow the goals set by persons will increase. As we develop our capacities to engage in genetic engineering not only of somatic cells but of the human germline, we will be able to shape and fashion human nature in the image and likeness of goals chosen by human persons, not by nature or God. In the end, this may mean so radically changing human nature that our descendants may be regarded by subsequent taxonomists as a new species. If there is nothing sacred about human nature (and no merely secular argument can reveal the sacred), no reason will be recognized as to why, with proper caution, human nature should not be radically changed.

In this secular reassessment of our nature, we gain a better understanding of the remark of Protagoras, "Man is the measure of all things, of existing things that they exist, and of non-existing things that they exist not."[6] It is persons who are the measure of all things, because there is no one else to do measuring but persons. We must be responsible to ourselves and in our own terms because we will not accept an independent, content-full, canonical claim on us by God and cannot find one in reason. We cannot recognize even a content to our responsibility to ourselves. We are left facing the project of redesigning ourselves without substantive virtues to steady us or a content-full canonical sense of responsibility to guide us. We have no canonical, content-full, normative vision of human nature and its meaning. Having become the measure of ourselves, we have no authoritative content-full measuring rod to guide us.

As a consequence, the possibilities are endless. There is an indefinite number of ways in which to envisage the human good, to improve the human condition and to reshape human nature. Once a univocal point of reference is lost, myriad possibilities emerge. As these possibilities entice, we are deprived of a common understanding of limits or purpose.

### Dr. Feelgood and the pursuit of health: drugs, treatments, artificial well-beings, and the realization of happiness

In "Regarding the End of Medicine and the Pursuit of Health," Leon Kass attempts to set limits to what is appropriately medical.[7] If medicine is primarily focused on the cure of somatic diseases, and if norms for somatic health can be discovered, the compass of medicine will not depend on individual desires or cultural vagaries. Then one would be able to know truly what medicine ought to be doing. By an appeal to the proper goals of somatic medicine, Kass wants to exclude from medicine proper all interventions not aimed at remedying individual somatic difficulties. He wishes to exclude everything from cosmetic repairs of sagging anatomies to artificial insemination and in vitro fertilization.[8] As chapter 5 has shown, such arguments cannot succeed (no matter how much I might wish that they would). Medicine has always been a collection of undertakings focused on the myriad complaints patients bring regarding disabilities, pains, deformities, and the threat of premature death. Medicine is directed to a heterogeneous range of diseases, disorders, difficulties, and problems, from acne, sagging buttocks, neuroses, and clogged coronary arteries to cancer of the lung, unwanted pregnancies, sterility, and migraine headaches. One cannot discover which requests one ought as a health professional to honor by an appeal to a canonical notion of somatic form or structure or to a somatic account of diseases, disorders, difficulties, and problems.

Some sorting of tasks between medicine and other social practices can take place on the basis of whether concern is directed to patients in terms of patho-anatomical and pathopsychological causal explanations rather than accounts of guilt, negligence, and liability. We find medicine marked off by our history from other major social endeavors, insofar as it is, (1) because of its focus on a range of special nonmoral values concerning human ability, freedom from pain, proper form, and scope of life, (2) because of the character of medical explanations, and (3) because of the character of the sick role versus the roles of criminal, sinner, and so on.[9] Although these considerations may in many circumstances be useful, they will not substitute for moral guidance in determining what ought not to be done by health care givers. After all, a Roman Catholic physician in a Roman Catholic hospital may be properly expected to give very particular religious advice regarding issues in bioethics.

A concern with wholeness, with health as other than the mere absence of disease, gives no deliverance from the ambiguities that result from a range of interests shaped by a wide range of values concerning human function, freedom from vexation, and human form. Here Christopher Boorse is correct. Positive concepts of health turn on specific goals, or clusters of goals, which are often mutually exclusive.[10] Boorse has in mind the incompatible types of functional excellence that make one physique better for Olympic marathon racing and another for Olympic weightlifting. Sports medicine, insofar as it is directed not simply to repairing athletic injuries but also to achieving particular athletic capacities, becomes a pursuit of special understandings of health—of particular constellations of physical and psychological capacities, of particular senses of wholeness.

One might note here that nothing can be made out in general secular moral terms as wrong in principle with attempting, by the use of drugs and hormones, to achieve particular goals in sports. It is rather that the use of such adjuvants would change the character of a sport that is expected to be pursued without the medical enhancement of physical capacities. In addition, such interventions might expose the users to risks of untoward side effects. Still, some might wish to employ medical interventions in order to climb a very difficult slope of a very dangerous mountain. Such a successful climb might still be approvingly noted in the record books. The point is that the answer to whether that is right or wrong, good or bad, cannot be discovered, at least in general moral secular terms. Answers exist only in particular practices, accounts, and value perspectives. Instead of discovering answers to such questions, answers must be forged, at least in general secular terms, by agreement regarding how to pursue particular excellences and goals and how to balance possible risks and benefits.

Because medicine is able not only to control pains and anxieties, but also enhance capacities and augment pleasures, the future of medicine is likely to be tied even more to making individuals perform well and feel good. After all, what slim bonds are there to unite cosmopolitans and yuppies, if not the pursuit of pleasure and the avoidance of pain? Even when they disagree about how to compare pleasures, pains, and sufferings, they may agree to develop the means to augment pleasures and avoid pains. Surely many of them will. Leon Kass condemns Dr. Feelgood, who ''devotes his entire practice to administering amphetamine injections to people seeking elevations of mood.''[11] However, it is difficult to mount a serious objection *in principle* in general secular moral terms to such activities, that is, if noxious physical and psychological side effects can be avoided. If such mood-elevating and controlling drugs had no serious side effects, but aided individuals in better realizing their goals, what would be the general secular moral grounds for objecting to their general use?

If one recognizes no final perspective, how can one show that it is in principle worse or inferior to have a life of virtual experiences well composed in a virtual experience machine?[12] What general secular moral criteria can show that life in a virtual experience machine is better or worse than one actually engaged in all the mire of reality?[13] If death is forever, why would one existence be less important than another, if all lives are in the end forever forgotten and thus finally equally without enduring significance?[14] Again, in the absence of recognizing the final point of moral reference, opinions will differ without a final resolution being available. But in a secular moral context, how can any of this be shown? Within particular views of the good life that hold that happiness won through self-discipline is to be preferred to tranquillity acquired by medical intervention, the dream machine could be condemned. Only those who understand that there is a canonical objective perspective can recognize that life in the dream machine is a colossal lie.[15]

This does not mean that one cannot criticize Dr. Feelgood within secular bioethics. Particular current interventions by Dr. Feelgood can be seen as seriously wrongheaded in the same way that certain diseases can be recognized as diseases across cultures, or the past attempts of physicians to cure inflammatory diseases through bleeding can now be recognized as harmful. Some side effects (e.g., forms of addiction) may undercut so many of the goals of persons that most communities and individuals across most cultures will be able to acknowledge them as harmful. In addition, the tranquillity or good feeling achieved medically may be superficial or stultifying. Many attempts to make life better, not just to cure disease, can often be shown to cause more harm than good. In contrast, when one is attempting to treat a disease rather than simply to augment human capacities, there are background harms to overcome that may outbalance the iatrogenic harms associated with the treatment. The goal of simply making people feel better cannot trade on the substantial known negative costs of failing to treat, as can interventions to cure arthritis or cancer. That is, when one tries to cure a serious disease with an established treatment, one may be able better to predict the benefits of a curative intervention than one of pure enhancement. Such considerations do not provide an argument in principle against the goals of Dr. Feelgood or the consummate virtual experience machine. One finds instead arguments on the basis of known benefits and harms as well as the dangers of particular modes of intervention and their possible side effects and failures. At most, this reinforces the old maxim *festina lente* (make haste slowly).

The pursuit of wholeness is the pursuit of some constellation of healths in the plural.[16] There are numerous visions of wholeness, health, and human fulfillment. This underscores a cardinal difficulty. Although finite men and women may have some of the aspirations of gods, their limited resources force them to choose among alternative goods. They do not have the capacities of an infinite being. It is not simply the limit on their purses, a limitation that plays a major role in choices among modes of allocating resources for health care. It is a limit set by the circumstance that they must choose between a body or a mind developed primarily to achieving one set of goods rather than another. To be finite means one can do only some things, but not all things. *Omnes determinatio est negatio.* Constraints make us what we are. Different biological abilities give us different destinies.

Increasingly, humans will not need so much to accept their destinies as to choose them, though all destinies will remain particular. As in Aldous Huxley's *Brave New World,* some could set aside the primary sexual differences between men and women that depend on the gestation and birth of children by the use of ever-more effective and less costly in vitro fertilization, in vitro gestation, and genetic engineering. Some might even refashion human secondary sexual characteristics to achieve a unisex Brave New World, or one populated by the numerous sexes of Kurt Vonnegut's *Slaughterhouse-Five*.[17] Such possibilities for genetic engineering raise prudential issues, as does the case of Dr. Feelgood. In general secular moral terms, all one can say is that one should be sure that the means for engineering will produce the desired goals without significant, undesired side effects. One must envisage with care the goals that one will seek, as well as the values and circumstances they presuppose. Since human capacities are integrated into a whole, it will be prudent to assess carefully the likely social and other changes that will result from redesigning human nature. In general secular morality, one will also need to make sure that particular individuals treated or produced through genetic engineering are not injured. However, it is unlikely that one can make out moral restrictions with respect to this last point, at least in general secular terms, that would be any more severe than those currently required for parents reproducing despite the risk of having defective newborns.

Nothing dramatic is likely to happen in the short run. For some time to come, genetic engineering will most likely be directed primarily to altering somatic cells in order to aid particular suffering individuals. However, if one looks to the long run, in any serious sense of the long run, major changes will be unavoidable if we remain a free and technologically advancing species. Humans, *Homo sapiens*, have been here for less than half a million years[18] and do not share a moral vision of the normatively human.[19] If we have descendants who survive over the next few millions of years (a short period in geological time), it is very likely that eventually some will decide to refashion themselves so as better to live in the transformed environments of this earth and perhaps in the environments of other planets. Others will simply be attracted by the diverse possibilities for enhancing and refashioning human nature. Some will understand the moral impropriety of certain possible changes. But what would hold all back from such genetic interventions, which over the long run will become both available and safe, since there are no secular moral grounds in principle forbidding such interventions? Over the long run, with the allure and temptations of new possibilities for adaptation and activity, there is no reason to presume that only one species would come from ours. There might be as many species as there are inviting opportunities for substantially refashioning human nature for this or new environments, as well as grounds for refusing to participate.

Here science fiction can be heuristic. In his 1931 novel, *Last and First Men*, Olaf Stapledon portrays the history of humans over a period of some two billion years from the present.[20] He pictures our descendants radically changing themselves during this period, so that they would no longer be members of our species, or perhaps even of our genus. As our descendants refashion themselves in diverse manners, they may no longer be recognizable as members of the same order of animals. However, they would be our descendants, no matter how nonhuman they might become. If one can envisage a conversation with extraterrestrials who have no bond to us in history and biology, but a common bond in the capacity to analyze and reason, one will be able to imagine an even greater kinship with those descendant individuals, and among the members of the diverse descendant species, genera, and orders, that might issue from ours, albeit they were no longer human. They would share a common past and likely many genes.

This science-fictional vision can give moral instruction on at least two points. First, it should remind us that there is nothing sacrosanct about human nature that can be understood in general secular terms. Or put more properly, the sacrosanct, the normatively human, cannot be appreciated in secular moral terms. As a consequence, second, persons will find themselves at secular moral liberty to refashion human nature as they wish, as long as they do so prudently, benevolently, and with consenting collaborators.

The allure of development, progress, and evolution without end provides a secular image of the traditional Christian understanding of theosis or deification.[21] But it is transmogrified and rendered polytheistic. In that the secular vision of progress has no final goal, the choices of futures and the possible visions to be realized are multiple. They fragment into diverse and incompatible options. Before such choices, perhaps the most momentous for the future of the human race, secular morality in general, and secular bioethics in particular, can offer no content-full canonical guidance.

### Virtues and vices

What are the virtues that should guide individuals engaged in the manipulation and the shaping of their very nature? What marks of character ought such individuals to have? What kinds of beings should they be? Having examined the principles of permission and beneficence, what can we say in general secular moral terms about the character of a good physician, a good nurse, or a good patient? What can one say of virtues within the secular morality this volume has explored? Aristotle held that virtue or excellence (*aretē*) has to do with the mean, and that it was indeed a sort of mean.[22] But what is the context within which we are to understand such a mean? The Schoolmen held that virtue is what makes a person good and a person's actions good (''quae bonum facit habentem, et opus eius bonum reddit''). But if a concrete view of the good is attainable only within a particular understanding of the good life, what can be said generally about virtue? Although Christians seek holiness and sanctity, and the pagans of the Mediterranean littoral pursued virtue, contemporary secular ethics seems at best able to raise questions concerning right conduct and the realization of the good. Secular ethics has no canonical content-full answers to offer unless it invokes a particular moral vision or ideology. Thus it should be no surprise that secular bioethics has failed to provide an account of virtue and character. It is unable to say anything about the content-full character one ought to have or the virtues one ought to develop without at the same time endorsing a particular moral understanding.

A general secular account of virtue and character, insofar as it is available, can be secured through a special interpretation of Kant's view that virtue is a strength of the moral will.[23] Secular virtue is the strength of the will to maintain a peaceable kingdom of ends, a community of moral strangers. But this will must be described without any particular commitment to any particular evaluation of peace. Nor can any such evaluation be presumed to be shared in common. Still, one can advance claims such as: The virtuous health care giver in a secular pluralist society is one who has a developed habit of the will to respect the freedom of others and to attempt to achieve their good, while taking due account of possible harms and benefits—indeed, in the face of intractable disagreements regarding the nature of the good and the significance of harms and benefits. Which is to say, each person's will may have a different concrete character and be moved by different concerns with maintaining a peaceable secular moral fabric. All that is required is a coincidence in this endeavor, although they may act from different grounds.

The cardinal secular virtues will then be tolerance, liberality, and prudence—but the first of these is tolerance. Tolerance is the primary cardinal virtue in the morality of mutual respect. Given the clash of conflicting views of the good life, each must have an established disposition to let other persons develop peaceably their own views of the good life, no matter how evil and depraved, insofar as such development is marked by similar tolerance. For a secular moral framework to endure, it must encourage a virtue that will sustain men and women in enduring commitments to tolerating the peaceful pursuit of many incompatible understandings of the good life and of good health care, even when the understandings are ultimately and profoundly misguided, even when they will lead to final, ultimate, and enduring ruin. The men and women who are exemplars in this moral context are those who are dedicated to avoiding all unconsented-to force against others. This dedication to toleration does not exclude condemning, vilifying, execrating, ostracizing, excommunicating, or attempting to convert those with whom one disagrees. Although one tolerates others in not using force against them and not invading their property, one is not constrained to agree with them. Indeed, tolerance is derived from the Latin *tolere*, to bear or endure. It is allied to *tolerabilis* (i.e., endurable, bearable) and is an attitude appropriate not to what one finds agreeable, but to what one finds disagreeable. Intolerance, because it is a disposition to use unconsented-to force against the secularly innocent, becomes the cardinal vice. The morality of welfare and of social sympathies for its part supports liberality, the developed moral disposition to give generously to the support of others. But what is given will usually be determined by the giver's vision of the good. Prudence will also be required so that one achieves a positive balance of benefits over harms. But again, prudence will in each case be directed by a particular vision of harms and benefits. In the face of such diversities, and restrained by the principle of permission, these latter two virtues will give practical issue only as expressed in the spontaneous orders they support and through agreements freely made. The vices that centrally undermine the morality that can bind moral strangers are intolerance, meanness, and imprudence.

Within actual, particular, concrete moral communities, the virtues, as well as the vices, have their substance and content-full fabric.[24] However, the singular task of a peaceable, secular morality spanning a pluralist society can in its own right only be sustained by persons with special marks of character and virtue. Here one must again recall Hegel's notion of civil servants as the universal class.[25] The good bureaucrat in a secular pluralist society (including the individuals overseeing endeavors in human genetic engineering) must at a minimum sustain tolerance and evenhandedness in caring for all who come for protection and welfare. All should receive their due, irrespective of their vision of the good life, their religious commitment, or their special ideological passions. To be a good bureaucrat in this sense requires special dedication to that tier of the moral life that is articulated in secular pluralist morality and that has as its core the sparse morality of mutual respect.

This special dedication cannot be understood in general secular terms. Bureaucrats and others who act to sustain the secular polity will do so for diverse reasons. Their activities will be understood in different ways in their various moral communities. If a secular pluralist polity is to be sustained, persons from disparate moral communities must in their own and differing ways, and for their own various purposes, see this undertaking as useful, valuable, or worthwhile. Each may have a different narrative or account of the need to sustain a common peaceable fabric of morality. Still, all citizens and all health care providers who do not closet themselves in special exclaves, as do the Amish, will need for different goals and motives to shoulder the virtues of the good bureaucrat.

Our traditions have given us little schooling in such austere virtues. We are faced with a moral world defined by procedures, agreements, and contracts. If one has anything of content to say, one is elaborating a particular account of virtue or character, one that can only be understood within a particular moral community and its commitments. It would not be an understanding of virtue and character open to all who wish to come to terms with moral controversies with moral authority in the face of a failure to hear God in the same way or to agree to a common moral vision, and despite the failure of reason to disclose *the* canonical content-full morality. What must be said to moral strangers as moral strangers about virtue must be said without calling on any particular moral sense, moral vision, or set of moral understandings. One must invoke the strengths of character that will sustain a secular moral framework out of common agreement within which there can even be divergent understandings of the goods and evils brought by peace.

## Postmodernity, pluralism, and secularity: the vision of secular bioethics

We are returned to where we began, to multiple interpretations of the good, to the dissociation of the grounds that motivate moral action from the justifications of morality, to our secular moral lack of final guidance, to the moral fragmentation that characterizes postmodernity, and which the modern philosophical project has not been able to heal. There are innumerable ways in which men and women may wish to come to terms with their diseases, disorders, and disabilities, and to pursue better control over their bodies so as to achieve their particular visions of the wholesome life. This heterogeneous range of moral visions can find its peaceable moral cement in a secular pluralist ethic, including a secular bio-ethics.[26] This volume has offered a vision of that ethic. This volume has shown that, in the face of the failure of the modern philosophical project to justify a canonical content-full morality or a content-full moral community binding all, and despite the failure of all to hear God in the same fashion, one can still justify a general secular morality. A thread of the Enlightenment hope can be secured. This volume has also shown that the success of practices such as consensual action, contract, the free market, and limited democracy can be appreciated in terms of this morality. Not only can one show that a portion of the Enlightenment project can be vindicated, but one can show that it is already realized in particular, indeed ubiquitous, practices.

This volume may seem to support propositions that are provocative, indeed offensive and morally repugnant. Rest assured, the author is distressed as well. Although the book has secured some moral communality in the face of the nihilism and relativism that postmodernity threatens, it surely has not sustained all the moral propositions that this author knows are necessary for the good life. It is simply that this is all that secular moral reasoning can provide. What is offered here is not the morality that guides the content-full life of the author. Indeed, it is far from it. The morality of secular bioethics is not one by which one should live a life. It is rather the morality that can bind moral strangers. It is that very little we share when we come from diverse moral communities and visions to meet and collaborate with a commonly justifiable moral authority. In such circumstances, much must be tolerated that one knows to be profoundly wrong. This wrongness cannot be remedied by rational analysis and argument, only by conversion to the moral community that will give proper guidance and moral substance.

My argument has not been that moral traditions, such as the Judeo-Christian, ought to be abandoned. Nothing could be further from the intentions of this

author or the force of the conclusions of this work. The propositions of a secular
pluralist morality, of a secular bioethics, are unavoidable, but not in the sense that
they must or should supplant the concrete moralities that individuals share with
consenting others. Secular morality offers the sparse language of peaceable communication with moral strangers. It provides that fabric of discourse that can be
shared, even with those with whom one profoundly disagrees. It is the language
that can be spoken in the ruins of the Enlightenment's failure and in the face of the
tragedy of fragmented moral commitment.

One is forced to live one's life within two dimensions of morality. On the one
hand, one will be committed to particular moral views concerning good health
care, by virtue of being a member of an actual and concrete moral community.
Here one will be a good Baptist, Hindu, Orthodox Catholic, Roman Catholic, or
Jew. However, insofar as one's community does not include all, one will need to
reach to others within the constraints of a secular pluralist morality. If one's only
contact with secular pluralist morality occurs when one walks to the property line
of one's peaceably established moral exclave (e.g., one's communist commune,
one's Amish community, or one's Orthodox desert), one can be seen as acknowledging secular moral constraints insofar as one does not carry the imposition of
one's viewpoint beyond that line and insofar as one expects reciprocal tolerance
of one's own way of life.

Secular morality, secular bioethics, is founded on limits: the limits of reason
and of authority. The limits of secular moral authority and their implications for
secular bioethics and health care policy are unavoidable not because they are
useful, good, or attractive, but because competing accounts cannot in general
secular terms establish the right to use force in controlling the lives of unconsenting innocent others. Because of our inability rationally to defend a canonical,
correct, concrete moral order or in general secular terms to establish the moral
authority coercively to impose a particular concrete moral vision, and because of
the ever-available moral standpoint of consensual association based on permission, we have a morality that allows many moralities to be and have their place.
In the ruins, even with moral strangers, we can meet and collaborate with moral
authority.

## Notes

1. To be oriented involves more than knowing one's temporal, spatial, social, and
personal context. Orientation is not simply to the immanent characteristics of one's
condition. More fundamentally, to be oriented is to look beyond this world to that
which gives ultimate place and significance. It is in this sense that Christians have
traditionally sought to be oriented in prayer, that is, always to face east. For example,
Origen observes: "the direction of the rising sun obviously indicates that we ought to
pray inclining in that direction, an act which symbolizes the soul looking towards

where *the true light* rises.'' *Prayer,* trans. J. J. O'Meara (New York: Newman Press, 1954), p. 136. See, also, St. Basil the Great, *On the Spirit* 27.66.

2. Albert Camus, *The Myth of Sisyphus* (New York: Alfred Knopf, 1961), p. 123.

3. Some rebellion is fundamental and enduring. Dostoevsky has the Elder Zosima give the following account:

> Oh, there are some who remain proud and fierce even in hell, in spite of their certain knowledge and contemplation of the absolute truth; there are some fearful ones who have given themselves over to Satan and his proud spirit entirely. For such, hell is voluntary and ever consuming; they are tortured by their own choice. For they have cursed themselves, cursing God and life. They live upon their vindictive pride like a starving man in the desert sucking blood out of his own body. But they are never satisfied, and they refuse forgiveness, they curse God Who calls them. They cannot behold the living God without hatred, and they cry out that the God of life should be annihilated, that God should destroy Himself and His own creation. And they will burn in the fire of their own wrath for ever and yearn for death and annihilation. But they will not attain to death.

Fyodor Dostoevsky, *The Brothers Karamazov* (New York: Norton, 1976), book 6, chap. 3, p. 302.

4. Nietzsche, in addressing "the nihilistic consequences of contemporary science," notes that "since Copernicus, man rolls from the center into the X." Friedrich Nietzsche, "Aus dem Nachlaß der Achtzigerjahre," in *Werke in drei Bänden* (Munich: Carl Hanser, 1960), vol. 3, p. 882.

5. The very character of modern lifestyles in which women are fully engaged in the workplace and fully sexually active, while planning when they will have children, and how many, depends on the reliability of modern contraceptive technology. In this the traditional view of the Roman Catholic church is correct: artificial contraception is a means for changing and directing nature, if one means by nature either the products of our past evolutionary history or the results of the Fall.

It should be noted that Orthodox Christianity does not oppose contraception, though it requires marriages to be open to the procreation of children. Paul Evdokimov remarks, for example, "Voluntary procreation is more noble than what is due blindly to chance, more often than not unforeseen and unwanted." *The Sacrament of Love* (Crestwood, N.Y.: St. Vladimir's Seminary Press, 1985), p. 179.

6. This fragment from Protagoras is preserved by Sextus Empiricus, *Outlines of Pyrrhonism,* trans. R. G. Bury (Cambridge, Mass.: Harvard University Press, 1976), 1.216, p. 131. Protagoras was interpreted by Sextus Empiricus as arguing for a moral relativism. Making persons the center of the moral life is not the same as making a particular person or a particular group of persons the center of the moral life. The second, not the first, constitutes a true moral relativism. Yet, without a canonical notion of human nature or a content-full vision of the significance of persons, (or some other source of canonical moral content) most elements of a relativism cannot be avoided.

7. Leon Kass, "Regarding the End of Medicine and the Pursuit of Health," *Public Interest* 40 (Summer 1975): 11–24. See, also, *Toward a More Natural Science* (New York: Free Press, 1985).

8. Leon Kass, "Babies by Means of *In Vitro* Fertilization: Unethical Experiments on the Unborn?" *New England Journal of Medicine* 285 (Nov. 18, 1971): 1174–79.

9. As we saw in chapter 5, a problem (e.g., alcoholism) need not be seen as either a

medical or a legal problem, but may be seen as a medical, legal, and religious problem.

10. Christopher Boorse, "Health as a Theoretical Concept," *Philosophy of Science* 44 (1977): 542–73.

11. Kass, "Regarding the End of Medicine and the Pursuit of Health," p. 13.

12. One might imagine a medically devised, computer-driven machine that creates virtual experiences, which are felt to be as real as any in actual life, but without any of the risks to life and health involved in "real" experiences.

    Once one is despoiled of a canonical perspective concerning reality and values, all becomes a fiction within a fiction. There is no final standpoint from which one vision of the good life can be recognized as ultimately better than the rest. All life becomes virtual life in lacking an enduring significance. The encounter with this ephemeral character of reality is presented by Jorge Luis Borges in his short story, "Las ruinas circulares," where the central character discovers: "Con alivio, con humillación, con terror, comprendió que él también era una apariencia, que otro estaba soñándolo." *Obras Completas* (Buenos Aires: Emecé, 1974), p. 455.

13. See Robert Nozick's attempt to show the superiority of having a real life. His argument depends on an unsecured premise that real experiences and actions have a value that full virtual experiences would not. *Anarchy, State, and Utopia* (New York: Basic Books, 1974).

14. The trisagion for the dead closes with the prayer, ". . . and make his memory to be eternal." Christianity promises not just the resurrection of the dead and immortality, but that the significance of each person's life will endure. *Service Book of the Holy Orthodox-Catholic Apostolic Church,* trans. Isabel Hapgood, 6th ed. (Englewood, N.J.: Antiochian Orthodox Christian Archdiocese, 1983), p. 391.

15. Once an ultimate perspective is lost, one cannot in a canonically normative fashion distinguish between the value of reality and illusion, truth and lie. It is for this reason among others that Christ reminds us that the Devil is "a liar and the father of lies" (John 8:44).

16. Chester R. Burns, "Diseases versus Healths: Some Legacies in the Philosophies of Modern Medical Science," in H. T. Engelhardt, Jr., and S. F. Spicker (eds.), *Evaluation and Explanation in the Biomedical Sciences* (Dordrecht: Reidel, 1975), pp. 29–47.

17. The Tralfamadorians, who communicate with Billy Pilgrim in *Slaughterhouse-Five,* have five sexes. They inform Billy that Earthlings come in seven sexes, though five of the seven sexes are sexually active only in the fourth dimension. Kurt Vonnegut, Jr., *Slaughterhouse-Five* (New York: Delacorte Press, 1969), pp. 98–99.

18. Linda Vigilant, Mark Stoneking, Henry Harpending, et al., "African Populations and the Evolution of Human Mitochondrial DNA," *Science* 253 (Sept. 1991): 1503–7.

19. Disputes regarding the character of the normatively human are expressed in controversies regarding the possibility of ordaining priestesses within the Christian religions. In great measure, these controversies are focused on the extent to which there is a normatively ontological core to being male or female, as well as to being human. See, for example, Kenneth Wesche, "Man and Woman in Orthodox Tradition: The Mystery of Gender," *St. Vladimir's Theological Quarterly* 37 (1993): 213–351.

20. Olaf Stapledon, *Last and First Men* (1931; repr. New York: Dover, 1968). For an exploration of many of the philosophical issues involved in "autoevolution," see Kurt Bayertz, *GenEthics,* trans. Sarah Kirkby (Cambridge: Cambridge University Press, 1994), especially chap. 13, "Process Without a Goal."

21. Orthodox Christianity takes seriously the Psalmist's statement, "I say, 'You are gods'" (Psalm 82:6). As St. Basil the Great understood, man is a creature who has been given the order to become a god. Or following St. Athanasius, God became incarnate that we might become "engodded." See Georgios Mantzaridis, *The Deification of Man,* trans. Liadain Sherrard (Crestwood, N.Y.: St. Vladimir's Seminary Press, 1984); Panayiotis Nellas, *Deification in Christ,* trans. Norman Russell (Crestwood, N.Y.: St. Vladimir's Seminary Press, 1987); and Vladimir Lossky, *The Mystical Theology of the Eastern Church* (Crestwood, N.Y.: St. Vladimir's Seminary Press, 1976). See, also, Gregory Palamas, *The Triads,* ed. John Meyendorff, trans. Nicholas Gendle (Mahway, N.J.: Paulist Press, 1983).

22. Aristotle, *Eudemian Ethics* 2.3.1220b 35.

23. Immanuel Kant, *The Metaphysical Principles of Virtue: Part II of The Metaphysics of Morals,* AK VI.

24. For a comprehensive treatment of the virtues in medicine, see Earl E. Shelp (ed.), *Virtue and Medicine* (Dordrecht: Reidel, 1985).

25. G. W. F. Hegel, *The Philosophy of Right,* sec. 303. See, also, H. T. Engelhardt, Jr., "Sittlichkeit and Post-Modernity: An Hegelian Reconsideration of the State," in H. T. Engelhardt, Jr., and T. Pinkard (eds.), *Hegel Reconsidered: Beyond Metaphysics and the Authoritarian State* (Dordrecht: Kluwer, 1994), pp. 211–24.

26. H. T. Engelhardt, Jr., *Bioethics and Secular Humanism: The Search for a Common Morality* (Philadelphia: Trinity Press International, 1991).

# Index